MEDICAL RADIOLOGY

Diagnostic Imaging and Radiation Oncology

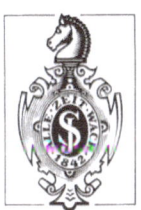

Concomitant Continuous Infusion Chemotherapy and Radiation

Contributors

J.D. Ahlgren · J.-P. Austin · H. Aziz · G.R. Blumenschein · M.A. Boileau
G.V. Burton · J.E. Byfield · W.H. Chapman · K. Choi · L.R. Coia · C.N. Coleman
M. Coleman · C. Collins · J. Crawford · I. Crocker · B.J. Cummings · R. DeConti
A. DiStefano · E.B. Douple · J. Dragovic · J. Dunst · P.F. Engstrom · R.G. Evans
B.A. Firstenberg · D. Glover · J.E. Gomez-Yeyille · S. Grabelsky · K. Griem
T.W. Griffin · P.W. Grigsby · G.E. Hanks · C.S. Higano · W. Hrushesky
S.L. Jampolis · M.J. John · E.L. Jones · D. Kaufman · T.J. Keane · J.P. Kelly
B.F. Kimler · T.J. Kinsella · W. Koh · R. Lanning · V. Liston · J.J. Lokich
N.L. Lowe · J.R. Marti · J.B. Mitchell · R.B. Mitchell · R.A. Morantz · M. Nuthakki
R.K. Oldham · A.R. Paul · C.A. Perez · L. Potters · L.R. Prosnitz · M.J. Ratain
A.M. Rauth · S. Reiner · T.A. Rich · C.J. Rosenthal · M. Rotman · A.H. Russell
K.J. Russell · A. Russo · L. Saltz · R. Sauer · L.E. Scheving · H.F. Seigler · B. Sischy
P. Stafford · R.S. Stark · S.G. Taylor · G.B. Thurman · A.T. Turrisi · T.S. Vats
N.J. Vogelzang · E.E. Vokes · R. von Roemeling · H. Wagner, Jr. · C. Weiler
M.L. Wills · W.G. Wolfe · P. Yi

Edited by

Marvin Rotman and C. Julian Rosenthal

Foreword by

Luther W. Brady and Hans-Peter Heilmann

Springer-Verlag
Berlin Heidelberg New York
London Paris Tokyo
Hong Kong Barcelona
Budapest

MARVIN ROTMAN, MD
Professor and Chairman, Dept. of Radiation Oncology

C. JULIAN ROSENTHAL, MD
Professor of Medicine and Oncology

State University of New York
SUNY Health Science Center at Brooklyn
450 Clarkson Ave. Box 1211
Brooklyn, 11203-2098
USA

MEDICAL RADIOLOGY · Diagnostic Imaging and Radiation Oncology

Continuation of
Handbuch der medizinischen Radiologie
Encyclopedia of Medical Radiology

With 42 Figures

ISBN-13: 978-3-642-84188-0   e-ISBN-13: 978-3-642-84186-6
DOI: 10.1007/978-3-642-84186-6

Library of Congress Cataloging-in-Publication Data. Concomitant continuous infusion chemotherapy and radiation / contributors, J.D. Ahlgren . . . [et al.]; edited by Marvin Rotman and C. Julian Rosenthal; foreword by Luther W. Brady and Hans-Peter Heilmann. p. cm. – (Medical radiology). Includes index.
ISBN-13: 978-3-642-84188-0. (alk. paper)
1. Cancer – Adjuvant treatment. 2. Cancer – Chemotherapy. 3. Cancer – Radiotherapy. 4. Infusion therapy.
I. Ahlgren, James D. II. Rotman, Marvin, 1933   . III. Rosenthal, C. Julian. IV. Series.
[DNLM: 1. Antineoplastic Agents, Combined – administration & dosage. 2. Cisplatin – administration & dosage. 3. Combined Modality Therapy. 4. Fluorouracil – administration & dosage. 5. Infusions, Intravenous. 6. Neoplasms – drug therapy. 7. Neoplasms – radiotherapy. 8. Radiation – Sensitizing Agents. QZ 269 C744] RC271.A35C65 1991
616.99'405 – dc20 DNLM/DCL

10/3130-543210 – Printed on acid-free paper

To Marsha, David, Sonny and Dolly
MARVIN ROTMAN

To Sandra, Lawrence and Irene
C. JULIAN ROSENTHAL

Foreword

The discovery of new drugs over the past decade has improved response rates to chemotherapy but has not significantly reduced local/regional recurrence rates. Attempts to increase antineoplastic activity by concentrating the drugs to the tumor site have included multiple routes of administration. Administration by continuous intravenous infusion has been encouraged by experimental in vitro data showing that the cytocidal effects of various antineoplastic of chemotherapeutic drugs as well as other biologic response modifiers depend not only on the concentration of the drugs but also on their duration of contact with the malignant cells.

These data have been reinforced by the clinical observations of NIGRO, BYFIELD, SISCHY, CUMMINGS, and ROTMAN indicating that squamous cell carcinomas of the anus and esophagus, adenocarcinomas of the rectum, and transitional cell carcinomas of the bladder regress when exposed to infusion of 5-fluorouracil and external beam radiotherapy. In addition, early phase II studies conducted by ROSENTHAL, ROTMAN, and others have suggested a synergistic antineoplastic effect of radiation therapy and continuous infusion of Adriamycin for selective soft tissue sarcomas and hepatomas, and of radiation therapy and infusion of cisplatin for some advanced squamous cell carcinomas.

The basic premise set forth by ROTMAN et al. regarding the value of continuous intravenous infusion of chemotherapeutic agents in combination with external beam radiation therapy has been confirmed by the work of several authors indicating that tumors regress more rapidly and that regressions are maintained more consistently when treated by continuous infusional chemotherapy and radiation therapy. The continuous intravenous infusion of chemotherapeutic agents not only improves the therapeutic index when compared with conventional intravenous bolus injection but also increases the potential for local/regional control and survival. The best results have been obtained when infusion is performed via central venous catheters, minimizing the risk of drug extravasation and peripheral vein thrombosis. This improvement in technology for intravenous access both reduces toxicity and permits agents to be administered on an outpatient basis using infusion pumps, making infusion more practical as a technique and more cost-effective. It is obvious that attention must be given to chemotherapy administration schedules and that studies are best performed within an appropriately controlled setting so as to permit accurate assessment of the clinical benefit in terms of increased antitumor efficacy. Therefore, the treatment technique which began as an experimental procedure best performed within those centers with the resources, facilities, and personnel to achieve the most effective exploration of the technique has now emerged as having potential for more active clinical application in the community setting.

This volume, edited by ROTMAN and colleagues, continues the tradition of the series in bringing to the community of practicing oncologists the latest in contemporary innovative cancer treatment. The significance of the observations set forth in this volume more than justifies the more widespread exploration of this technique in terms of its potential for improved local/regional control and ultimately improved survival.

LUTHER W. BRADY   HANS-PETER HEILMANN
Philadelphia   Hamburg

Preface

This publication offers a detailed review of continuous infusion chemotherapy and radiation as described by some of the foremost pioneers in the field. Emphasis is given to the rationale of treatment, procedures, and ongoing clinical and basic research.

The reader will note that the clinical experience of concomitant continuous infusion chemotherapy and radiation (CCIC & RT) has been of a relatively short duration. However, with the treatment of a variety of tumor sites, we have been able to arrive at significant observations. The most striking of these is an improved degree of tumor clearance and a high complete response rate which has allowed for organ-sparing treatment in all but the most advanced cancers of esophagus, anus, and bladder. The use of CCIC & RT is becoming a viable therapeutic alternative to radiation or chemotherapy alone for the treatment of gastrointestinal tumors, as well as their hepatic metastases. These results infer that the potential of such therapy could be utilized in an adjuvant setting for patients at risk of developing liver and intraperitoneal metastases from ovarian and endometrial cancers. In other historically radioresistant malignancies, such as those with large tumor deposits, bone infiltration, or sarcomatous histology, the amount of radiation required for sterilization is reduced by at least 30%. This has become the case not only for advanced epithelial cancers of the head and neck, in particular the paranasal sinuses with adjacent bone destruction, but also with the response of certain soft tissue sarcomas. Further evaluation is required to determine which sarcomas would be most responsive to this treatment.

The concentrations of drugs, whether or nor these drugs can be combined with radiation, the proper scheduling of the drug infusion, and the required total dose and fractionation of radiation still needs to be identified. Since the improved local control of regional disease does not preclude the occurrence of hematogenous disease, it may be unrealistic to expect that only two or three courses of infused chemotherapeutic agents with limited efficacy as single agents, will have a marked effect against occult metastasis. In certain instances, it may be necessary to combine CCIC and RT with effective systemic therapy.

This mode of therapy offers considerable hope for increasing organ preservation and decreasing the need for radical surgery. It has yet to be determined if radiation must be combined with chemotherapy in all cases to be optimally effective. Whether long-term toxicity arises from this type of treatment will only become apparent with the passage of time. However, we feel the reader must reserve judgement on this treatment data since the results described in this publication need to be confirmed by larger prospective randomized trials, before becoming accepted as treatment of choice.

MARVIN ROTMAN, MD
C. JULIAN ROSENTHAL, MD

Contents

Section III   5-Fluorouracil Radiopotentiation and Its Modulation by Other Agents

**Section VI   Efficacy of Continuous Infusion Adriamycin
as a Radiation Potentiator**

The Development of Chemotherapy Drugs as Radiosensitizers: an Overview

C. Julian Rosenthal and Marvin Rotman

CONTENTS

1 Introduction

The last three decades have seen the development of chemotherapy from being a means of palliating cancer symptoms and occasionally prolonging survival times, to being a means of effecting a cure. However, even now, only 15% of patients with advanced cancer can be cured by the use of chemotherapy alone.

A major reason for these poor results is the failure to completely eradicate malignant cells in the primary site while the disease is still localized. Where surgical resection has been used as the preliminary treatment, limitations in diagnostic technique may be responsible for this failure. Where surgery is inapplicable and the primary mode of treatment is irradiation, the innate radio-resistance of malignant cells may be the limiting factor. It was in an effort to overcome this resistance that the idea was developed of using chemotherapy to enhance the effectiveness of radiation.

C. Julian Rosenthal, MD, Professor of Medicine and Oncology, Marvin Rotman, MD, Professor and Chairman Department of Radiation Oncology, Suny Health Science Center at Brooklyn, 450 Clarkson Avenue, Brooklyn, NY 11203, USA

The first attempt to implement this idea was made more than 30 years ago (Heidelberg et al. 1958), but the successful use of this approach awaited better understanding regarding the synchronization of timing of the two modalities. Another problem was the inability to administer chemotherapy agents at a constant rate throughout most of the radiation treatment. This problem was overcome during the last decade with the introduction and rapid development of the technology of portable pumps and indwelling central ports and catheters.

2 Impact on Cytotoxicity of Protracted Contact Between Neoplastic Cells and Antineoplastic Agents

Prolonging the time over which tumor cells are exposed to drugs was tried early in the development of chemotherapy in the hope of enhancing the effectiveness of the drugs and, at the same time, of reducing their side-effects because of the need for lower concentrations.

Shimoyama (1975), in the course of in vitro studies on Yoshida ascites sarcoma cells, delineated two different groups among the antineoplastic agents whose performance was enhanced by prolonged contact with malignant cells. Drugs in the first group (Adriamycin, bleomycin, mitomycin C, dactinomycin, etc.) are cytotoxic to malignant cells when kept in contact for 24–96 hrs. at concentrations 100–500 times lower than when kept in contact with the same cells for just 30 min. Lower concentrations of the drugs decrease their cytotoxic effect on normal cells. These in vitro findings were confirmed by clinical studies of continuous infusion Adriamycin and bleomycin. There were significant reductions in myocardial toxicity from continuously infused Adriamycin, and in lung toxicity from proctracted infusion of bleomycin.

For the second group of antineoplastic agents (5-fluorouracil, cytosine arabinoside, methotrexate, L-asparaginase, vinblastine, vincristine, cisplatin, etc.), protracted contact with malignant cells for more than 2 days increases their cytotoxic activity by 2–3 logs as compared with only 30 min of contract. This is of particular importance since these drugs rapidly reach a plateau level beyond which an increase in concentration is no longer reflected by an increase in cytotoxicity (SHIMOYAMA 1975). Clinical evidence, again, confirmed the benefits of prolonged infusion for all these drugs with the exception of methotrexate. Another group of antineoplastic agents can be distinguished which includes nitrosoureas and most of the alkylating agents with the exception of cisplatin and cyclophosphamide. Only minimal improvements in cytotoxicity are achieved by prolonging contact between Yoshida ascites sarcoma cells and this group of agents. The cell-killing curve with these drugs is exponential, as it is with radiation therapy (SHIMOYAMA 1975). Increasing the time period over which malignant cells are in contact with these agents has no clinical benefit: in this case, toxicity levels can only be maintained over time using increased drug concentration and, hence, increasing the potential for side-effects.

In the early 1960s, 5-fluorouracil (5-FU) was the only drug being used concomitantly with radiation therapy. Since then, the growth in experimental data has led to an increasing understanding of the rationale behind this approach. This, in turn, has led to a growing amount of clinical investigation in the last decade into the multimodal use of a variety of other neoplastic agents, including cisplatin, Adriamycin, dacarbazine, and bleomycin.

3 Mechanism of Radiopotentiation by Chemotherapeutic Agents

The exact mechanism by which these chemotherapeutic agents potentiate the radiation therapy effect is, in most cases, poorly understood. Following the schematic classification of chemical modifiers of cancer treatment recently reviewed by COLEMAN et al. (1988), most of these drugs (i.e., anthracyclines, bleomycin, dacarbazine) could be considered to be acting as hypoxic cell sensitizers primarily through their interference with the repair of the DNA injury inflicted on neoplastic cells by radiation therapy. 5-FU belongs to another class of radiosensitizers, the thymidine analogs, that are incorporated into the DNA of cycling cells and make them more sensitive to irradiation. None of the chemotherapeutic agents appear to belong to a third major class of radiosensitizers that enhance the radiation effect through glutathione depletion of neoplastic cells like that induced by L-buthiomine sulfoxide or diethylimaleate.

3.1 5-Fluorouracil as Radiopotentiator

5-Fluorouracil is a pyrimidine analog that inhibits de novo synthesis of DNA by binding thymidylate synthetase. It also leads to synthesis of defective DNA due to its combination with an RNA precursor nucleotide. Its effects as a radiopotentiator could be due to its inhibition of the repair of sublethal damage produced by radiation (VIETTI et al. 1971).

The use of 5-FU in continuous infusion with concomitant chemotherapy began fortuitously in 1974 with NIGRO et al. working at Wayne State University with SEIFERT. SEIFERT was the first investigator of the benefits of administration of 5-FU by continuous infusion (SEIFERT et al. 1975). NIGRO tested the effect of administering 5-FU in this new way (combined with mitomycin C or porfiromycin) while giving concomitant radiation therapy to three patients with squamous cell carcinoma of the anus. All three patients achieved a complete and durable remission. This was documented in two of the cases by careful microscopic scrutiny of the anal canal, which had been removed through anteroposterior resection after the preoperative administration of 5-FU and radiation therapy. This initial favorable experience was followed by systematic preclinical studies carried out by BYFIELD and associates (1977) which established the scheduling requisites for the effective use of infused 5-FU as a radiosensitizer of human tumors; these findings are extensively reviewed in this book, in Chap. 13. In 1979, BRUCKNER et al. reported on the successful use of a similar concomitant bimodality therapy. Complete remission was achieved in three patients with advanced squamous cell carcinoma of the anus after failure of attempted curative resection.

In 1980, BYFIELD et al. expanded the use of concomitant irradiation with 5-FU infusion at a dose of 20 mg/kg/day for 5 consecutive days every 2 weeks to the treatment of unresectable squamous cell carcinoma of the esophagus. A complete clinical response was achieved in five out of six cases. It was, however, only in 1982 that two reports of somewhat larger series of patients (SISCHY et al. 1982; CUMMINGS et al. 1982) clearly documented the curative effect of concomitant combined modality therapy. Radiosensitization was achieved by the use of 5-FU at a dose of 1000 mg/m^2/day administered by continuous infusion for 96–120 h every 2 weeks with one dose of mitomycin C (10 mg/m^2) on the 1st day of therapy only. All patients in these two series (a total of 32 patients) achieved complete remissions which were maintained at the time of reporting (2–36 months). Based on these results, combined concomitant modality therapy had replaced surgical resection in the treatment of squamous cell carcinoma of the anus; this represents, to date, the most successful application of concomitant modality therapy in the treatment of malignant tumors. It is a clear indication of the effectiveness of 5-FU infusion in enhancing the effects of radiation, which was found to be capable of inducing complete lasting remissions by itself. However, in cases with advanced T_3 and T_4 lesions (UICC classification) in which external radiation was complemented by interstitial radiotherapy, up to 25% failure rates have been reported (PAPILLON 1984).

During the following years, similar combined modality therapy was administered with varying degrees of success to other squamous cell carcinomas. COIA et al. reported in 1984 a 17-month median survival in patients with stage I and II squamous cell carcinoma of the esophagus. The regimen used was two cycles of 5-day infusion 5-FU with concomitant radiation therapy to a total dose of 60 Gy over a 6-week period. Recurrences in previously irradiated areas were reported in only 10% of cases.

KEANE et al. (1985) and CUMMINGS et al. (1986) reported on a similar combined modality treatment administered to 35 patients with locally advanced esophageal squamous cell carcinoma (lesion larger than 5 cm in diameter), circumferential or extending outside the esophagus; 15 patients received just one cycle of 5-FU infusion while 20 received two cycles. The results of this pilot study were compared with matched controls from a previous series of patients with esophageal

squamous cell carcinoma who received irradiation alone. In 18 out of 35 patients receiving the combined concomitant therapy, the tumor remained locally controlled. The 2-year acturial rate of 30% and the local relapse-free rate of 47% compared favorably with the rates of 15% and 20%, respectively, noted in the patients receiving irradiation alone. Continuous course therapy resulted in better survival at 2 years (48% vs 13%) and in better local relapse-free rates (73% vs 29%) than the split-course irradiation. However, the slope of the survival curve was not changed for responding patients, indicating that the noted improvement may represent just a delay in death for those patients with advanced unresectable tumors. This was not the case for patients treated in the early stages by COIA et al. Here, responders did not relapse after 5 years, as reported elsewhere in this volume.

The results obtained by COIA et al. (1984) using 60 Gy irradiation compare favorably with the complete remission rate of 25% reported by LEICHMAN et al. in the same year among twenty-five patients with squamous cell carcinoma of the esophagus who were treated preoperatively with 5-FU infusion and mitomycin C with concomitant irradiation (FUMIR) for only 3 weeks to a total dose of 30 Gy. Results were even less favorable in patients with esophageal carcinoma receiving 30 Gy radiation therapy alone (LEICHMAN et al. 1984), in whom complete remission was achieved in only 3% of cases. A similar response rate of 22% was achieved with a group of squamous cell carcinoma patients receiving 60 Gy to the primary lesion and another group of patients receiving 5-FU, cisplatin, and 30 Gy radiation. The risk of distant metastases, the failure to improve cure rates when residual tumor was still present after preoperative 5-FU–mitomycin C (LEICHMAN et al. 1984), and the relatively high mortality rates following resection of residual esophageal cancer (CAIN et al. 1985; CUMMINGS et al. 1986) suggest that patients in whom symptomatic residual tumor remains after treatment with FUMIR would do better with a palliative bypass rather than a radical esophageal resection. However, in early-stage patients achieving a complete response, survival is clearly improved. It remains to be determined whether or not surgical resection of the esophageal segment is necessary after complete remission is obtained through the administration of 5-FU with or without mitomycin C.

Similar results were reported in two early studies (Kaplan et al. 1985; Cain et al. 1985) of Fumir administered to patients with advanced stages (more than 80% with T_3 and T_4 tumors) of head and neck squamous cell carcinoma. In the Kaplan et al. series (1985), Fumir was administered only at the beginning of a 30 Gy irradiation course followed 2 weeks later by a 20 Gy course administered alone. In the Cain et al. series (1985), a split-course Fumir regimen was used, identical to that administered to patients with squamous cell carcinoma of the esophagus. Complete clinical responses were noted in 61% of the 42 cases entered in the first study and in 62% of the 57 patients with carcinoma of the larynx and pharynx entered in the second study. At 2 years, only 51% of cases were free of local recurrence (Cummings et al. 1986).

The Fumir combined concomitant modality therapy was also used in the therapy of locally advanced squamous cell carcinoma of the cervix with disease expanding to both pelvic side walls or to the rectum and bladder. In these cases, irradiation alone is followed by a 75% risk of pelvic failure (Cummings et al. 1986). Twenty-seven patients were treated by Thomas et al. (1984) at Princess Margaret Cancer Institute with split-course radiation therapy with hyperfractionation. Two daily doses of 1.5 Gy were administered for 4 days together with 5-FU infusion and one dose of 6 mg/m^2 mitomycin C followed by single doses of 1.8 Gy radiation for another 6 days. This course was repeated once after a 24-day interval and was complemented by an intracavitary cesium 137 line source delivering a dose of 40 Gy at 2 cm from the applicator. Seventy-four percent of patients achieved complete remission (CR); in 65% of cases the CR was maintained at 3 years, but long-term follow-up results are not yet available. The Fumir combination was also used successfully in the therapy of locally advanced transitional cell carcinoma and squamous cell carcinoma of the bladder, initially by Rotman et al. (1986, 1987) and more recently by Russell et al. (1988); both studies are presented together with additional data elsewhere in this volume. Of the 20 evaluable patients in the Rotman et al. (1988) study, 86% achieved CR after receiving 40–45 Gy in daily fractions for 5 days a week and an additional 20–25 Gy as a pelvic boost or a 30 Gy interstitial implant with concomitant 5-FU infusion at 25 mg/kg/24 h for 5 days and one dose of mitomycin C of 10 mg/m^2 as i.v. bolus. These results compare favorably with CR rates of 31%–49% reported by various investigators after the preoperative administration of 40–50 Gy alone (Bloom et al. 1982; Van Der Werf Messing 1982). The adjusted overall 5-year survival rate (Rotman et al. 1986, 1988, 1990) was projected at 53%, with better rates for stages A_2 and B_1 (80%) than for B_2, C, and D (40%).

Finally, the Fumir combined concomitant modality therapy was also tested in a few studies in patients with adenocarcinoma at various sites, particularly the rectum and stomach. There were encouraging results from the rectal adenocarcinoma study (Hagbin et al. 1988). Among 64 patients with locally advanced disease (ulcerated, fixed lesions at least 4 cm in diameter), complete response was attained in 12.5% of cases; operations were performed after a total tumor dose of 40 Gy was given over a period of 4 weeks with two cycles of 96 h infusion of 5-FU at a dose of 1000 mg/m^2/day and one bolus injection of mitomycin C (10 mg/m^2). No nodal involvement was seen in 73.5% of cases while in historical control studies less than 50% of the patients are free of nodal involvement. The projected survival at 5 years of 64% was slightly better than in historical control studies. However, the data of Fumir effectiveness in patients with adenocarcinoma are less convincing than those in patients with squamous cell carcinoma at various sites and transitional cell carcinoma of the bladder. In the latter groups of patients, previously reviewed, there is convincing evidence that 5-FU alone or in combination with mitomycin C leads to statistically significant better results than those seen after the administration of radiation therapy alone. The contribution of mitomycin C to the radiosensitizing effect of 5-FU is, to date, unknown. It is undergoing analysis in an RTOG study in which patients with squamous cell carcinoma of the anus are receiving radiation therapy and concomitant infusional 5-FU alone or in combination with mitomycin C.

Recent data have suggested that the radiosensitizing effect of infusion 5-FU could be further enhanced by its combination with cisplatin, an alkylating agent which has been found to have a radiosensitizing effect when used alone in some experimental animal models as well as in a few cases of human malignancy.

3.2 Cisplatin as Radiopotentiator

CIS-Diamminedichloroplatinum II (*cis*-DDP or cisplatin), the first of the group of platinum co-ordination complexes used effectively against some human malignancies, was found in 1974 (WADINSKY et al.) to potentiate irradiation effects on a rat experimental tumor. In the late 1970s, studies by DOUPLE and RICHMOND on *E. coli* bacteria, V-79 Chinese hamster cells, and mouse mammary carcinoma showed that cisplatin sensitized hypoxic cells to radiation by increasing DNA susceptibility to radiation damage. The effect can be seen in the abrogation of the shoulder and the steepening of the exponential portion of the single cell survival curve. At the same time, cisplatin inhibits the repair of potentially lethal radiation-induced damage to the DNA (DOUPLE et al. 1977; DOUPLE 1988; DEWITT 1987). In order to produce these two major effects, however, it was found that cisplatin must be present at the time of irradiation as well as shortly after irradiation at a concentration of at least 10 M (DOUPLE et al. 1988a). It was these findings that led to a number of experimental studies by FU et al. starting in 1984, and more recently by DOUPLE et al. (see Chap. 22, this volume), into the kinetics and the efficacy of cisplatin and paraplatin (a second generation platinum compound) in potentiating radiation effects. A convincing experimental demonstration of the radiosensitizing effect of cisplatin was performed by KYRIAZIS et al. (1983) on human bladder carcinoma implanted in nude mice. The mice receiving both modalities of therapy had a statistically significant improvement in response and survival over those receiving radiation alone. Other experimental data suggested that the cisplatin–radiation interaction is enhanced when radiation is administered by multiple fractions (DRITSCHILO et al. 1979).

All the early clinical studies on the cisplatin–radiation interactions used only bolus intravenous administration of the drug (REIMER et al. 1981; SOLOWAY et al. 1982). While indicating a favorable trend, the results have been inconclusive in proving a cisplatin radiosensitizing effect. Better results were reported in studies using higher intermittent doses of cisplatin. A phase II trial by the Radiation Therapy Oncology Group (RTOG) administered 100 mg/m^2 cisplatin every 3 weeks with appropriate hydration and antiemetics, to patients with stage III and IV head and neck neoplasms. Results from this study were an improvement when compared

with those from studies using fractionated smaller doses of 15–20 mg/m^2. Survival at 1 year of 66% and median survival of just over 2 years (AL-SARRAF et al. 1987) was encouraging. In a recently reported pilot study (WHEELER et al. 1988) of patients with squamous cell carcinoma of the lung and head and neck who received high dose cisplatin (40 mg/m^2/day) for 5 consecutive days for three cycles during radiation therapy, a complete response rate of 100% was achieved. This suggests that dose may be important for cisplatin synergy with radiation. However the toxicity of this regimen was significant and no information is available from this study concerning survival or duration of response.

Other recent therapeutic trials with carcinoma of the bladder have used cisplatin bolus injection every 3 weeks with concomitant irradiation to the bladder given to a total dose of 60 Gy in a split course (JASKE et al. 1986) or nonsplit course (COPPIN and BROWN 1986; SHIPLEY et al. 1987). Results indicate an improvement of approximately 20% in CR rate for patients with macroscopic residual tumor when compared with historical control studies in which cisplatin was administered sequentially after radiation therapy.

However, it was not until the phase I-II study by ROSENTHAL et al. (1986) that the maximum tolerated dose and the overall toxicity of cisplatin as a potential radiosensitizer were assessed. Trials were set up in patients with squamous cell carcinoma of the lung, head and neck, and eso-phasgus (ROSENTHAL et al. 1986), transitional cell carcinoma of the bladder (SAUER et al. 1988), and advanced paranasal sinus and esophageal squamous cell carcinoma (ROTMAN et al., 1968; CHOI et al., Chap. 23, this volume). The phase I study on protracted continuous infusion (ROSEN-THAL et al. 1986) indicated that a daily dose of 5 mg/m^2/day was well tolerated for a mean of 18 consecutive days. Increasing the daily dose led within a few days to intolerable gastrointestinal toxicity, while prolonging the duration of the cisplatin infusion beyond 18 days led to unacceptable thrombocytopenia (85 $\pm$ 12 $\times$ 10^3/liter). However, this same study, as well as SAUER's study (1988), found that cisplatin can be administered by continuous infusion over a shorter period of only 5 days up to a dose of 25 mg/m^2/day with only moderate gastrointestinal toxicity.

Ongoing clinical trials are attempting to define further the role of continuous infusion cisplatin as a radiosensitizer in the treatment of other primary tumors. However, data suggesting that a combination of infusional cisplatin and infusional 5-FU administered with concomitant radiation therapy produces somewhat better results than those obtained with either of the two drugs administered alone, have directed many investigators towards the use of this combination infusional chemotherapy. This trend was reinforced by early results from AL-SARRAF et al. (1987) indicating that the cisplatin–5-FU infusion achieves twice the complete response rate of any previously reported regimen in advanced head and neck squamous cell carcinomas.

4 Radiation Potentiation by Cisplatin-5-FU Combination Infusional Chemotherapy

Three studies in patients with advanced head and neck squamous cell carcinoma using infusional 5-FU and cisplatin with concomitant radiation therapy have reported excellent results (TAYLOR et al. 1985 and Chap. 27, this volume). Cisplatin $60 \, mg/m^2$ was administered on day 1, 5-FU $800 \, mg/m^2/day$ on days 1–5, and split-course radiation therapy also on days 1–5, with the cycle repeated every 2 weeks. A 98% overall response rate was reported and a CR rate of 55% with a median survival of 37 months. A different regimen in which cisplatin was given at $75 \, mg/m^2$ on days 1 and 43 with 5-FU administered by continuous nonsplit course of radiation therapy for 3 weeks led to an overall response rate of 100% with 94% CR and 64% survival at 21 months (ADELSTEIN et al. 1988). These results were similar to those of WENDT et al. (1987), who administered a nonsplit course of radiation therapy following a hyperfractionation schema (twice daily $0.18 \, Gy$ per 8-day therapy) and a lower dose of 5-FU ($350 \, mg/m^2/day$ by continuous infusion on days 2–5). It is notable that in respect to advanced head and neck squamous cell carcinoma, survival is not significantly better in patients achieving complete clinical remission than in good partial responders (TAYLOR et al. 1985). This indicates the difficulties encountered in determining complete responses by clinical evaluation or random endoscopic biopsies.

A similar experience concerning potentiation of radiation therapy by concomitant chemotherapy was reported by JOHN et al. (1987a, 1989). Infusional 5-FU was administered in combination with cisplatin or mitomycin C or high dose methotrexate with calcium leucovorin rescue. These sequential studies indicated that an increase in the total dose of radiation delivered to the primary lesion together with an increase in the number of drugs administered in combination with 5-FU led to a parallel increase in the complete response rate from 57% to 72% and finally to 100% and a decrease in the local failure rate from 50% to 15%. As in head and neck carcinomas, achieving complete clinical and histological responses documented by a random endoscopic biopsy does not preclude local recurrences nor does it have a significant impact on 5-year survival rates as projected by the analysis of the two early studies by JOHN et al. It is of note that in the studies concerning locally advanced esophageal carcinoma approximately 25% of all cases were adenocarcinomas and that in these cases and those with squamous cell carcinoma histology results were similar.

The improved response rates of adenocarcinoma of the esophagus to a combination of infusional 5-FU with cisplatin and concomitant radiation was confirmed by a study of 21 patients with adenocarcinoma of the gastroesophageal junction. These patients received three cycles of 5-FU ($1000 \, mg/m^2/day$) and cisplatin ($20 \, mg/m^2/day$) infusion for 96 h concomitantly with $5 \, Gy$ radiation therapy (VON BURTON et al., Chap. 31, this volume). In 16 cases, the treatment was followed by radical surgery which revealed complete histological responses in five cases, microscopic tumors in six, and gross tumors in five. This is better than the response found in historical controls but inferior to that reported for cases of squamous cell carcinoma of the esophagus. In the same study, while patients' median survival was improved vis-à-vis that of historical controls, no improvement in long-term survival was noted.

Finally, the infusional 5-FU–cisplatin combination was successfully used in patients with squamous cell carcinoma of the cervix (JOHN et al. 1987b; KRUSKER et al. 1989; GRISBY and PEREZ, Chap. 32, this volume). This led to a decrease in the rate of recurrence at 3 years from 60% in historical controls in whom radiation therapy was administered with concomitant 5-FU alone to 35% in the relatively small series of patients who received cisplatin as well as 5-FU infusion with concomitant irradiation.

Despite significant progress in the rate and duration of response, these studies of combined cisplatin–5-FU infusional therapy with concomitant radiation therapy indicate that in squamous cell carcinoma of the head and neck, esophagus, and cervix, as well as in the few adenocarcinomas tested, cure is not yet achievable at a statistically significant rate. The challenge of clinical research in the near future is to capitalize further on the apparent radiopotentiating effect of various chemotherapeutic agents that have a cytocidal effect on tumor cells to the point of achieving complete tumor erradication.

5 Radiopotentiation by Doxorubicin (Adriamycin)

The effect of in vitro interaction between doxorubicin (Adriamycin) and irradiation in mammalian tumor cells has been studied since 1977 (BYFIELD et al). The combination was found to be synergistic at lower doses and additive when the Adriamycin dose was increased to more than 0.15 mg/kg body weight. Despite this finding, and despite early clinical trials showing that single pulses of Adriamycin in conventional doses (40–60 mg/m^2/q 3 weeks) were well tolerated (BYFIELD et al. 1975), the predominant view for many years was that Adriamycin administered concomitantly with radiation therapy led to increased toxicity represented by enteritis, esophagitis (REED et al. 1976), cardiomyopathy (ROSEN et al. 1975), and a skin recall phenomenon (CASSIDY 1975).

The radiopotentiating effects on certain neoplasms (sarcomas and some hepatocellular carcinomas) of Adriamycin administered by continuous infusion concomitantly with irradiation and the clinical feasibility of this approach were first reported by ROSENTHAL et al. (1986). The use of this regime was based on prior reports (LEGHA et al. 1982) showing a significant reduction in Adriamycin cardiotoxicity when administered over periods of 96 h as compared with a bolus intravenous administration of an equal dose. The kinetics of the Adriamycin infusion (ROSENTHAL et al. 1986) indicate an initial delay of approximately 16 h in reaching maximum serum level, probably due to Adriamycin's initial diffusion to various tissues from where it is subsequently released. A steady level is reached after 30 h of the 120 h infusion (see also ROSENTHAL et al., Chap 33, this volume).

In the preliminary pilot study (ROSENTHAL and ROTMAN 1988), four out of nine patients with locally advanced or metastatic soft tissue sarcomas achieved complete response at the level of all lesions that received radiation therapy concomitantly with the 5-day cycle of continuous infusion doxorubicin at a concentration of 12 mg/m^2/day. The cycles were repeated every 3–4 weeks (split-course therapy). Two out of the original three patients with advanced locoregional recurrent disease without distant metastases who achieved complete remission have maintained their remission longer than 5 years and are probably cured. The same regime was followed in a further 14 cases with similarly beneficial results (see elsewhere in this volume). It is interesting to note that complete remission and maximum tumor size reduction in patients with only partial remissions are achieved at a significantly lower total dose of radiation therapy (mean 38 Gy) than the amount needed in historical controls to achieve equal results using conventional nonsplit-course radiation therapy (mean 65 Gy).

A similar regime of combined concomitant irradiation with doxorubicin infusion has been reported to produce some benefits in patients with hepatocellular carcinomas limited to one hepatic lobe (ROSENTHAL et al. 1986), as further documented by STARK et al. (Chap. 34, this volume).

In summary, then, concomitant combined modality therapy involving radiation therapy and various chemotherapy agents administered by continuous infusion appears to offer significant promise for achieving cures in patients with locally advanced malignancies that are beyond the scope of surgical resection. It has the potential, also, of being successfully used in the therapy of early malignant primary lesions as an alternative to surgical resection that provides significant advantages in preserving the function of the affected organ. To date, this has been successfully implemented only in patients with squamous cell carcinoma of the anus.

References

Adelstein D, Sharan V, Earle A et al. (1988). Simultaneous radiotherapy and chemotherapy with 5 Fluorouracil and cisplatin for locally confined squamous cell head and neck cancer. NCI Monogr. 6: 347–351

Al-Sarraf M, Pajak TF, Marciol VA et al. (1987). Concurrent radiotherapy and chemotherapy with cis platin in inoperable squamous cell carcinoma of the head and neck. Cancer 59: 259–265

Bloom HJD, Henry W, Wallace D, Skeet R (1982). Treatment of T3 bladder cancer: A controlled trial of preoperative radiotherapy and radical castectomy versus radical radiotherapy. Brit J Urol 54: 136–151

Bruckner HW, Spiegelman MK, Mandel E et al. (1979). Carcinoma of the anus, treated with a combination of radiotherapy and chemotherapy. Cancer Treatment Re 44: 437–45

Byfield JE, Watring WG, Kemkin SR et al. (1975). Adriamycin: a useful adjuvant drug for combination radiation therapy. Proc Am Assoc Cancer Res – Am Soc Clin Onc 16: 253 (Abstr.)

Byfield JE, Chan PYM, Seargran SL (1977). Radiosensitization of 5 FU: molecular origins and clinical scheduling implications. Proc Amer Assoc Can Res 18: 74 (abstr.)

Byfield JE, Lynch M, Kulhaman I, Chan PYM (1977). Cellular effects of combined Adriamycin and x-ray irradiation in human tumor cells. Cancer 19: 194–204

Byfield JE, Barone R, Mendelsohn J et al. (1980). Infusional 5-Fluorourical and x-ray therapy for nonresectable esophageal cancer. Cancer 45: 703–708

Cassidy JR (1975). Radiation-Adriamycin interaction; preliminary clinical observations. Cancer 36: 946–948

Coia LR, Eugstrom PF, Paul A et al. (1984). A pilot study of combined radiotherapy and chemotherapy for esophageal carcinoma. Am J Clin Oncol 7: 653

Coleman NA, Bump EA and Kramer RA (1988). Chemical modifiers of cancer treatment. J Clinic Oncol 6: 709–733

Coppin C and Brown E (1986). Concurrent cisplatin with radiation for locally advanced bladder cancer: a pilot study suggesting improved survival. Proc Am Soc Clin Oncol 5: 99

Cummings BJ, Rider WD, Harwood AR (1982). Combined radical radiation therapy and chemotherapy for esophageal carcinoma. Am J Clin Oncol 7: 653

Cummings BJ, Keane TJ, Harwood AR and Thomas GM (1986). Combined modality therapy with 5-Fluorouracil, Mitomycin C and Radiation Therapy for squamous cell cancers in Clinical Applications of Continuous Infusion Chemotherapy and Concomitant Radiation Therapy. CJ Rosenthal and M Rotman (ed.) pp 133–147

DeWitt L (1987). Combined treatment of radiation and cisdiammine dichloroplatinum (11). A review of experimental and clinical data. Int J Rad Oncol Biol Phys 13: 403–426

Douple EB (1988). Keynote address: platinum-radiation interactions. NCI Monogr. 6: 315–319

Douple EB, Richmond RC, Logan ME (1977). J Clinic Hematol Oncol 7: 585–603

Douple EB, ToHen MD, Spencer F. (1988a). Platinum levels in murine tumor following intraperitoneal administration of Cisplatin or paraplatin. NCI Monogr. 6: 129–132

Dritschilo A, Piro AJ, Kelman AD (1979). The effect of cisplatin on the repair of radiation damage in plateau phase chinese hamster (V-79) cells. Int J Radiat Oncol Biol Phys 5: 1345–1349

Fu KK, Rayner PA, Lam KN (1984). Modification of Continuous low dose rate irradiation by concurrent chemotherapy infusion. Int J Radiat Oncol Biol Phys 10: 1473–1478

Greco AA, Brereton HD, Kent H et al. (1976). Adriamycin and enhanced radiation reaction in normal esophagus and skin. Ann Int Med 85: 294–298

Haghbin M, Sishy B, Hinson EJ (1988). Combined modality preoperative therapy in poor prognostic rectal adenocarcinoma. Rad Oncol 13: 75–81

Heidelberger C, Greisbach C, Montag BJ et al. (1958). Studies in fluorinated pyrimidin: II. Effects of transplanted tumor: Cancer Res 18: 305–317

Jakse G, Rauschmeier H, Fritsch E et al. (1986). Die Intergrier te radiotherapie and chemotherapie des lokal fortgeschritteneu harnblasenkarinomas. Akt Urel 17: 68–73

John M, Flam M, Wittlinger P and Mowry PA (1987). Inoperable esophageal carcinoma: results of aggressive synchronous radiotherapy and chemotherapy a pilot study. Am J Clin Oncol 10: 310–316

John M, Cooke K, Flam M, et al. (1987b). Preliminary results of concomitant radiotherapy and chemotherapy in advanced cervical carcinoma. Gynecol Oncol 28: 101–110

John MJ, Flam M, Mowry PA et al. (1989). Radiotherapy alone and chemoradiation for nonmetastatic esophageal carcinoma. A critical review of chemoradiation. Cancer 63: 2397–2403

Kaplan MJ, Hahn SS, Johns ME et al. (1985). Mitomycin and fluorouracil with concomitant radiation therapy in head and neck cancer. Arch Otolaryngol 111: 220

Keane TJ, Harwood AR, Beale FA et al. (1985). A pilot study of mitomycin C and 5 Fluorouracil infusion combined with split course radiation therapy for advanced carcinoma of the larynx and hypopharynx. J Otolaryn 15: 286–288

Keane TJ, Harwood AR, Elhakim T et al. (1985). Radical radiation therapy with 5-fluorouracil infusion and mitomycin C for esophageal squamous cell carcinoma. Radiother Onc 4: 205–210

Kuske R, Perez G, Grisby P et al. (1900 in press). Phase I/II study of definitive radiotherapy and chemotherapy (cisplatin and 5 Fluorouracil) for advanced or recurrent gynecologic malignancies, preliminary report. Am J Clin Oncol

Kyriazis AP, Yagoda A, Kereiasker JG et al. (1983). Experimental studies on the radiation modifying effect of Cis-diamminedichloroplatinum II (DDP) in human bladder transitional cell carcinomas grown in nude mice. Cancer 52: 452–457

Legha SS, Benjamin RS, Mackay B et al. (1982). Reduction of doxorubicin cardiotoxicity by prolonged continuous intravenous infusion. Ann Int Med 96: 133–139

Leichman L, Steiger Z, Seydel HG and Vaitkevicius VK (1984). Combined preoperative chemotherapy and radiation therapy for cancer of the esophagus: the Wayne State University, Southwest Oncology Group and Radiation Therapy Oncology Group experience. Sem Oncol 11: 178–185

Nigro ND, Vaitkevicius VK, Basil Considine Jr., MD (1974). Combined therapy for cancer of the Anal Canal: a preliminary report. Dis Col-Rectum 17: 354–36

Papillon J (1974). Radiation Therapy in the Management of the Epidermoid Carcinoma of the anal region. Dis Colon 17: 181–187

Reimer RR, Gahbauer R, Bukowski RM (1981). Simultaneous treatment with cisplatin and radiation therapy for advanced solid tumors: a pilot study. Cancer Treat Rep 6: 19–222

Rosen G, Tefft M, Martinez A et al. (1975). Combination chemotherapy and radiation therapy in the treatment of metastatic osteogenic sarcoma. Cancer 35: 622–630

Rosenthal CJ and Rotman M (1988). Pilot study of interaction of radiation therapy with doxorubicin by continuous infusion. NCI Monographs 6: 285–290

Rosenthal CJ, Rotman M, Choi K and Sand J (1986). Cisplatin by continuous infusion with concurrent radiation in malignant tumors (a phase I–II study) In: Rosenthal CJ and Rotman M. (eds.) Clinical Applications of Continuous Infusion Chemotherapy and Concomitant Radiation Therapy. Plenum Press. New York and London, pp 177–180

Rosenthal CJ, Rotman M and Bhutiani M (1986a) Concomitant radiation therapy and doxorubicin by continuous infusion in advanced malignancies – A phase I–II study: Evidence of synergistic effects in soft tissue sarcomas and hepatomas in "Clinical Applications of Continuous Infusion Chemotherapy and Concomitant Radiation Therapy. Rosenthal CJ, Rotman M (eds). Plenum Press, New York and London (publ) pp 159–176

Rotman M, Choi K, Isaacson S et al. (1986). Treatment of occurent carcinoma of the paranasal sinuses using concomitant infusion cis-platinum and radiation therapy. In: Rosenthal CJ, Rotman M (eds) Clinical applications of continueus infusion chemotherapy and concomitant radiation therapy. Plenum Press, New York and London, pp 189–194

Rotman M, Macchia R, Silverstein M et al. (1986). Treatment of bladder carcinoma with concomitant infusion chemotherapy and irradiation. In: Clinical Applications of Continuous Infusion Chemotherapy and Concomitant Radiation Therapy. CJ Rosenthal and M Rotman eds. Plenum Press (publ), New York and London, pp 149–153

Rotman M, Macchia R, Silverstein M et al. (1987). Treatment of advanced bladder carcinoma with irradiation and concomitant 5-fluorouracil infusion. Cancer 59: 710–714

Rotman M, Aziz H, Parruzzo M et al. (1990). Treatment of advanced transitional cell Ca of the bladder with irradiation and concomitant 5-Fluorouracil infusion. Int J Rad Oncol Biol Phys 19: 1131–1137

Russell KJ, Boileou MA, Tretori RC et al. (1988). Transitional cell carcinoma of the urinary bladder: histologic clearance with combined 5-FU chemotherapy and radiation therapy. Preliminary results of bladder preservation study. Radiology 167: 848

Sauer R, Schrott KM, Dunst J et al. (1988). Preliminary results in the treatment of invasive bladder carcinoma with radiotherapy and cisplatinum. Int J Rad Oncol Biol Phys 15: 871–875

Seifert P, Baker LH, Reed ML and Vantkevicius VK (1975). Comparison of continuously infused 5-Fluorouracil with bolus injection in patients with colorectal adenocarcinoma. Cancer 36: 123–128

Shimoyama M (1975). The cytocidal action of alkylating agents and anticancer antibodies against in vitro cultured Yoshida ascites sarcoma cells. Jpn Soc Cancer Ther 10: 63–72

Shipley WU, Prant GR, Einstein AB et al. (1987). Treatment of invasive bladder cancer by cisplatin and radiation in patients unsuited for surgery. J Am Med Assoc 258: 931–935

Sishy B, Remington JH, Hinson J et al. (1982). Definitive treatment of anal-canal carcinoma by menas of radiation therapy and chemotherapy. Dis Colon Rectum 25: 686–688

Soloway MS, Kard M, Scheinberryu M et al. (1982). Concurrent radiation and cisplatin in the treatment of advanced bladder cancer: a preliminary report. J Urol 128: 1031–1033

Taylor SG IV, Murthy AK, Caldarelli DD et al. (1985). Improved control in advanced head and neck cancer with simultaneous radiation and cisplatin/5-FU chemotherapy. Cancer Treat Rep 69: 938–939

Taylor SG IV, Murthy AK, Showel JL et al. (1985). Improved control in advanced head and neck cancer with simultaneous radiation and cisplatin/5-FU chemotherapy. Cancer Treat Rep 69: 938–939

Thomas G, Dembo A, Beale F et al. (1984). Concurrent radiation mitomycin C and 5-Fluorouracil in poor prognosis carcinoma of the cervix: preliminary results of a phase I–II study. Int J Radiat Oncol Biol Phys 10: 1785

van der Werf-Messing G, Friedall GH, Menon RS et al. (1982). Carcinoma of the urinary bladder T2 Nx Mo treated by preoperative irradiation followed by cystectomy. Int J Rad Oncol Biol Phys 8: 1849–1855

Vietti J, Eggerding F, Voleriote E (1971). Combined effect of radiation and 5-FU on survival on transplanted leukemia cells. J Nat Cancer Inst 47: 865–870

Wendt TC, Wustrow TPU, Hortenstein RC et al. (1987). Accelerated split course radiotherapy and simultaneous cis-dichloro diammine platinum and 5 Fluorouracil chemotherapy with folinic acid enhancement for unresectable carcinoma of the head and neck. Radiation Oncol. 10: 277–284

Wheeler P, Salter M, Stephans S et al (1988). Simultaneous therapy with high dose cisplatin and radiation for unresectable squamous cell cancer of the head and neck: a phase I–II study. NCI Monogr. 6: 339–341

Wolinsky I, Swiniorsky J, Kensler CI, Venditi JM (1974). Combination radiotherapy and chemotherapy for P388 lymphocytic leukemia in vitro. Cancer Treat Rep 4: 73–76

Section I
Principles of Infusion Chemotherapy

1 Experimental Rationale for Continuous Infusion Chemotherapy

R. Brian Mitchell, Mark J. Ratain, and Nicolas J. Vogelzang

CONTENTS

1.1 Introduction

The optimal schedule has not been established for the administration of most antineoplastic agents. Schabel et al. (1984), using murine tumor models, have demonstrated the importance of dose intensity for optimal antineoplastic effect. The administration schedule required to achieve maximal dose

R. Brian Mitchell, MD, Mark J. Ratain, MD, Assistant Professor of Medicine and Clinical Pharmacology, Nicholas J. Vogelzang, MD, Associate Professor of Medicine, Joint Section of Hematology/Oncology, The University of Chicago, 5841 S. Maryland Avenue, Box 420, Chicago, IL 60637, USA

intensity, however, is not the same for every drug. The pharmacodynamic response to any drug is a function of concentration and duration of exposure. The simplest function is the concentration–time product ($C \times T$) or area under the (concentration) curve (AUC) (Powis 1985). Many antineoplastic agents, however, demonstrate a marked schedule dependency – i.e., at equivalent AUCs, a prolonged infusion will yield much greater tumor cell kill than a shorter infusion or bolus. Other anticancer drugs may exhibit a marked concentration dependency, such that the reverse is true.

The relative cell cycle or phase specificity of a drug in vitro is often the most important determinant of its in vivo schedule dependency. The strongest theoretical argument for continuous infusion chemotherapy is that most chemotherapeutic agents are, to some degree, phase specific or cycle specific, and most tumors have a very low growth fraction (i.e., most cells resting in G_0) (Simpson-Herren and Lloyd 1970; Lira 1966). In general, a better response to chemotherapy with cell cycle specific agents is obtained in experimental tumor systems with high proliferative

Table 1.1. Determinants of schedule dependency

In favor of continuous infusion	In favor of bolus dosing
Short half-life	Long half-life
Antimetabolite	Alkylating agent
Drug has reversible action	Drug has irreversible action
Phase specific	Non-cycle specific
Slow uptake into cells	Rapid uptake into cells
Rapid cellular excretion	Prolonged cellular retention
Activation slow compared to excretion	No drug activation required
Low growth fraction	High growth fraction
Dose-limiting toxicity is related to peak serum concentration	Dose-limiting toxicity is related to length of exposure
Stable drug	Unstable drug
Plateau in dose–response curve	Steep dose–response curve

Table 1.2. Concentration vs time dependency of antineoplastic agents (adapted from MATSUSHIMA et al. 1985)

Drug	$IC_{50}(\mu g/ml)$[a]		
	1-h exposure	24-h exposure	SDR[b]
5-Fluorouracil	220	0.23	957
Methotrexate	97	0.32	303
Bleomycin	3.5	0.012	292
Etoposide	3.3	0.032	103
Cisplatin	19	0.30	63
Teniposide	0.45	0.012	38
Melphalan	1.3	0.13	10
Nimustine	14	1.5	9.3
Daunomycin	0.05	0.0055	9.1
Mitomycin C	0.48	0.06	8.0
Actinomycin D	0.052	0.0081	6.4
Doxorubicin	0.13	0.022	5.9

[a] IC = concentration which allows only 50% colony growth compared with control cultures
[b] SDR = schedule dependency ratio: < 24 implies concentration dependency; > 24 implies time dependency

fractions. Table 1.1 lists the variables that may affect the schedule dependency of a drug.

A variety of classification systems have been developed to group antineoplastic agents based on in vitro survival curves of tumor cell lines (BRUCE et al. 1966; DREWINKO et al. 1979; SHIMOYAMA 1975; MATSUSHIMA et al. 1985). Two of the simplest, yet most useful, are those of SHIMOYAMA and MATSUSHIMA et al. SHIMOYAMA found three types of action: Ia – concentration dependent, II – time dependent, and Ib – AUC dependent. However, studies by MATSUSHIMA et al. suggest a continuum between types Ia and II, as shown in Table 1.2.

In vitro assays to determine the advantage of prolonged exposure do not account for other biological variables such as half-life, threshold concentration, intracellular metabolism, active metabolites, tissue distribution and storage, tissue penetration, differential in vivo toxicities, development of resistance, or drug stability. In vivo experiments, however, can be difficult to interpret because of these variables. In vivo experiments can be performed in at least three ways: (a) direct measurement of tumor size or total tumor burden, ignoring toxicity to the animal; (b) assessment of overall survival, which should account for different therapeutic ratios of various schedules; and (c) the use of "equitoxic doses" in an attempt to correct for differences in toxicity between bolus and infusion schedules. In vivo studies suggesting that divided frequent doses of a drug are more effective

than single bolus doses are considered to favor the use of infusion chemotherapy.

Unfortunately, both in vitro and in vivo data may predict only the response in that tumor system. This chapter attempts to assess the potential advantage of continuous infusion for those antineoplastic agents which have been found to or might possibly potentiate radiation therapy. Other agents, such as the vinca alkaloids (vincristine, vinblastine, vindesine) may exhibit schedule dependency, but are not thought to be useful in combination with radiation therapy. Clinical data are presented in succeeding chapters.

1.2 Antimetabolites

The antimetabolites were among the first antineoplastic agents, and are probably the best-studied class of anticancer drugs. These compounds are either analogs of nucleotides [cytosine arabinoside, 5-azacytidine, 6-mercaptopurine, 6-thioguanine, 5-fluorouracil (5-FU)] or inhibit the synthesis of nucleotides (methotrexate, hydroxyurea) that are required for DNA synthesis. Most of these drugs have short elimination half-lives (ALBERTS and CHEN 1980) and are phase specific (BRUCE et al. 1966; SHIMOYAMA 1975), making them good theoretical candidates for continuous infusion chemotherapy. In fact, most antimetabolites have been employed by continuous infusion in clinical trials (VOGELZANG 1984), and continuous infusion of cytosine arabinoside is part of many standard treatment regimens for acute nonlymphocytic leukemias (LISTER and ROHATINER 1983) and preleukemic syndromes (WISCH et al. 1983). Unlike alkylating agents, which show a steep dose–response curve when cell lines are incubated for 1 h, antimetabolites such as methotrexate and cytosine arabinoside show a plateau in the dose–response curve even with 24-h exposures. Added therapeutic effectiveness requires the use of prolonged exposure (FREI et al. 1988).

1.2.1 Cytosine Arabinoside

Cytosine arabinoside (ara-C) is well suited for continuous infusion because: (a) intracellular metabolism to the active form (ara-CTP) appears to be saturable (PLUNKETT et al. 1987), (b) the terminal half-life is short due to rapid deamination by plasma cytidine deaminase (α = 7–20 min; β = 0.5–2.6 h) (CHABNER 1982a) and (c) it is stable in solution for several days.

In Vitro Data. MUUS et al. (1987), using fresh bone marrow cells from patients with acute myelocytic leukemia (AML), have demonstrated the schedule dependency of ara-C in vitro. Exposure to ara-C at a concentration of 100 µM for 1 h ($C \times T$ = 100 µM · h) allows 80% colony survival compared to controls, while exposure at 0.1 µM for 240 h ($C \times T$ = 24 µM · h) allowed 0% colony survival.

In Vivo Data. KLINE et al. (1966) found that a single dose of 1.4 g/kg ara-C had little effect on L1210 leukemia in mice, whereas divided doses were quite effective. A 3 mg/kg dose was required on a four times daily schedule, whereas a 500 mg/ kg dose was necessary when the mice were treated every 4 days. Several subsequent reports have concluded that ara-C is optimally administered in frequent divided doses (SHACKNEY 1970; SKIPPER et al. 1967, 1970; VENDITTI 1971). SKIPPER et al. (1970) found that the only curative schedule was administration every 3 h (for eight doses) on every 4th day. Using a 512 mg/kg total dose, they obtained a cure rate of over 80%. A single dose of 3000 mg/kg was equitoxic to the animals, and induced a modest (60%) increase in life span, but no cures. Interestingly, daily administration of ara-C (total dose 510 mg/kg) produced an increase in life span, but there were no cures. No in vivo experiments using long-term infusions, similar to those used clinically, have been reported.

1.2.2 Fluorinated Pyrimidines

The rationale for infusion of these drugs is strong because they are cell cycle specific antimetabolites with very short elimination half-lives (10–20 min for 5-FU) (EL SAYED and SADEE 1983). Despite the strong theoretical rationale for the administration of these agents by continuous infusion, and the frequent use of this schedule clinically, there is sparse and conflicting data concerning the schedule dependency of 5-FU.

In Vitro Data. The data of CALABRO-JONES et al. (1982) suggest that the pharmacodynamic effect of 5-FU exposure in vitro is proportional to $C \times T$. They found that a 240-h exposure at 1 µg/ml was as effective as a 2-h exposure at 100 µg/ml. On the

other hand, MATSUSHIMA et al. (1985) found that either 220 µg/ml for 1 h (AUC = 220 h · µg/ml) or 0.23 µg/ml for 24 h (AUC = 5.5 h · µg/ml) achieved 50% cytotoxicity in PC-7 lung carcinoma. This latter finding suggests that the exposure time is much more important, and argues against the use of the concentration–time product to compare dosing schedules.

In Vivo Data. There are no conclusive in vivo data on the use of 5-FU or FUDR by infusion. SKIPPER et al. (1970), using a murine L1210 leukemia model, found the total LD_{10} for a single dose or for 15 daily doses to be 250 mg/kg and 338 mg/kg, respectively. Using equitoxic doses (0.7–1.0 of the LD_{10} for each schedule), they demonstrated a 50% increase in life span over that of control animals for the single dose, but a >100% increase in life span for the daily × 15 schedule. There were no cures using 5-FU in this tumor system.

Recently, calcium leucovorin has been shown to potentiate the effect of 5-FU in several tumor systems (KEYOMARSI and MORAN 1985; RUSTUM et al. 1987), suggesting that combination dosing schedules should be studied.

1.2.3 Methotrexate

Methotrexate (MTX) inhibits purine and pyrimidine synthesis by rapidly reversible competitive inhibition of dihydrofolate reductase (SCHILSKY 1983). MTX is a rational candidate for continuous infusion because: (a) its effect upon tumor cells is reversible (cytostatic), (b) it exerts its effect only on cells in cycle (JOHNSON et al. 1978), and (c) its elimination half-life is only 8–10 h in man (SCHILSKY 1983). However, continuous infusion may not be superior to oral daily doses.

In Vitro Data. Although MTX activity and toxicity are dependent on both dose and duration of treatment, EICHOLTZ and TROTT (1985) and KEEFE et al. (1982) have developed mathematical models of MTX cytotoxicity which show that cell survival is affected to a greater extent by exposure duration than by exposure dose. In the first of these studies, doubling the duration of exposure resulted in a four- to tenfold decrease in tumor cell survival, while a tenfold increase in concentration caused less than a tenfold decrease in cell survival. MATSUSHIMA et al. (1985) showed that either a 1-h exposure at 97 µg/ml (AUC = 97 h · µg/ml) or a

24-h exposure at $0.32 \mu g/ml$ (AUC = $7.7 h \cdot \mu g/ml$) resulted in 50% cytotoxicity. MTX would likely be more dependent on exposure duration were it not for the intracellular accumulation of MTX polyglutamates. In some tumor systems, polyglutamates efflux from the cell much more slowly than MTX itself, resulting in prolonged inhibition of dihydrofolate reductase (JOLIVET et al. 1982). Different rates of formation and efflux of these polyglutames would be expected to alter the schedule dependency of MTX in various tumor systems.

In Vivo Data. PINEDO and CHABNER (1977) demonstrated that MTX toxicity cannot be related to the $C \times T$ in vivo, as continuous infusion at plasma concentrations of $0.05 \mu M$ for 72 h (AUC = $3.6 \mu M \cdot h$) was equitoxic to $10 \mu M$ for 12 h (AUC = $120 \mu M \cdot h$). Divided doses or prolonged infusions of MTX are more toxic to normal cells than intermittent bolus treatments (PINEDO and CHABNER 1977; ZAHARKO et al. 1974). Toxicity varies from tissue to tissue (small intestine > marrow > Lewis lung tumor) (ZAHARKO et al. 1974). There have been no in vivo studies comparing the therapeutic index of MTX by continuous infusion to intermittent bolus therapy. VENDITTI et al. (1964) assessed the therapeutic index (survival) of a variety of schedules of MTX in murine L1210 leukemia. The schedules ranged from twice daily to weekly, and once daily appeared to be optimal. Thus, it is not clear that continuous intravenous infusion of MTX would be superior to oral daily doses.

1.2.4 Hydroxyurea

Hydroxyurea (HYD), an older antineoplastic agent, interferes with DNA synthesis by inhibiting ribonucleotide reductase (KRAKOFF et al. 1968). Because it is rapidly eliminated (FISHBEIN 1967), it is usually given as multiple daily oral doses. As was stated above for MTX, continuous infusion of HYD may not be superior to divided oral daily doses.

In Vitro Data. RUPNIAK et al. (1983) suggested that prolonged exposure to HYD is required for cytoxicity. Both 1- and 6-h exposures were ineffective at a concentration of 1 mg/ml (13 mM) against both ovarian carcinoma cells and the COLO 205 cell line. In contrast, there was less than 10% survival using $50 \mu g/ml$ (0.66 mM) continuously,

although the length of the incubation was not stated.

In Vivo Data. Both SKIPPER et al. (1970) and VENDITTI (1971) compared the effectiveness of a range of treatment schedules of HYD against L1210 leukemia in vivo. Both studies demonstrated that administering the drug every 3 h on every 4th day was optimal. This was the only schedule that was curative, although the effect of continuous infusion or continuous multiple daily doses was not assessed.

1.3 Plant Alkaloids

Plant alkaloids are a diverse group of antineoplastic agents. The vinca alkaloids are believed to cause mitotic arrest via their interactions with tubulin (BENDER and CHABNER 1982). Because they do not interact with DNA, there is little reason to suspect that they would be useful in concomitant therapy, and they will not be discussed further except to mention that there are some data to support the administration of vinca alkaloids by continuous infusion. Recent experimental data suggest that the epipodophyllotoxins (VP-16, VM-26) are cytotoxic due to their ability to inhibit topoisomerase II (ROSS et al. 1984; MINOCHA and LONG 1984). In contrast to the antimetabolites, these agents generally have long half-lives in man, ranging from 8 h for VP-16 to 85 h for vincristine (VCR) (CREASEY 1981; NELSON 1982), suggesting that intermittent bolus dosing may provide nearly equivalent activity. These drugs are usually administered by bolus i.v. injections or short infusions, although an oral form of VP-16 has recently become available (LAU et al. 1979).

1.3.1 Epipodophyllotoxins

Two epipodophyllotoxins are in clinical use – etoposide (VP-16) and teniposide (VM-26). VP-16 has a shorter half-life (8–11 h) than the vinca alkaloids and VM-26. Fairly strong experimental evidence supports the use of divided doses of these drugs, although the superiority of continuous infusion has not been established. Because these agents are highly insoluble (JACKSON and BENDER 1978) and relatively unstable (LUDWIG and

ALBERTS 1984), dilutions for continuous infusion must be made with care.

In Vitro Data. DREWINKO and BARLOGIE (1976) showed that at a VP-16 concentration of 1 μg/ml, doubling the exposure time produced a tenfold increase in cytotoxicity. LUDWIG et al. (1984) tested fresh human tumor explants, and found that 5% were sensitive (≤ 30% cell survival) to a 1-h exposure to VP-16, but 15% were sensitive to a continuous exposure (200 h at 1/200th of the 1-h dose). Interestingly, none of the tumors were sensitive to both 1-h and continuous exposure. This is especially interesting in light of these same investigators' results regarding the instability (60% decay over 72 h) of VP-16 in solution (LUDWIG and ALBERTS 1984). MATSUSHIMA et al. (1985) achieved 50% cytotoxicity with a 1-h exposure to VP-16 at 3.3 μg/ml ($C \times T = 3.3$ μg · h/ml) or a 24-h exposure at 0.032 μg/ml ($C \times T = 0.77$ μg · h/ml).

In Vivo Data. VIETTI et al. (1978) assessed the in vivo cytotoxicity of VM-26 in mice bearing L1210 leukemia using both an i.v. bolus and 24-h infusion. The systemic toxicities of the two schedules were comparable, but there was a tenfold or greater increase in tumor cytotoxicity with the infusion schedule. BROGGINI et al. (1983) found that 6.5 mg/kg of VM-26 every 3 days × 3 was more effective and less toxic than 20 mg/kg as a single bolus dose in treating mice injected intramuscularly with Lewis lung carcinoma cells.

DOMBERNOWSKY and NISSEN (1973) compared various schedules of VP-16 administration in L1210-bearing mice. They did not use continuous infusion, but assessed the effect of frequent (every 3 h) small doses on survival. Some cures were achieved with all 16 schedules, but a 100% cure rate was achieved only by using 3.75 mg/kg every 3 h on days 1 and 5. Further studies of these drugs are needed to compare frequent dosing to continuous infusion. The availability of an oral form may obviate the need for continuous infusion, although the absorption of oral etoposide is highly variable.

1.4 Alkylating Agents

The alkylating agents are a diverse group of drugs with a final common pathway – the covalent bind-ing of alkyl groups of the drug to DNA, and with many agents, the formation of intrastrand, inter-strand, and protein–DNA cross-links (COLVIN 1981). The alkylating agents are not phase specific, but may have an increased effect on cells in cycle. They are usually classified as Ia (Shimoyama) agents, showing steep, exponential dose–response curves in vitro (BRUCE et al. 1966; SHIMOYAMA 1975; FREI et al. 1988). Although most alkylating agents have short half-lives, they are generally small molecules that penetrate rapidly into tissues and cells and rapidly bind to DNA (FRIBERG et al. 1987). These agents do not show increased activity with continuous infusion, although the therapeutic index may be improved.

1.4.1 Cyclophosphamide

Cyclophosphamide (CTX) is a widely used anti-neoplastic agent, available in both oral and parenteral forms, although the bioavailability of the oral form may have significant interindividual variation (GROCHOW and COLVIN 1983). CTX is eliminated fairly rapidly by metabolism and urin-ary excretion, with a half-life of approximately 7 h. The activated metabolites appear to have an even shorter half-life. CTX must be metabolized in vivo to the active compound 4-hydroxycyclopho-sphamide (4-HC) (COLVIN 1982). FREI et al. (1988) have shown that in vitro 4-HC exhibits a steep dose–response curve against a human breast ade-nocarcinoma cell line (MCF-7). There are no in vitro data directly assessing the schedule de-pendency of 4-HC. Early in vivo studies in L1210-bearing mice compared single (or weekly) doses to frequent intermittent dosing (SKIPPER et al. 1970; VENDITTI 1971; VENDITTI et al. 1964). In all stu-dies, a single or weekly dose was optimal. SKIPPER et al. (1970) cured 44 of 79 animals with a single dose of 300 mg/kg i.p., compared to no cures in 30 mice treated with 26 mg/kg daily for 15 days. The latter schedule had only minimal activity, with an 8% improvement in survival.

1.4.2 Ifosfamide

Ifosfamide is an alkylating agent similar to CTX. There are few data concerning its schedule de-pendency, although it is frequently given as a 3- to 5-day infusion. KLEIN et al. (1984) treated mice inoculated with Ehrlich-ascites tumor cells with a single i.v. bolus of 250 mg/kg or with 60 mg/kg every 6 h for four doses. The animals which received fractionated doses experienced a 1-log greater tumor cell kill.

1.4.3 Nitrogen Mustard

Like CTX, nitrogen mustard has been classified as a type 1 or Ia agent, i.e., prolonged exposure causes little increase in cell kill at any given concentration in vitro (BRUCE et al. 1966; SHIMOYAMA 1975). There have been few studies of the pharmacokinetics of nitrogen mustard, but it appears to have a half-life of approximately 9 min (WILLIAMSON et al. 1966).

In Vitro Data. SHIMOYAMA (1975) compared 30-min and 48-h exposures to nitrogen mustard in four different cell lines. There was only a slight decrease (ranging from 23% to 72%) in the drug concentration required for 1-log cytotoxicity when the exposure time was lengthened 100-fold. This is the expected in vitro pattern for an alkylating agent.

In Vivo Data. BRUCE et al. (1966) compared the in vivo effects of bolus and divided (every 6 h × 4) doses of nitrogen mustard in lymphoma-bearing mice. Using bolus dosing (0.1–0.4 mg/mouse), there was an equal effect of the drug on both normal and malignant cells (using colony-forming assays). However, when the same total dose was administered in four doses (every 6 h), there was a five- to ninefold therapeutic advantage versus the malignant cells. Toxicity to normal cells was slightly less, but significantly increased toxicity to malignant colony-forming units was observed. This result is somewhat surprising, and it has not been duplicated in other tumor systems.

1.4.4 Melphalan

Melphalan (MEL) is a nitrogen mustard analogue that is usually administered orally. There have been no in vivo studies of the schedule dependency of MEL, but the in vitro data do not favor the use of infusion for administration. WU et al. (1982) compared the effects of 1-h and 14-day exposures of MEL on Raji lymphoma cells in vitro. Prolonged exposure did not increase the cytotoxicity of MEL, although it appears to be unstable at

37°C. MATSUSHIMA et al. (1985) showed that an increase in incubation time from 1 h to 24 h allows a tenfold decrease in dose.

1.4.5 Nitrosoureas

The nitrosoureas are unique among the alkylating agents because of their lipophilicity, ability to cross the blood–brain barrier, and delayed toxicity (COLVIN 1981). They are type Ia agents, with no expected advantage to continuous infusion. In addition, drug stability is a practical obstacle, particularly for carmustine (BCNU) (DREWINKO et al. 1972; WHEELER et al. 1975).

In Vitro Data. WHEELER et al. (1975) evaluated the importance of exposure time on curmustine cytotoxicity. The instability of the drug in solution was a major problem, but they were able to show that the survival fraction is related to the area under the curve of extracellular BCNU:

$$SF = Ne^{-K \cdot AUC}$$

This would suggest that prolonged infusion might have equivalent activity to a single bolus (if the elimination of BCNU is first order), but does not suggest any advantage to infusion.

In Vivo Data. VENDITTI et al. (1964) compared the effects of a variety of schedules of BCNU administration on murine L1210 leukemia. A single dose of 96 mg/kg cured five of eight mice, and was the optimal schedule. Low dose daily administration was active, with an increase in survival of 460%, but was not curative. On the other hand, SCHMIDT et al. (1972) showed that continuous exposure could be quite effective. They used implanted silicone rubber capsules to administer BCNU dissolved in either ethanol or sesame oil. This allows for the slow release of the drug over a 16-h period. Capsules were inserted both subcutaneously and intraperitoneally and were compared with standard intraperitoneal injections. The delivery of BCNU by slow diffusion was quite effective, with 80% of mice surviving 30 days compared with none receiving intraperitoneal bolus injections.

1.4.6 Mitomycin C

Although mitomycin C (MIT) is an antitumor antibiotic, it acts as an alkylating agent, probably by reduction of its quinone group intracellularly (CROOKE 1981). MIT is rapidly metabolized in vivo, with a terminal half-life of 40–120 min. Only 15% of the administered dose is recovered in the urine (DEN HARTIGH et al. 1983). Because of its short half-life, MIT would, a priori, be a good candidate for continuous infusion; however, the experimental data thus far do not support this.

In Vitro Data. SHIMOYAMA (1975) placed MIT in group Ib – implying some time-dependent cytotoxicity. WU et al. (1982) and BARLOGIE and DREWINKO (1980) independently demonstrated that the tumoricidal effect of MIT was equivalent for long and short exposures at equivalent $C \times T$. On the other hand, MATSUSHIMA et al. (1985) found that a 1-h exposure required a lower $C \times T$ than a 24-h exposure to achieve 50% inhibition of tumor cell growth ($0.48 \, \mu g \cdot h/ml$ vs $1.44 \, \mu g \cdot h/ml$).

In Vivo Data. ROCKWELL et al. (1987), using an EMT6 murine mammary tumor model, showed that the cytotoxicity of MIT is proportional to AUC regardless of schedule, ranging from a single i.v. bolus to a daily $\times$ 5 schedule. A prolonged course of daily injections, while less toxic, was also less effective.

1.4.7 Cisplatin

Although cisplatin is similar to other alkylating agents in its ability to bind DNA, it blocks LoVo cells in the S and G_2 phases, suggesting that at least in some tumor systems the drug may be phase specific (BERGERAT et al. 1979b).

In Vitro Data. The pharmacodynamics of cisplatin in vitro are complex. RUPNIAK et al. (1983) demonstrated that the slope of the dose–response curve is increased as the exposure time is increased, for both ovarian and colon carcinoma cell lines. For example, a 1-h exposure of COLO 205 cells to $3 \, \mu g/ml$ cisplatin permitted 40% survival compared with controls, whereas a 6-h exposure to $0.5 \, \mu g/ml$ cisplatin permitted 10% survival. For the ovarian cell line, there was a similar decrease in cell survival with prolonged incubation (at equal $C \times T$), although this cell line was sensitive at much higher concentrations. Most other in vitro studies do not suggest any advantage for prolonged exposure (DREWINKO et al. 1973; BERGERAT et al. 1979a; NIELL et al. 1982), and there may be a

disadvantage to prolonged exposure for some cell lines (WU et al. 1982; LUDWIG et al. 1984). However, there are no in vitro studies that take into account nonspecific protein binding (e.g., to albumin, etc.), assuring that there is a continuous supply of free (ultrafilterable) cisplatin, as would be the case with in vivo continuous infusion.

In Vivo Data. Although there are multiple human studies of continuous infusion, some of which suggest decreased toxicity (and therefore, perhaps, increased therapeutic ratio) of continuous infusion cisplatin, there has been only one in vivo animal study of the schedule dependency of cisplatin (MORAN and STRAUS 1981). Using the murine L1210 leukemia model, treatment schedules were varied from bolus infusion (12 mg/kg) to a 72-h infusion (12 mg/kg/day). There was no significant cytotoxic advantage to any schedule when the optimal dose (in terms of prolonged survival of the animals) was used, although a 24-h infusion was inferior to bolus injection when an equivalent dose was used.

1.4.8 Carboplatin

Carboplatin is a new cisplatin analogue that causes minimal renal, neuro- and ototoxicity. It is believed to have the same mechanism of action as cisplatin–DNA interstrand and protein cross-linking, although the occurrence of these changes takes longer than after exposure to cisplatin (WAGSTAFF et al. 1989). Gradual tissue accumulation of carboplatin has been demonstrated, and in some cases levels are higher in tumor than in surrounding normal tissue (NEWELL et al. 1987). The relatively short half-life and the evidence for tissue accumulation of carboplatin suggest that repetitive dosing or prolonged infusion should be investigated. There have been no preclinical studies of the schedule dependency of carboplatin.

1.4.9 Dacarbazine

Dacarbazine (DTIC) was originally designed as a purine antimetabolite, but subsequent studies have shown it to be metabolized to an alkylating agent (CHABNER 1982b). DTIC is largely inactive in vitro, so there are few data addressing its schedule dependency in vitro.

None of the in vivo experiments were designed specifically to assess the schedule dependency of DTIC, but it appears to be as active against L1210 leukemia as a bolus dose or as a daily dose (SHIRAKAWA and FREI 1970). MONTGOMERY (1976) showed that a single dose of 480 mg/kg intraperitoneally on day 1 after inoculation prolonged survival of mice with L1210 leukemia by 93% while 100 mg/kg/day on days 1–30 (total dose 3000 mg/kg) prolonged survival by 80%. VENDITTI (1971) also showed that a single dose of 300–600 mg/kg i.p. is as effective as 100 mg/kg i.p. on days 1–9.

1.4.10 Thiotepa

Thiotepa is an alkylating agent which exhibits a steep dose–response curve through several logs (TEICHER et al. 1988). It is well tolerated when given as an intravenous bolus, and the dose-limiting toxicity is myelosuppression. The schedule dependency of thiotepa has not been investigated, but it is likely to be a concentration-dependent rather than a time-dependent agent, as are the other alkylating agents.

1.5 Antineoplastic Antibiotics

The group of agents generally classified as antibiotics is a diverse, complex set of agents that vary substantially in their schedule dependency in experimental systems. This group includes (a) classical anthracycline antibiotics; (b) anthracenes, which although not anthracycline antibiotics, share the planar ring structure with the anthracyclines; (c) bleomycin and its analogues; and (d) antinomycin D and other agents, such as neocarzinostatin. The benefit of continuous infusion of antibiotic agents must be assessed for each agent independently.

1.5.1 Doxorubicin

Doxorubicin (DOX) has a terminal half-life of approximately 30 h (GREEN et al. 1983), and it is taken up by cells, resulting in intracellular concentrations 30–100 times plasma concentrations (SPETH et al. 1987a, b).

In Vitro Data. MATSUSHIMA et al. (1985) showed that an increase in exposure time from 1 h to 24 h allowed only a sixfold decrease in median inhibitory concentration for DOX and a ninefold decrease for daunomycin. DOX was the least time-dependent drug of the 17 they tested. LUDWIG et al. (1984), using the human tumor clonogenic assay, found that five of six sensitive tumors were only sensitive to the 1-h exposure and not to the continuous exposure (equivalent $C \times T$). DREWINKO et al. (1983), using the LoVo human colon adenocarcinoma cell line, found that cytotoxicity was maximal (90%) by 2 h of DOX exposure. No increase in cytotoxicity was observed with drug exposure up to duration of 50 h. WU et al. (1982), using Raji lymphoma cells, showed that while prolonged exposure could kill more tumor cells than a 1-h exposure, the $C \times T$ product required was much greater. Multiple other studies support the classification of DOX as AUC dependent, with concentration being more important than length of exposure (NGUYEN-NGOC et al. 1984; KRISHAN and FREI 1976; EICHHOLTZ-WIRTH 1980).

In Vivo Data. ENSMINGER et al. (1979) compared a 3-day continuous infusion with a bolus schedule in rats with acute myelogenous leukemia. In this model system, the infusion was slightly more effective, but also more toxic. GOLDIN and JOHNSON (1975) concluded that DOX had no schedule dependency in either L1210 or P388 murine leukemia, B-16 melanoma, or Lewis lung carcinoma. A single bolus on day 1 was as effective as a daily × 9 days administration schedule.

SANDBERG et al. (1970), in the L1210 model, concluded that a single bolus of DOX was therapeutically equivalent to injections every 3 h. However, the greatest number of survivors occurred when animals were given injections every 3 h for the first day only. PACCIARINI et al. (1978) treated mice bearing murine mammary carcinoma or Lewis lung carcinoma with either a single i.v. bolus dose or the same dose of DOX divided over 4 days. They found both an increased survival and slightly decreased toxicity (20% early deaths vs 0% early deaths) with divided dose schedules. The intracardiac DOX concentration was lower in the animals treated daily × 4. JENSEN et al. (1984) and SOLCIA et al. (1981) both reported that cardiotoxicity was more severe in animals given bolus DOX than in animals receiving either long-term infusion or low-dose daily injections.

1.5.2 Mitoxantrone

Mitoxantrone is the first anthracene derivative to enter clinical trials, and it appears to have activity in breast cancer, acute leukemia, and lymphoma (HENDERSON et al. 1989; PRENTICE et al. 1984; GEMS et al. 1984). FOUNTZILAS et al. (1984), using human pancreatic adenocarcinoma cells, found that increasing exposure time did not increase cytotoxicity.

1.5.3 Bleomycin

Bleomycin (BLM) is a unique antineoplastic agent isolated from a soil *Streptomyces* by UMEZAWA in the 1960s (UMEZAWA et al. 1966); it acts as a mininuclease, causing DNA strand scissions and release of thymidine from the DNA strand (SAUSVILLE et al. 1978; PRATT and RUDDON 1979). The terminal half-life of BLM is 2.5–9 h (BROUGHTON et al. 1977; YEE et al. 1983; HALL et al. 1982).

In Vitro Data. DREWINKO et al. (1972), using a lymphocytic lymphoma cell line, showed that the dose–response curve for BLM has an upward concavity: progressively higher doses causes proportionately less cytotoxicity. However, with an increase in BLM exposure from 5 h to 35 h (sevenfold increase in $C \times T$) there was a 3-log decrease in survival using the same cell line. MATSUSHIMA et al. (1985) achieved 50% cytotoxicity with either a 1-h exposure at 3.5 µg/ml ($C \times T = 3.5\,\mu\text{g} \cdot \text{h/ml}$) or a 24-h exposure at 0.0112 µg/ml ($C \times T = 0.27\,\mu\text{g} \cdot \text{h/ml}$). LUDWIG et al. (1984) found that, of 25 clinical tumor specimens tested against BLM, only six were sensitive to the drug. However, four of these six were sensitive only at the 200-h exposure (equivalent $C \times T$). Using cell lines, they found a 200-fold increase in incubation time allowed a 900-fold decrease in BLM concentration.

In Vivo Data. The in vivo data concerning BLM scheduling are contradictory. PENG et al. (1980), using P388 leukemic spleen colony-forming units in mice, demonstrated a 0.5 greater log cell kill ($P < 0.01$) with a 6-day intraperitoneal (i.p.) infusion compared with daily i.p. injections. SIKIC et al. (1978), using a Lewis lung carcinoma model, compared the effect of continuous subcutaneous (s.c.)

infusion, s.c. injection twice weekly, and s.c. injection ten times weekly using the same total dose for all three groups. There was significantly ($P < 0.05$) greater inhibition of tumor growth with the continuous s.c. route as compared with the twice weekly s.c. route. Although the advantage was modest (<0.5 log difference), this was a relatively insensitive tumor, in that the highest dose (80 mg/kg) resulted in only a 0.5 log inhibition as compared with untreated controls. At tolerable doses (40 mg/kg and less), s.c. injection twice weekly was not significantly different from continuous s.c. infusion.

Two other groups, using human tumor xenografts of human testicular (OSIEKA et al. 1984) and squamous cell cancer of the nasal cavity (WAHLBERG et al. 1987), have been unable to show a therapeutic advantage to continuous infusion i.p. compared to daily injections or bolus administration of the same total dose.

1.5.4 Actinomycin D

Actinomycin D binds to DNA between complementary pairs of deoxyguanosine residues (GLAUBIGER and RAMU 1982). This intercalation into the DNA helix probably blocks the progression of RNA polymerases along the DNA. The tight binding to DNA may explain why early studies found that actinomycin D is cytotoxic at any phase of the cell cycle (BHUYAN et al. 1977). It is usually given as a daily i.v. bolus × 5 days, but recent data suggest that a single i.v. bolus may be equally effective because of the prolonged tissue phase (GLAUBIGER and RAMU 1982).

In Vitro Data. None of the studies addressing the schedule dependency of antinomycin D have shown any significant increase in cytotoxicity for prolonged exposure compared with 1-h exposure at an equivalent $C \times T$. Against Raji lymphoma cells, WU et al. (1982) showed that a 1-h exposure to 0.5 µg/ml ($C \times T = 0.5\,\mu\text{g} \cdot \text{h/ml}$) permitted 0% tumor cell survival while a 336-h exposure to 0.001 µg/ml ($C \times T = 0.34\,\mu\text{g} \cdot \text{h/ml}$) permitted 0% survival. Using PC-7 cells, MATSUSHIMA et al. (1985) showed that an increase in exposure time from 1 h to 24 h allowed only a sixfold reduction in drug concentration. LUDWIG et al. (1984), using a fresh tumor clonogenic assay and four human tumor cell lines, were unable to show any advantage for prolonged exposure (200 h) compared with a 1-h exposure.

In Vivo Data. VALERIOTE et al. (1973), using AKR murine leukemia, found that cytotoxicity to leukemia cells and normal cells was concentration dependent, but recommended frequent small doses of the drug since they found that a single bolus dose was more toxic than a daily × 5 bolus schedule. GALBRAITH and MELLETT (1976) Ridgeway found that a single nonlethal dose of actinomycin D cured osteogenic sarcoma, and that all animals receiving daily doses (continuous schedule) died.

1.6 Biological Agents

1.6.1 Interferon

In vitro the interferons (IFNs) are cytostatic. An antiproliferative effect has been demonstrated against a variety of cell lines (BELLARDELLI et al. 1982; NICKLOFF et al. 1985; BORDEN et al. 1984) and fresh malignant tumors in vitro using the human tumor clonogenic assay (SALMON et al. 1983). The exact mechanisms, yet to be clarified in each tumor system, involve interaction with specific high affinity receptors leading to inhibition of protein synthesis and/or gene expression (PESTKA et al. 1987).

The in vivo effects of the IFNs may be due to their antiproliferative action or to immune modulation via induction of class I MHC antigens (α, β, γ), class II MHC antigens (γ), or tumor-associated antigens (SALMON et al. 1983; PESTKA et al. 1987; STEINIGER et al. 1987). KATAOKA et al. (1985) demonstrated that the in vivo effect of human purified IFN-α (hybrid A/D) on various tumors inoculated into BALB/c mice was not correlated with the in vitro sensitivity of the tumor to IFN. BELLARDELLI et al. (1982) and LEE et al. (1983) have demonstrated that mouse IFN-α/β is effective in vivo against both IFN-sensitive and IFN-resistant Friend erythroleukemia cells injected into DBA/2 mice.

In Vitro Data. There are few studies addressing the schedule dependency of the IFNs in vitro. Most studies have utilized a continuous exposure to IFN, and have found that 4 days of incubation are usually needed to exert an antiproliferative effect (BORDEN et al. 1984; SALMON et al. 1983).

On the other hand, NICKLOFF et al. (1985) found that a 30-min exposure of SCL-1 to IFN-γ was as effective in inhibiting cell proliferation as prolonged exposure to the same concentration.

In Vivo Data. There are also few in vivo studies comparing various schedules of IFN administration at equivalent AUCs. GRESSER et al. (1986) injected 6-week-old male DBA/2 mice with 2.2 × 10^5 Friend leukemia cells and then treated all animals with a total dose of 6.4 × 10^6 units of mouse IFN-α/β. Animals treated every 4 days survived no longer than control animals, whereas animals treated daily or with three injections per week survived significantly longer than control animals (58 days compared with 28 days).

1.6.2 Tumor Necrosis Factor

Human recombinant tumor necrosis factor (TNF) has recently become available for clinical investigation. Produced by macrophages in response to endotoxin and various other stimuli, it binds to a specific membrane receptor on target cells and is then internalized (TSUJIMOTO et al. 1985). In some tumor systems TNF is directly cytotoxic, while in others hemorrhagic necrosis occurs, perhaps because of a procoagulant effect of TNF (ASHER et al. 1987). It has a brief half-life of 15–30 min (CHAPMAN et al. 1987). HARANAKA and SATOMI (1981) used 48-h exposures to show that TNF was cytotoxic for tumor cells but not for normal cells. However, others have shown that the therapeutic ratio is not as great as these early in vitro data suggested (ASHER et al. 1987). DARZYNKIEWICZ et al. (1984) have shown that mouse L-cells treated with TNF are blocked in G_2, but subsequently enter mitosis and lyse. The G_2 block can be detected within 4 h, but cell lysis does not occur for 7–12 h. ROSENBLUM et al. (1988) have also suggested that in vitro exposures of 12–36 h are more cytotoxic than brief exposures. On the other hand, ASHER et al. (1981) have shown that single doses of TNF administered subcutaneously can cure some mice with transplanted murine sarcomas and adenocarcinomas. Unfortunately, the doses necessary (6–10 µg) were near the LD_{50} (10 µg). CHAPMAN et al. (1987) found the dose-limiting side-effect of subcutaneous administration to be local inflammation. Although the above data suggest a role for continuous infusion in the clinical use of TNF, much work remains to be done to define the

Table 1.3. Experimental rationale for continuous infusion: classification of antineoplastic agents

Agent	Data supporting classification		
	Theoretical	In vitro	In vivo
Bolus infusion superior			
CTX/4-HC	++		
Nitrogen mustard	++	+	±
MEL	++	±	
Nitrosoureas	++	±	+
MIT	+	+	±
DTIC	+	±	±
Actinomycin D	+	+	+
Continuous infusion superior			
Ara-C	++	++	++
5-FU	++		
HYD[a]	++		
VP-16[a]	+	+	+
BLM[a]	+	++	±
IFN[a]	++	±	+
TNF	++	±	
Vinca alkaloids	+	±	±
MTX[a]	++	++	±
AUC dependent			
CDDP	+	+	+
Carboplatin	+		
DOX	±	++	++
Mitoxantrone	±		

Abbreviations as defined in the text
[a] Oral or subcutaneous administration may substitute for continuous infusion

usefulness of TNF as an anticancer agent and to define the optimal schedule of administration.

1.7 Conclusion

The optimal scheduling of antineoplastic drugs is a complex subject. Direct, empirical data supporting a dosing schedule are always desirable, but are not available for many agents. Based on the available experimental data, antineoplastic agents can be divided into three groups, as shown in Table 1.3: (a) agents for which there is a pharmacodynamic advantage (i.e., increased tumor cell kill) to bolus infusion; (b) agents for which there is a pharmacodynamic advantage to continuous infusion; and (c) agents whose cytotoxicity is roughly proportional to AUC. These three groups roughly parallel Shimoyama's types Ia, II, and Ib. For many agents, the classification may be based more on theoretical than on empirical grounds because of the lack of data. As therapy for certain diseases

becomes more refined, it becomes more important to use preclinical studies in planning dose schedules, but schedule dependency may need to be reassessed when concomitant therapy is employed.

References

Alberts DS, Chen H-SG (1980) Tabular summary of pharmacokinetic parameters relevant to in vitro drug assay. In: Salmon SE (ed) Cloning of human tumor stem cells. Alan R. Liss, New York, pp 351–359

Asher A, Mulc JJ, Reichert CM, Shiloni E, Rosenberg SA (1987) Studies on the anti-tumor efficacy of systemically administered recombinant tumor necrosis factor against several murine tumors in vivo. J Immunol 138: 963–974

Barlogie B, Drewinko B (1980) Lethal and cytokinetic effects of mitomycin-C on cultured human colon cancer cells. Cancer Res 40: 1973–1980

Barlogie B, Drewinko B, Johnston DA, Freireich EJ (1976) The effect of adriamycin on the cell cycle traverse of a human lymphoid cell line. Cancer Res 36: 1975–1979

Bellardelli F, Gresser I, Maury C, Maunoury MT (1982) Anti-tumor effects of interferon in mice injected with interferon-sensitive and interferon-resistant Friend leukemia cells. Int J Cancer 30: 813–820

Bender RA, Chabner BA (1982) Tubulin binding agents. In: Chabner BA (ed) Pharmacologic principles of cancer treatment. W.B. Saunders, Philadelphia, pp 256–262

Bergerat J-P, Barlogie B, Drewinko B (1979a) Effects of cis-dichlorodiammineplatinum (II) on human colon carcinoma cells in vitro. Cancer Res 39: 1334–1338

Bergerat J-P, Barlogie B, Golde W, Johnston DA, Drewinko B (1979b) In vitro cytokinetic response of human colon cancer cells to cis-dichlorodiammineplatinum (II). Cancer Res 39: 4356–4363

Bhuyan BK, Fraser TJ, Day KJ (1977) Cell proliferation kinetics and drug sensitivity of exponential and stationary populations of cultured L1210 cells. Cancer Res 37: 1057–1062

Borden EC, Groveman DS, Nasu T, Reznikoff C, Bryan GT (1984) Antiproliferative activities of interferons against human bladder carcinoma cell lines in vitro. J Urol 132: 800–803

Bosanquet AG, Bird MC (1988) Degradation of melphalan in vitro: rationale for the use of continuous exposure in chemosensitivity assays. Cancer Chemother Pharmacol 21: 211–215

Broggini M, Colombo T, D'Incali M (1983) Activity and pharmacokinetics of teniposide in Lewis lung carcinoma-bearing mice. Cancer Treat Rep 67: 555–559

Broughton A, Strong JE, Holoye PY, Bedrossian WM (1977) Clinical pharmacology of blemoycin following intravenous infusion as determined by radioimmunoassay. Cancer 40: 2772–2778

Bruce WR, Meeker BE, Valeriote FA (1966) Comparison of the sensitivity of normal hematopoietic and transplanted lymphoma colony-forming cells to chemotherapeutic agents administered in vivo. J Natl Cancer Inst 37: 233–245

Calabro-Jones PM, Byfield JE, Ward JF, Sharp TR (1982) Time-dose relationships for 5-fluorouracil cytotoxicity against human epithelial cancer cells in vitro. Cancer Res 42: 4413–4420

Cantrell DA, Smith KA (1984) The interleukin-2 T cell system: a new cell growth model. Science 224: 1312

Chabner BA (1982a) Cytosine arabinoside. In: Chabner BA (ed) Pharmacologic principles of cancer treatment. W.B. Saunders, Philadelphia, pp 387–401

Chabner BA (1982b) DTIC (dacarbazine). In: Chabner BA (ed) Pharmacologic principles of cancer treatment. W.B. Saunders, Philadelphia, pp 350–354

Chapman PB, Lester TJ, Casper ES et al. (1987) Clinical pharmacology of recombinant human tumor necrosis factor in patients with advanced cancer. J Clin Oncol 5: 1942–1951

Cheever MA, Greenberg PD, Irle C et al. (1984) Interleukin-2 administered in vivo induces the growth of cultured T cells in vivo. J Immunol 132: 2259

Colburn WA, Hakimi J, Bekersky I (1987) Plasma concentration profiles of human recombinant interleukin-2 (HrIL-2) in the rat following administration by various systemic routes. Drug Metab Dispos 15: 429–430

Colvin M (1981) Molecular pharmacology of alkylating agents. In: Crooke ST, Prestayko AW (eds) Cancer and chemotherapy, vol III. Antineoplastic agents. Academic, New York, pp 287–302

Colvin M (1982) Alkylating agents. In: Chabner BA (ed) Pharmacologic principles of cancer treatment. W.B. Saunders, Philadelphia, pp 276–308

Creasey WA (1981) The vinca alkaloids and similar compounds. In: Crooke ST, Prestayko AW (eds) Cancer and chemotherapy, vol III. Antineoplastic agents. Academic, New York, pp 79–96

Crooke ST (1981) Mitomycin C – an overview. In: Crooke ST, Prestayko AW (eds) Cancer and chemotherapy, vol III. Antineoplastic agents. Academic, New York, pp 49–60

Darzynkiewicz Z, Williamson B, Carswell EA, Old LJ (1984) Cell cycle-specific effects of tumor necrosis factor. Cancer Res 44: 83–90

den Hartigh J, McVie JG, van Oort WJ, Penedo HM (1983) Pharmacokinetics of mitomycin C in humans. Cancer Res 43: 5017–5021

Dombernowsky P, Nissen NI (1973) Schedule dependency of the antileukemic activity of the podophyllotoxin-derivative VP-16-213 (NSC-141540) in L1210 leukemia. Acta Pathol Microbiol Scand 81: 715–724

Donohue JH, Rosenberg SA (1983) The fate of interleukin-2 after in vivo administration. J Immunol 130: 2203–2208

Drewinko B, Barlogie B (1976) Survival and cycle-progression delay of human lymphoma cells in vitro exposed to VP-16-213. Cancer Treat Rep 60: 1295–1306

Drewinko B, Novak JK, Barranco SC (1972) The response of human lymphoma cells in vitro to bleomycin and 1,3-bis(2-chloroethyl)-1-nitrosourea. Cancer Res 32: 1206–1208

Drewinko B, Brown BW, Gottlieb JA (1973) The effect of cis-diamminedichloroplatinum (II) on cultured human lymphoma cells and its therapeutic implications. Cancer Res 33: 3091–3095

Drewinko B, Roper PR, Barlogie B (1979) Patterns of cell survival following treatment with anticancer agents in vitro. Eur J Cancer 15: 93–99

Drewinko B, Yang L-Y, Barlogie B, Trujillo JM (1983) Comparative cytotoxicity of bisantrene, mitoxantrone, ametantrone, dihydroxyanthracenedione, dihydroxyanthracenedione diacetate, and doxorubicin on human cells in vitro. Cancer Res 43: 2648–2653

Eichholtz H, Trott KR (1985) Effect of methotrexate concentration and exposure time on mammalian cell survival in vitro. Br J Cancer 41: 277–284

Eichholtz-Wirth H (1980) Dependence of the cytostatic effect of adriamycin on drug concentration and exposure time in vitro. Br J Cancer 41: 886–891

El Sayed YM, Sadee W (1983) In: Ames MM, Powis G, Kovach JS (eds) Pharmacokinetics of anticancer agents in humans. Elsevier, New York, pp 209–227

Ensminger WD, Greenberger JS, Egan EM, Muse MB, Moloney WC (1979) Technique for preclinical evaluation of continuous infusion chemotherapy with the use of WF rat acute myelogenous leukemia. JNCI 62: 1265–1268

Ettinghausen SE, Rosenberg SA (1986) Immunotherapy of murine sarcomas using lymphokine activated killer cells: optimization of the schedule and route of administration of recombinant interleukin-2. Cancer Res 46: 2784–2792

Ferguson T (1980) Prevention and delay of spontaneous mammary and pituitary tumors by long- and short-term ingestion of 5-fluorouracil in Wistar-Furth rats. Oncology 37: 353–356

Fishbein WN (1967) Excretion and hematologic effects of single intravenous hydroxyurea infusions in patients with chronic myeloid leukemia. Johns Hopkins Med J 121: 1–8

Fountzilas G, Gratzner H, Lim LO, Yunis AA (1984) Sensitivity of cultured human pancreatic carcinoma cells to dihydroxyanthracenedione. Int J Cancer 33: 347–353

Frei E, Teicher BA, Holden SA, Cathcart KNS, Wang Y (1988) Preclinical studies and clinical correlation of the effect of alkylating dose. Cancer Res 48: 6417–6423

Friberg S, Ehrsson H, Eksborg S, Carenfeldt C (1987) Intratumoral measurement and plasma pharmacokinetics of intravenously administered melphalan: report of a patient with plasmacytoma. Cancer Chemother Pharmacol 20: 342–343

Glabraith WM, Mellett LB (1976) Disposition of [^{3}H]actinomycin D in tumor-bearing mice. Cancer Res 36: 1242–1245

Gems RA, Steinberg J, Posner L (1984) Mitoxantrone in malignant lymphoma. Semin Oncol 11(3) [Suppl 1]: 47–49

Glaubiger D, Ramu A (1982) Anti-tumor antibiotics. In: Chabner BA (ed) Pharmalogic principles of cancer treatment. W.B. Saunders, Philadelphia, pp. 402–415

Goldin A, Johnson RK (1975) Experimental tumor activity of adriamycin (NSC-123127). Cancer Chemother Rep 6: 137–145

Green RF, Collins JM, Jenkins JF, Speyer JL, Myers CE (1983) Plasma pharmacokinetics of adriamycin and adriamycinol: implications for the design of in vitro experiments and treatment protocols. Cancer Res 43: 3417–3421

Gresser I, Belardelli F, Maury C, Tovey MG, Maunoury M-T (1986) Anti-tumor effects of interferon in mice injected with interferon-sensitive and interferon-resistant Friend leukemia cells. IV. Definition of optimal treatment regimens. Int J Cancer 38: 251–257

Grochow LB, Colvin M (1983) Clinical pharmacokinetics of cyclophosphamide. In: Ames MM, Powis G, Kovach JS (eds) Pharmacokinetics of anticancer agents in humans. Elsevier, New York, pp 135–154

Hall SW, Strong JE, Broughton A, Frazier ML, Benjamin

RS (1982) Bleomycin clinical pharmacology by radioimmunoassay. Cancer Chemother Pharmacol 9: 22–25

Haranaka K, Satomi N (1981) Cytotoxic activity of tumor necrosis factor (TNF) on human cancer cells in vitro. Jpn J Exp Med 51: 191–194

Henderson IC, Allegra JC, Woodcock T et al. (1989) Randomized clinical trial comparing mitoxantrone with doxorubicin in previously treated patients with metastatic breast cancer. J Clin Oncol 7: 560–571

Hortobagyi GN, Frye D, Buzdar AU et al. (1989) Decreased cardiac toxicity of doxorubicin administered by continuous intravenous infusion in combination chemotherapy for metastatic breast carcinoma. Cancer 63: 37–45

Jackson DV, Bender RA (1978) The clinical pharmacology of the vinca alkaloids, epipodophyllotoxins, and maytansine. In: Pinedo HM (ed) Clinical pharmacology of anti-neoplastic drugs. Elsevier, Amsterdam, pp 277–293

Jensen RA, Acton EM, Peters JH (1984) Doxorubicin cardiotoxicity in the rat: comparison of electrocardiogram, transmembrane potential, and structural effects. J Cardiovasc Pharmacol 6: 186–200

Johnson LF, Fuhrman CL, Abelson HT (1978) Resistance of resting 3T6 mouse fibroblasts to methotrexate cytotoxicity. Cancer Res 38: 2408–2412

Jolivet J, Schilsky RL, Baily BD, Drake JC, Chabner BA (1982) Synthesis, retention and biological activity of methotrexate polyglutamates in cultured human breast cancer cells. J Clin Invest 70: 351–360

Kataoka T, Matsuura N, Oh-hashi F, Suhara Y (1985) Treatment regimen and host T-cell dependent therapeutic effect of interferon in mouse solid tumors. Cancer Res 45: 3548–3553

Keefe DA, Capizzi RL, Rudnick SA (1982) Methotrexate cytotoxicity for L5178Y/Asn- lymphoblasts: relationship of dose and duration of exposure to tumor cell viability. Cancer Res 42: 1614–1645

Keyomarsi K, Moran RG (1985) Folinic acid augmentation of the effects of fluoropyrimidines on murine and human leukemic cells. Cancer Res 46: 5229–5235

Klein HO, Wickramanayake PD, Christian E, Coerper C (1984) Therapeutic effects of single-push or fractionated injections or continuous infusion of oxazaphosphorines (cyclophosphamide, ifosfamide, asta Z 7557). Cancer 54: 1193–1203

Kline I, Venditti JM, Tyrer DD, Goldin A (1966) Chemotherapy of leukemia L1210 in mice with 1-β-D-arabinofuranosylcytosine hydrochloride. I. Influence of treatment schedules. Cancer Res 26: 853–859

Krakoff IH, Brown NC, Reichard P (1968) Inhibition of ribonucleoside diphosphate reductase by hydroxyurea. Cancer Res 28: 1559–1565

Krishan A, Frei E (1976) Effect of adriamycin on the cell cycle traverse and kinetics of cultured human lymphoblasts. Cancer Res 36: 143–150

Lau ME, Hansen HH, Niessen NI, Pedersen H (1979) Phase 1 trial of a new form of an oral administration of VP-16-213. Cancer Treat Rep 63: 485–487

Lee SH, Chiu H, Rinderknecht E, Sabo W, Stebbing N (1983) Importance of treatment regimen of interferon as an antitumor agent. Cancer Res 43: 4172–4175

Lira AK (1966) The dynamics of tumor growth. Br J Cancer 28: 490–502

Lister Ta, Rohatiner AZS (1983) The treatment of acute myelogenous leukemia in adults. Semin Hematol 19: 172–192

Ludwig R, Alberts DS (1984) Chemical and biological stability of anticancer drugs used in a human tumor clonogenic assay. Cancer Chemother Pharmacol 12: 142–145

Ludwig R, Alberts DS, Miller TP, Salmon SE (1984) Evaluation of anticancer drug schedule dependency using an in vitro human tumor clonogenic assay. Cancer Chemother Pharmacol 12: 135–141

Matsushima Y, Kanzawa F, Hoshi A et al. (1985) Time-schedule dependency of the inhibiting activity of various anticancer drugs in the clonogenic assay. Cancer Chemother Pharmacol 14: 104–107

Minocha A, Long BH (1984) Inhibition of the DNA catenation activity of type II topoisomerase by VP-16-213 and VM-26. Biochem Biophys Res Commun 122: 165–170

Montgomery JA (1976) Experimental studies at southern research institute with DTIC (NSC-45388) Cancer Treat Rep 60: 125–134

Moran RE, Straus MJ (1981) Effects of pulse and continuous intravenous infusion of cis-diamminedichloroplatinum on L1210 leukemia in vivo. Cancer Res 41: 4993–4996

Muus P, Haanen C, Raijmakers R et al. (1987) Influence of dose and duration of exposure on the cytotoxic effect of cytarabine toward human hematopoietic clonogenic cells. Semin Oncol 14(2) [Suppl 1]: 238–244

Nelson RL (1982) The comparative clinical pharmacology and pharmacokinetics of vindesine, vincristine, and vinblastine in human patients with cancer. Med Pediatr Oncol 10: 115–127

Newell DR, Siddik ZH, Gumbrell LA et al. (1987) Plasma free platinum pharmacokinetics in patients treated with high dose carboplatin. Eur J Cancer Clin Oncol 25: 1399–1405

Nguyen-Ngoc T, Vrignaud P, Robert J (1984) Cellular pharmacokinetics of doxorubicin in cultured mouse sarcoma cells originating from autochthonous tumors. Oncology 41: 55–60

Nickloff BJ, Basham TY, Merigan TC, Morhenn VB (1985) Immunomodulatory and antiproliferative effect of recombinant alpha, beta, and gamma interferons on cultured human malignant squamous cell lines, SCL-1 and SW-1271. J Invest Dermatol 84: 487–490

Niell HB, Wood CA, Mickey DD, Soloway MS (1982) Time- and concentration-dependent inhibition of the clonogenic growth of N-[4-(5-nitro-2-furyl)-2-thiazoly] formamide-induced murine bladder tumor cell lines by cis-diamminedichloroplatinum (II). Cancer Res 42: 807–811

Osieka R, Glatte P, Schmidt C-G (1984) Continuous infusion versus intermittent bolus injection of bleomycin in a human embryonal testicular cancer xenograft. Cancer Treat Rep 68: 799–801

Pacciarini MA, Barbieri B, Colombo T, Broggini M, Garattini S, Donelli MG (1978) Distribution and antitumor activity of adriamycin given in a high-dose and a repeated low-dose schedule to mice. Cancer Treat Rep 62: 791–800

Peng YM, Alberts DS, Cheng H-SG, Mason N, Moon TE (1980) Antitumor activity and plasma kinetics of bleomycin by continuous and intermittent administration. Br J Cancer 41: 644–647

Pestka S, Langer JA, Zoon KC, Samuel CE (1987) Interferons and their actions. Ann Rev Biochem 56: 727–777

Pinedo HM, Chabner BA (1977) Role of drug concentration, duration of exposure, and endogenous metabolites in determining methotrexate cytotoxicity. Cancer Treat Rep 61: 709–719

Plunkett W, Liliemark JO, Estey E, Keating MJ (1987) Saturation of ara-CTP accumulation during high-dose ara-C therapy: pharmacologic rationale for intermediate-dose ara-C. Semin Oncol 14(2) [Suppl 1]: 159–166

Powis G (1985) Anticancer drug pharmacodynamics. Cancer Chemother Pharmacol 1985: 14: 177–183

Pratt WB, Ruddon RW (1979) The anticancer drugs. Oxford University Press, Oxford

Prentice HG, Robbins G, Ma DDF, Ho AD (1984) Mitoxantrone in relapsed and refractory acute leukemia. Semin Oncol 11(3) [Suppl 1]: 32–35

Rockwell S, Nierenburg M, Irvin CG (1987) Effects of the mode of administration of mitomycin on tumor and marow response and on the therapeutic ratio. Cancer Treat Rep 71: 927–934

Rosenberg SA, Mule JJ, Spiess PJ, Reichert CM, Schwarz SL (1985) Regression of established pulmonary metastases and subcutaneous tumor mediated by the systemic administration of high-dose recombinant interleukin-2. J Exp Med 161: 1169–1188

Rosenblum MG, Donato NJ, Gutterman JU (1988) Characterization of human tumor necrosis factor alpha antiproliferative effects on human cells in culture. Lymphokine Res 7: 107–117

Rosenstein M, Yron I, Kaufmann Y, Rosenberg SA (1984) Lymphokine-activated killer cells: lysis of fresh syngeneic natural killer-resistant murine tumor cells by lymphocytes cultured in interleukin-2. Cancer Res 44: 1946–1953

Ross W, Rowe T, Glisson B, Yalowich J, Liu L (1984) Role of topoisomerase II in mediating epipodophyllotoxin-induced DNA cleavage. Cancer Res 44: 5857–5860

Rupniak HT, Whelan RDH, Hill BT (1983) Concentration and time-dependent inter-relationships for antitumor drug cytotoxicities against tumor cells in vitro. Int J Cancer 32: 7–12

Rustum YM, Trave F, Zakrzewski SF et al. (1987) Biochemical and pharmacologic basis for potentiation of 5-fluorouracil by leucovorin. NCI Monogr 5: 165–170

Salmon SE, Durie BGM, Young L, Liu RM, Trown PW, Stebbing N (1983) Effects of cloned human leukocyte interferons in the human tumor stem cell assay. J Clin Oncol 3: 217–225

Sandberg JS, Howsden FL, DiMarco A, Goldin A (1970) Comparison of the antileukemic effect in mice of adriamycin (NSC-123127) with daunomycin (NSC-82151). Cancer Chemother Rep 54: 1–7

Sausville EA, Stein RW, Peisach J, Horwitz SB (1978) Properties and products of the degradation of DNA by bleomycin and iron. Biochemistry 17: 2746–2754

Schabel FM, Griswold DP, Corbett TH, Laster WR (1984) Increasing the therapeutic response rates to anticancer drugs by applying the basic principles of pharmacology. Cancer 54 [Suppl]: 1160–1167

Schilsky RL (1983) Clinical pharmacology of methotrexate. In: Ames MM, Powis G, Kovach JS (eds) Pharmacokinetics of anticancer agents in humans. Elsevier, New York, pp 187–208

Schmidt V, Zapol W, Prenoky W, Wonders T, Wodinsky I, Kitz R (1972) Continuous cancer chemotherapy: nitrosourea diffusion through implanted silicone rubber capsules. Trans Am Soc Artif Int Organs 18: 45–52

Shackney SE (1970) A computer model for tumor growth and chemotherapy, and its application to L1210 leukemia treated with cytosine arabinoside (NSC-63878). Cancer Chemother Rep 54: 399–429

Shimoyama M (1975) Cytocidal action of anticancer agents: evaluation of the sensitivity of cultured animal and human cancer cells. Bibl Haemat 40: 711–722

Shirakawa S, Frei E (1970) Comparative effects of the antitumor agents 5-(dimethyltriazeno)-imidazole-4-carboxamide and 1,3-bis(2-chloroethyl)-1-nitrosourea on cell cycle of L1210 leukemia cells in vivo. Cancer Res 30: 2173–2179

Sikic BI, Collins JM, Mimnaugh EG, Gram TE (1978) Improved therapeutic index of bleomycin when administered by continuous infusion in mice. Cancer Treat Rep 62: 2011–2017

Simpson-Herren L, Lloyd HH (1970) Kinetic parameters and growth curves for experimental tumor systems. Cancer Chemother Rep 54: 143–174

Skipper HE, Schabel FM, Wilcox WS (1967) Experimental evaluation of potential anticancer agents. XXI. Scheduling of arabinosylcytosine to take advantage of its S-phase specificity against leukemia cells. Cancer Chemother Rep 51: 125–165

Skipper HE, Schabel FM, Mellett LB et al. (1970) Implications of biochemical, cytokinetic, pharmacologic, and toxicologic relationships in the design of optimal therapeutic schedules. Cancer Chemother Rep 54: 431–450

Solcia E, Ballerini L, Bellini O et al. (1981) Cardiomyopathy of doxorubicin in experimental animals. Factors affecting the severity, distribution and evolution of myocardial lesions. Tumori 67: 461–472

Speth PAJ, Linssen PCM, Boezeman JBM, Wessels HMC, Haanen C (1987a) Cellular and plasma adriamycin concentrations in long-term infusion therapy of leukemia patients. Cancer Chemother Pharmacol 20: 305–310

Speth PAJ, Linssen PCM, Holdrinet RSG, Haanen C (1987b) Plasma and cellular adriamycin concentrations in patients with myeloma treated with ninety-six-hour continuous infusion. Clin Pharmacol Ther 41: 661–665

Steiniger B, van der Meide PH, Westermann J, Klempnauer J (1987) Systemic induction of class II MHC antigens after continuous intravenous infusion of recombinant gamma interferon in rats. Transplant Proc 5: 4322–4324

Teicher BA, Holden SA, Cucchi CA, et al (1988) Combination of N,N',N''-triethylenethiophosphoramide and cyclophosphamide in vitro and in vivo. Cancer Res 48: 94–100

Tsujimoto M, Yip YK, Vilcek J (1985) Tumor necrosis factor: specific binding and internalization in sensitive and resistant cells. Proc Natl Acad Sci USA 82: 7626–7630

Umezawa H, Meada K, Takeuchi T, Toshioka O (1966) New antibiotics: bleomycin A and B. J Antibiot (Tokyo) 19: 200–206

Valeriote F, Vietti T, Tolen S (1973) Kinetics of the lethal effect of antinomycin D on normal and leukemic cells. Cancer Res 33: 2658–2661

Venditti JM (1971) Treatment schedule dependency of experimentally active antileukemic (L1210) drugs. Cancer Chemother Rep 2: 35–59

Venditti JM, Kline I, Goldin A (1964) Evaluation of antileukemic agents employing advanced leukemia L1210 in mice. VIII. Cancer Res 24: 827–879

Vietti TJ, Valeriote FA, Kalish R, Coulter D (1978) Kinetics of cytotoxicity of VM-26 and VP-16-213 on L1210 leukemia and hematopoietic stem cells. Cancer Treat Rep 62: 1313–1320

Vogelzang NJ (1984) Continuous infusion chemotherapy: a critical review. J Clin Oncol 2: 1289–1304

Wagstaff AJ, Ward A, Benfield P, Heel RC (1989) Carboplatin: a preliminary review of its pharmacodynamic and pharmacokinetic properties and therapeutic efficacy in the treatment of cancer. Drugs 37: 162–190

Wahlberg P, Wennerberg J, Alm P, Blörklund A, Tropé C (1987) The effect of continuous bleomycin infusion on the growth and cell kinetics of heterotransplanted squamous cell carcinoma of the head and neck. Anticancer Res 7: 55–58

Wheeler KT, Tel N, Williams ME, Sheppard S, Levin VA, Kabra PM (1975) Factors influencing the survival of rat brain tumor cells after in vitro treatment with 1,3-bis(2-chloroethyl)-1-nitrosourea. Cancer Res 35: 1464–1469

Williamson CE, Kirby JG, Miller JI et al. (1966) Enzyme-alterable alkylating agents. IX. The enzymatic transformation of some nitrogen respiratory. Cancer Res 26: 323–330

Wisch JS, Griffin JD, Kufe DW (1983) Response of pre-leukemic syndromes to continuous infusion low-dose cytarabine. N Engl J Med 309: 1599–1602

Wu P-C, Ozols RF, Hatanaka M, Boone OW (1982) Anti-cancer drugs: effect on the cloning of Raji lymphoma cells. J Natl Cancer Inst 68: 115–121

Yee GC, Crom WR, Lee FH, Smyth RD, Evans WE (1983) Bleomycin disposition in children with cancer. Clin Pharmacol Ther 33: 668–673

Zaharko DS, Dedrick RL, Peale AL, Drake JC, Lutz RJ (1974) Relative toxicity of methotrexate in several tissues of mice bearing Lewis lung carcinoma. J Pharmacol Exp Ther 189: 585–592

2 Combination Chemotherapy by Infusion in Hematological Malignancies

LEONARD SALTZ, MORTON COLEMAN, and PETER YI

CONTENTS

2.1 Introduction

Continuous intravenous infusions of antineoplastic agents have been incorporated into a number of chemotherapeutic strategies employed in the management of hematological malignancies. For the past decade our group has been interested in the use of infusional chemotherapy in the treatment of lymphomas. The following discussion will review our experiences and those of others in this area. We will also comment on work by other investigators on the use of infusional chemotherapy in multiple myeloma. Infusional therapy for the acute leukemias has been considered standard therapy for some time now and as such is regarded as beyond the limits of this review.

2.2 Infusional Therapy for the Lymphomas

In 1977 we in the division of hematology–oncology at the New York Hospital/Cornell University Medical Center began to investigate a new chemotherapeutic regimen for large cell lymphoma (LAURENCE et al. 1982). This six drug regimen,

LEONARD SALTZ, MD,* Division of Hematology-Oncology
MORTON COLEMAN, MD, Clinical Professor of Medicine,
PETER YI, MD, Cornell University Medical Center,
407 East 70th Street, New York, NY 10021, USA

* Present address: Division of Medical Oncology, Memorial Sloan Kettering Cancer Center, 1275 York Avenue, New York, NY 10021, USA

commonly referred to by the acronym "COPBLAM" [cyclophosphamide, Oncovin (vincristine), prednisone, bleomycin, Adriamycin, Matulane (procarbazine)], incorporated several then state of the art concepts in combination chemotherapy. These included the use of six putatively non-cross-resistant drugs in keeping with the rationale of combination chemotherapies as outlined by GOLDIE, COLDMAN, and GUDAUSKAS (GOLDIE et al. 1982), the incorporation of procarbazine, an agent with good central nervous system penetration and activity in large cell lymphoma (DEVITA et al. 1975), the use of 3-week treatment cycles instead of the conventional 4-week period, and the provision for dose escalation of cyclophosphamide and Adriamycin as tolerated to maximum intensity. Among previously untreated patients 73% achieved a complete remission and 55% remained alive and disease free with a minimum follow-up in excess of 8 years.

These early results and reports of similar progress with other combination chemotherapies in large cell lymphoma (SCHEIN et al. 1976; MCKELVEY et al. 1976; SKARIN et al. 1977) encouraged exploration for further improved results using recently evolved concepts in large cell lymphoma treatment. Our group was particularly interested in the utility of incorporating infusional chemotherapy into treatment regimens.

Two qualities which make a drug theoretically more efficacious when given by infusion are a relatively short plasma half-life and a phase specific activity. Also the drug must be adequately stable in solution over time (LOKICH 1987). Bleomycin and vincristine, two drugs used in bolus fashion in the original COPBLAM regimen, were considered particularly ideal for infusional administration. They were both putatively minimally myelosuppressive and considerable experimental evidence existed to suggest that they had the aforementioned desirable characteristics.

The plasma half-life of bleomycin in human circulation is less than 2 h when administered by bolus. It is a phase specific agent with greatest activity in the G_2 and M phases (CARLSON and SIKIC 1983). DREWINKO et al. had demonstrated that an increase in duration of exposure to bleomycin from 4 h to 35 h decreased the survival fraction of human lymphoma cell in culture from 10% to 0.06% (DREWINKO et al. 1972). Subsequently it was reported that both improved therapeutic efficacy and reduced pulmonary toxicity of bleomycin were seen in mice bearing Lewis lung carcinoma when the drug was administered by continuous infusion (SIKIC et al. 1978). A prospective study of 15 patients given bleomycin with a bolus dose followed by 7-day continuous infusion, with a mean total of 227 units, further supported the theory that infusional bleomycin may be less toxic than intermittent bolus injection (COOPER and HONG 1981).

Vincristine also has a short plasma half-life and is M phase specific (VOGELZANG 1984). In vitro work (JACKSON and BENDER 1979) had suggested improved efficacy of vincristine by infusion and phase I trials had demonstrated the safety of this mode of administration (JACKSON et al. 1981a). Further pharmacokinetic studies demonstrated the ability of continuous infusions to sustain blood concentrations of vincristine in man beyond those seen in conventional bolus administration (JACKSON et al. 1981b).

Given much of this experimental underpinning, our group in 1979 began a study on the effects of continuous infusion vincristine and bleomycin in 16 patients with resistant non-Hodgkin's lymphoma (HOLLISTER et al. 1982). Patients received a 48-h infusion of vincristine, a bolus followed by a 120-h infusion of bleomycin, and oral prednisone for 5 days. Responding patients received midcycle treatments of high dose methotrexate with leukovorin rescue. Treatment cycles were repeated every 6 weeks. Three complete responses and five partial responses were noted for a total response rate of 50%. All eight responders were resistant to bolus vincristine and seven were resistant to bolus bleomycin. Though response and survival duration were short (median duration 29 weeks), the results indicated responsiveness based on the manner of administration rather than on the drug itself. The vincristine and bleomycin infusions were therefore incorporated into a revision of the COPBLAM regimen for the initial treatment of non-Hodgkin's lymphoma.

Between 1981 and 1984 our group treated 51 patients with diffuse large cell lymphoma with this modified "COPBLAM III" (BOYD et al. 1988). Treatments consisted of six cycles of 6 weeks' duration each. Each cycle included an inpatient portion containing a 48-h vincristine infusion and a 120-h bleomycin infusion, as well as intravenous boluses of Adriamycin and cyclophosphamide, and 5 days of oral procarbazine and prednisone. The dose of bleomycin was reduced compared with the doses used in the pilot study on resistant lymphoma in an attempt to reduce the risk of pulmonary toxicity in this group of patients in whom long-term survival and multiple treatments were anticipated. On day 22 patients received the outpatient portion of the protocol, which was the same as the inpatient treatment with the exceptions that bleomycin was not given and vincristine was given by bolus. Doses of Adriamycin were escalated by 5 mg in each treatment portion and cyclophosphamide was increased by 50 mg in each treatment portion as tolerated to a maximum dose of 50 mg and 500 mg respectively. The protocol also allowed for dose reduction of Adriamycin, cyclophosphamide, and procarbazine for supervening leukopenia or thrombocytopenia.

There were 51 evaluable patients. Of these, 43 (84%) achieved a complete response and six (12%) achieved a partial response, yielding an overall response of 96%. Clinical complete remissions were noted after a median of two treatment cycles. Of note, response did not differ significantly between stages II bulky, III, and IV. Complete remissions were achieved in 23 of 26 patients (88%) with extranodal involvement, in 24 of 25 patients (96%) less than age 60, and 19 of 26 patients (73%) greater than age 60.

Of the 51 patients, 33 (65%) remain alive and free of disease with a minimum follow-up of greater than 2 years. Of the other 18 patients, five died due to toxicity of therapy, eight failed to achieve a complete response and have subsequently died, one patient died of unrelated causes while in complete remission, and four patients have relapsed, the relapses occurring at 4, 11, 13, and 24 months. It is noteworthy that 92% of patients under the age of 60, as contrasted to 42% of patients over the age of 60, remain alive and free of disease. Thus advanced age proved in this study to be a poor prognostic factor. It is possible that the elderly patients may have had less ability to withstand intensive treatment.

Although a comparison of the COPBLAM III study with COPBLAM shows the COPBLAM III data to be superior, the additional treatment time, expense, and toxicity of COPBLAM III must be considered. The major limiting toxicity in COPB-LAM III was pulmonary toxicity due to bleomycin. This occurred in 39% of patients and resulted in two toxic deaths. This prompted a dose reduction of bleomycin from $7.5 \, mg/m^2$ to $4 \, mg/m^2$ in our current approach. This lower dose level in our hands still retains antitumor activity while reducing the likelihood of pulmonary toxicity.

Several other observations regarding responses and toxicity have led to additional modifications. Bleomycin toxicity was rarely seen before the third or fourth cycle of treatment, whereas those patients destined to obtain a complete response usually did so rapidly, within a median of two cycles. This, taken with the widespread observation that complete remission is necessary for long-term survival, is consistent with reports by Armit-age et al. that patients with early response to treatment have a better long-term prognosis (Armitage et al. 1986). Further, those few early progressions or early recurrences that did occur had a strong propensity to happen during the outpatient (noninfusional) phases of therapy. We therefore believe that "up front" exposure to sequential infusion cycles will be of benefit. These observations have been incorporated into our newer approaches (Coleman et al. 1987).

The CODBLAM IV schema is designed with four sequential infusion cycles similar to the inpatient cycles of COPBLAM III, with the exceptions that the reduced bleomycin dose is used and dexamethasone is substituted for prednisone. Following these infusion cycles patients are fully restaged. They are then treated with single cycles of high dose Adriamycin and then high dose cyclophosphamide, each with bolus vincristine and oral dexamethasone. The remaining six cycles consist of methotrexate with citrovorum rescue, cytarabine, and etoposide. These noninfusional cycles are given in a manner patterned after the COMLA regimen (Gaynor et al. 1985). Results with CODBLAM IV remain preliminary; however, the complete response rate of 82% in a cohort of 61 patients is comparable to the results of COPB-LAM III. No treatment-related deaths occurred and all patients who achieved complete remission did so by the end of the four infusion cycles. The postinfusional intensified phase failed to induce any further complete responses.

Currently we are pursuing further modifications in our approach. Our COPBLAM V program utilizes the infusional cycles of CODBLAM IV

given every 21 days for a minimum of four and a maximum of six cycles. Patients are restaged after each cycle until a complete response is documented and then treated for an additional three cycles, or up to a maximum of six cycles. If complete remission is not obtained after four cycles the patient is considered a treatment failure and is removed from protocol.

The COPBLAM V regimen utilizes six of the eight most active, putatively non-cross-resistant drugs for Hodgkin's disease. Our group has begun to investigate the efficacy of this approach in patients with high risk, refractory, or relapsed Hodgkin's disease. In our initial trials 18 of 26 patients have achieved a complete remission (75%) and four a partial remission. The durability of these responses appears to be shortlived; however, given the poor prognosis of this patient cohort these preliminary results have encouraged further exploration of this approach to Hodgkin's disease.

2.3 Infusional Therapy in Multiple Myeloma

Since the advent of melphalan and other alkylating agents the median survival of patients with multiple myeloma has improved from 7 months in the 1950s to approximately 30 months today (Berg-sagel 1988). A major factor contributing to this benefit is the improved supportive care for infectious and other medical complications of the disease. Despite these improved results, multiple myeloma remains uniformly fatal. In an attempt to improve survival in patients with myeloma refractory to standard chemotherapies the use of infusional chemotherapy protocols has been investigated.

The standard chemotherapeutic approached to multiple myeloma is the use of melphalan and prednisone, which produces an objective response in 50%–60% of patients (Durie et al. 1985). Attempts to improve on these results have centered around the use of multiple chemotherapeutic agents (Case et al. 1977). Randomized studies, however, have failed to demonstrate a clear survival advantage for patients treated with multiple agents over those treated with standard melphalan and prednisone (Cohen et al. 1984).

In 1981 a study of plasma cell growth kinetics demonstrated that the growth fractions of tumor cells were different in different clinical phases of the disease (DREWINKO et al. 1981). Specifically, relapsing patients who had had a good prior response to treatment were shown to have rapid tumor doubling times, with growth fractions of plasma cells ranging from 14% to 83%, as opposed to those of untreated, remission, or primary refractory patients, in whom the growth fraction of plasma cells was consistently below 4%. These data suggested that patients with relapsed myeloma might have disease which would be relatively more susceptible to cycle specific agents, and that the increased exposure time offered by infusion of such agents might be of benefit.

With this background information a study was initiated to investigate the effects of infusional vincristine, Adriamycin, and high dose dexamethasone, the so-called VAD regimen (BARLOGIE et al. 1984). Patients were given vincristine 0.4 mg/day and Adriamycin 9 mg/m²/day by continuous infusion for 96 h, along with daily dexamethasone 40 mg for 4 days, starting on days 1, 9, and 17 of each cycle.

A rapid response, defined as at least a 75% reduction in tumor burden as measured by M protein spike, was seen in 14 of 20 patients (70%) with disease refractory to alkylating agents and in three of nine patients with disease refractory to the bolus administration of Adriamycin. The response rate for patients refractory to alkylating agents was significantly higher than the 23% response reported for a comparable group of refractory patients treated with vincristine, Adriamycin, and prednisone in a noninfusional regimen, and was higher than the response rate for other previously reported salvage regimens (BUZAID and DURIE 1986).

The two unique features of the VAD treatment are the administration of chemotherapy (vincristine and Adriamycin) by infusion and the use of very high dose glucocorticoids. To separate out the contributions of these two modalities a study was undertaken to compare VAD with high dose dexamethasone alone (ALEXANIAN et al. 1986). In this study the response rate to high dose steroids alone was comparable to that for VAD in patients with primary refractory disease. Given the known small growth fraction of myeloma cells in such patients it is not surprising that infusional chemotherapy offered little benefit. However, in patients with relapsed disease, in whom a high plasma cell growth fraction would be expected, a 65% response rate to VAD was noted, compared with a 21% response rate for high dose dexamethasone alone. No other salvage regimen has been reported to achieve comparable response rates to those reported for VAD in relapsed disease. It should be noted, however, that these results represent sequential rather than randomized trials. The implications nevertheless are sufficiently encouraging to warrant further study.

More recently the results of applying infusional chemotherapy in front line treatment of myeloma have been reported (ALEXANIAN and BARLOGIE 1988). Patients received cycles of VAD with and without oral cyclophosphamide. The complete response rate (63%) was comparable to rates seen in other noninfusional, multiagent regimens, and no survival advantage was seen over melphalan and prednisone. Rapidity of response and correction of anemia, however, were greater with infusional regimens than with standard or bolus treatment.

The above results suggest a role for infusional chemotherapy in a select group of myeloma patients. In addition to a potential therapeutic advantage, infusional administration is likely to reduce the cardiotoxicity of Adriamycin (LEGHA et al. 1982). Indeed, measurement of plasma cell and blood plasma concentrations of Adriamycin in myeloma patients showed comparable levels of Adriamycin in the plasma cells with either bolus or infusional administration, but markedly lower peak plasma concentrations by infusion (SPETH et al. 1987). Peak plasma Adriamycin levels are thought to correlate with cardiotoxicity.

Despite improvements in the management of myeloma, all patients ultimately die of their disease. Though response rates to salvage therapy have been improved, all patients ultimately will develop refractory disease, assuming they do not first succumb to some other intervening complication. Investigations are continuing into ways to increase further the responsiveness of multiple myeloma to chemotherapy. One such approach is to attempt to overcome multiple drug resistance by the use of verapamil, a calcium channel blocker. Calcium channel blockers have been shown to interfere with multiple drug resistance of some tumor cells in vitro (TSURUO et al. 1983). An Adriamycin-resistant myeloma plasma cell line has been shown to become sensitive to continued exposure to Adriamycin in the presence of levels of verapamil which are easily achieved clinically (DURIE and DALTON 1988). These levels are lower than those reported necessary for verapamil-induced sensitization of other tumor cells. Mentioned in the same report is the case of one patient whose disease was resistant to VAD, who subsequently responded to VAD after verapamil was begun for treatment of a supraventricular tachycardia. Prospective trials of verapamil–VAD combinations are currently underway.

2.4 Summary

The use of infusional chemotherapy in the hematological malignancies is based on considerable theoretical and laboratory groundings. Clinical trials have so far yielded some encouraging results, and optimism for further therapeutic advances in this field is fully justified. Many clinical investigations are actively underway.

References

Alexanian R, Barlogie B (1988) VCAD-VAD as initial chemotherapy for multiple myeloma (abstr). Am Soc Hematol 859

Alexanian R, Barlogie B, Dixon D (1986) High-dose glucocorticoid treatment of resistant myeloma. Ann Intern Med 105: 8–11

Armitage JO, Weisenburger DD, Hutchins M et al. (1986) Chemotherapy for diffuse large-cell lymphoma: rapidly responding patients have more durable remissions. J Clin Oncol 4: 160–164

Barlogie B, Smith L, Alexanian R (1984) Effective treatment of advanced multiple myeloma refractory to alkylating agents. N Engl J Med 310: 1353–1356

Bergsagel DE (editorial) (1988) Use a gentle approach for refractory myeloma patients. J Clin Oncol 6: 757–758

Boyd DB, Coelman M, Papish SW et al. (1988) COPB-LAM III: infusional combination chemotherapy for diffuse large-cell lymphoma. J Clin Oncol 6: 425–433

Buzaid AC, Durie BGM (1986) Management of refractory myeloma: a review. J Clin Oncol 6: 889–905

Carlson RW, Sikic BI (1983) Continuous infusion or bolus injection in cancer chemotherapy. Ann Intern Med 99: 823–833

Case DC Jr, Lee BJ III, Clarkson BD (1977) Improved survival times in multiple myeloma treated with melphalan, prednisone, cyclophosphamide, vincristine, and BCNU: M-2 protocol. Am J Med 63: 897–903

Cohen HJ, Silberman HR, Tornyos K et al. (1984) Comparison of two long term chemotherapy regimens, with or without agents to modify skeletal repair, in multiple myeloma. Blood 63: 639–648

Coleman M, Gerstein G, Topilow A et al. (1987) Advances in chemotherapy for large-cell lymphoma. Semin Hematol [Suppl 1]: 8–20

Cooper KR, Hong WK (1981) Prospective study of the pulmonary toxicity of continuously infused bleomycin. Cancer Treat Rep 65: 419–425

DeVita VT Jr, Canellos GP, Chabner B, Schein P, Hubbard SP, Young RC (1975) Advanced diffuse histiocytic lymphoma, a potentially curable disease. Results with combination chemotherapy. Lancet I: 248–250

Drewinko B, Novak JK, Barrabco SC (1972) The response of human lymphoma cells in vitro to bleomycin and 1, 3-bis (2-chloroethyl)-1-nitrosourea. Cancer Res 32: 1206–1208

Drewinko B, Alexanian R, Boyer H, Barlogie B, Rbinow SI (1981) The growth fraction of human myeloma cells. Blood 57: 333–338

Durie BGM, Dalton WS (1988) Reversal of drug-resistance in multiple myeloma with verapamil. Br J Haematol 68: 203–206

Durie BGM, Barlogie B, Kyle RA (1985) Current approaches to multiple myeloma and related diseases. Education Program, American Society of Hematology

Gaynor ER, Ultmann JE, Golomb HM et al. (1985) Treatment of diffuse histiocytic lymphoma (DHL) with (cyclophooshamide, Oncovin, methotrexate, leulovorin, cytosine arabinodise): a 10 year experience in a single institution. J Clin Oncol 12: 1596–1604

Goldie JH, Coldman AJ, Gudauskas GA (1982) Rationale for the use of alternating non-cross-resistant chemotherapy. Cancer Treat Rep 66: 439–449

Hollister D Jr, Silver RT, Gordon B, Coleman M (1982) Continuous infusion vincristine and bleomycin with high dose methotrexate for resistant non-Hodgkin's lymphoma. Cancer 50:1690–1694

Jackson DV Jr, Bender RA (1979) Cytotoxic thresholds of vincristine in a murine and a human leukemia cell line in vitro. Cancer Res 39: 4346–4349

Jackson DV Jr, Sethi VS, Spurr CL (1981a) Intravenous vincristine infusion: phase I trial. Cancer 48: 2559–2564

Jackson DV Jr, Sethi VS, Spurr CL et al. (1981b) Pharmacokinetics of vincristine infusion. Cancer Treat Rep 65: 1043–1048

Laurence J, Coleman M, Allen SL, Silver RT, Pasmantier M (1982) Combination chemotherapy of advanced diffuse histiocytic lymphoma with six-drug COP-BLAM regimen. Ann Intern Med 97: 190–195

Legha SS, Banjamin RS, Mackay B et al. (1982) Reduction of doxorubicin cardiotoxicity by prolonged continuous intravenous infusion. Ann Intern Med 96: 133–139

Lokich JJ (1987) Cancer chemotherapy by infusion. Precept, Chicago, pp 3–11

McKelvey EM, Gottlieb JA, Wilson HE et al. (1976) Hydroxyldaunomycin (Adriamycin) combination chemotherapy in malignant lymphoma. Cancer 38: 1484–1493

Schein PS, DeVita VT Jr, Hubbard S et al. (1976) Bleomycin, adriamycin, cyclophosphamide, vincristine, and prednisone (BACOP) combination chemotherapy in the treatment of advanced diffuse histiocytic lymphoma. Ann Intern Med 85: 417–422

Sikic BI, Collins JM, Mimnaugh EG, Gram TE (1978) Improved therapeutic index of bleomycin when administered by continuous infusion in mice. Cancer Treat Rep 62: 2011–2017

Skarin AT, Rosenthal DS, Noloney WC, Frei E III (1977) Combination chemotherapy of advanced non-Hodgkin's lymphoma with bleomycin, adriamycin, cyclophosphamide, vincristine, and prednisone (BACOP). Blood 49: 759–770

Speth PAJ, Linssen PCM, Holdrinet RSG, Haanen C
  (1987) Plasma and cellular Adriamycin concentrations in
  patients with myeloma treated with ninety-six-hour
  continuous infusion. Clin Pharmacol Ther 41: 661–665
Tsuruo T, Lida H, Norjiri M, Tsukagoshi S, Sakurai Y

(1983) Circumvention of vincristine and doxorubicin
  resistance in vitro and in vivo by calcium influx blockers.
  Cancer Res 43: 2905–2910
Vogelzang NJ (1984) Continuous infusion chemotherapy: a
  critical review. J Clin Oncol 2: 1289–1304

3 Combination Chemotherapy by Infusion in Solid Tumors

JAMES D. AHLGREN

CONTENTS

Drug delivery by infusion is a promising avenue for improving the therapeutic index of several classes of drugs. Although the pharmacological rationale for infusional therapy has been long appreciated, relevant clinical trials have only recently begun to emerge, and only in a relatively few forms of cancer.

Infusional drug delivery can be used either to increase therapeutic efficacy or to reduce certain forms of toxicity; in some cases both objectives can be achieved simultaneously. Efficacy can be improved in the case of cycle specific drugs (e.g., antimetabolites) which have short plasma half-lives: increased exposure of cells during the sensitive part of the cell cycle increase killing. Another avenue for increasing efficacy is possible in synergistic combinations requiring increased duration of exposure. An example would be infusional schedules of a short-acting drug capable of inhibiting repair of alkylation damage of DNA, as has been suggested for bleomycin or etoposide. Some drug-related toxicities are related to peak

JAMES D. AHLGREN, MD, Associate Professor of Medicine, Division of Hematology-Oncology, The George Washington University, Medical Center, 2150 Pennsylvania Avenue, NW, Washington, DC 20037, USA

drug levels rather than to area under the curve (AUC). If efficacy is related to AUC, equivalent doses delivered by infusion can reduce toxicity without sacrificing efficacy.

Thus, combination chemotherapy in which one or more drugs are given by infusion can be designed either based upon the infusional advantages of the drug by itself (in terms of efficacy or toxicity) or upon increased synergy resulting from the infusional schedule. This chapter will discuss such combination chemotherapy in the solid tumors.

3.1 Combinations Based on Infusional 5-Fluorouracil

The pharmacological and clinical advantages of infusional schedules over bolus schedules of 5-FU are irrefutably established. 5-FU, an S phase specific agent, has a plasma half-life of only 11 min (MACMILLAN et al. 1978). Yet solid tumors typically have only a small fraction of cells in S phase at any time. For example, thymidine pulse labeling studies in most human solid tumors show labeling indices of only 2%–10% (SHACKNEY 1985). Thus, a bolus dose of 5-FU reaches only a small fraction of cells during the susceptible period. Infusional schedules increase the fraction of cells exposed during S phase. Both long-term continuous infusion schedules and shorter-term (typically 5-day) infusions have been utilized for this purpose. A recent example of the striking advantage of infusional over bolus schedules of 5-FU comes from the Mid-Atlantic Oncology Program (MAOP) prospective randomized trial in 179 patients with metastatic colorectal cancer. In this study an aggressive bolus schedule of 5-FU ($500 \, mg/m^2$ qd × 5 every 5 weeks) was compared with protracted continuous infusion 5-FU at $300 \, mg/m^2$/day. There was a fourfold increase in objective response rate (30% vs 7%, $P < 0.001$) favoring the infusional arm, and complete responses (5%) were seen only in the infusional arm (LOKICH et al. 1989). The reduction in toxicity with the infusional schedule was equally impressive. Whereas there was a 13% incidence of serious (grade 3) and a 7% incidence of life-threatening (grade 4) hematological toxicity with the bolus schedule (and four drug-related neutropenic deaths), only one patient on the infusional schedule experienced any degree of myelosuppression, and there was no grade 4 toxicity of any cause on the infusional arm.

Regimens in which one or more additional drugs are combined with infusional 5-FU have been investigated in a number of malignancies. The most frequently investigated drugs have been cisplatin and mitomycin C, but methotrexate, bleomycin, and others have also been studied.

3.1.1 Cisplatin and 5-Fluorouracil

Preclinical studies have shown a high degree of synergy between cisplatin and 5-FU in sensitive cell lines. Even on a single-dose schedule marked synergy was noted in L1210-implanted mice (DIONET and VERRELLE 1984; SCHABEL et al. 1979). These results have led to the use of cisplatin with infusional 5-FU in a variety of tumors, and an impressive clinical benefit has been observed in some.

3.1.1.1 Cisplatin/Infusional 5-FU in Squamous Carcinoma of the Head and Neck

Little attention has been given to protracted infusion schedules of 5-FU in head and neck cancer, but shorter infusion schedules, typically 5 days at doses of the order of $1 g/m^2$/day given in combination with cisplatin, have been widely investigated. This combination yields response rates of the order of 80%–90% when given as initial therapy (Table 3.1), with complete response rates in the range 20%–50%, and probably represents the most widely used chemotherapy regimen in head and neck cancer today. When administered to patients with recurrent disease after radiotherapy or chemotherapy, a wider range of response rates, 10%–70%, has been reported (Table 3.2). Even in recurrent disease some complete responses, up to 20% in some series, are reported.

Because of the high response rate of head and neck cancer to cisplatin/infusional 5-FU, it has been speculated that induction chemotherapy with this regimen may improve survival and/or cure rate when it is given prior to surgery or radiotherapy. However, to date, no randomized trial has yet demonstrated such an advantage. Randomized trials in the past using other less active chemotherapy regimens have been consistently negative (TANNOCK and BROWMAN 1986). Trials are underway to test cisplatin/infusional 5-FU as induction therapy in a prospective randomized setting. One comparison of three successive pilot studies suggests that superior induction chemotherapy may influence survival irrespective of subsequent radiotherapy or surgery (ROONEY et al. 1985).

Cisplatin/infusional 5-FU has also been studied in combination with simultaneous radiotherapy, both preoperatively and as definitive treatment in head and neck cancer. TAYLOR, MURTHY, and co-workers (MURTHY et al. 1987; TAYLOR et al. 1985, 1988a) combined cisplatin ($60 mg/m^2$), 5-FU ($800 mg/m^2$/day $\times$ 5), and radiotherapy ($2 Gy \times 5$) in cycles repeated every 2 weeks. Seven cycles were given to M_0 patients, with a lesser number of cycles given palliatively to patients with distant

Table 3.1. Trials of cisplatin/infusional 5-FU in previously untreated squamous carcinoma of the head and neck

Cisplatin dose	5-FU dose	Frequency	CR + PR	CR	Patients	References
$100 mg/m^2$	$1000 mg/m^2$/day $\times$ 5	q 3 wk	93%	54%	61[a]	ROONEY et al. 1985
$100 mg/m^2$	$1000 mg/m^2$/day $\times$ 4	q 3 wk	88%	19%	26[b]	ROONEY et al. 1985
$100 mg/m^2$	$1000 mg/m^2$/day $\times$ 4	q 3 wk	88%	19%	26[b]	KISH et al. 1982
$80 mg/m^2$	$800 mg/m^2$/day $\times$ 5	q 3 wk	84%	23%	31	AMREIN and WEITZMAN 1985
$100 mg/m^2$	$1000 mg/m^2$/day $\times$ 5	q 3 wk	83%	33%	30[a,c]	JACOBS et al. 1987
$100 mg/m^2$	$1000 mg/m^2$/day $\times$ 5	q 4 wk	84%	26%	19[b]	DASMAHAPATRA et al. 1985
$100 mg/m^2$	$1000 mg/m^2$/day $\times$ 5	q 3 wk	87%	37%	70[a]	KIES et al. 1985
$100 mg/m^2$	$1000 mg/m^2$/day $\times$ 5	q 3 wk	77%	17%	23[a]	HAAS et al. 1985

[a] Response rate evaluated after three cycles of therapy
[b] Response rate evaluated after two cycles of therapy
[c] Six patients received bleomycin rather than 5-FU

Table 3.2. Trials of cisplatin/infusional 5-FU in patients with recurrent squamous carcinoma of the head and neck

Cisplatin dose	5-FU dose	Frequency	CR + PR	CR	Patients	Reference
80 mg/m^2	800 mg/m^2/day × 5	q 3 wk	46%	14%	39	AMREIN and WEITZMAN 1985
100 mg/m^2	1000 mg/m^2/day × 5	q 4 wk	11%	0%	18	DASMAHAPATRA et al. 1985
120 mg/m^2	1000 mg/m^2/day × 5	q 3 wk	41%	7%	29	PAREDES et al. 1988
100 mg/m^2	1000 mg/m^2/day × 5	q 3 wk	25%	10%	20	CHOKSI et al. 1988
100 mg/m^2	1000 mg/m^2/day × 4	q 3 wk	55%	18%	23[a]	KISH et al. 1984
100 mg/m^2	1000 mg/m^2/day × 4	q 3 wk	72%	22%	18[b,c]	KISH et al. 1984
100 mg/m^2	1000 mg/m^2/day × 4	q 3 wk	31%	NS	32	JACOBS et al. 1988
100 mg/m^2	1000 mg/m^2/day × 5	q 3–4 wk	71%	24%	21	ROWLAND et al. 1984

[a] Twelve patients without prior radiotherapy or chemotherapy deleted from results
[b] Includes three patients without prior radiotherapy or chemotherapy
[c] Randomized trial. Infusional 5-FU superior to bolus ($P < 0.01$)

metastases. Local control was achieved in 98% of 44 patients. Of 34 patients treated with curative intent, three died during treatment but only four more suffered local recurrences with follow-up of 24–58 months (MURTHY et al. 1987). Median survival had not been reached at last publication; 3-year actuarial survival was 63% (TAYLOR et al. 1988a). Using a different sequence but with 60 Gy and surgery in some patients, ADELSTEIN and colleagues (ADELSTEIN et al. 1986, 1988) have reported similar results.

3.1.1.2 Cisplatin/Infusional 5-FU in Esophageal Carcinoma

Squamous carcinoma of the esophagus has also been shown to be responsive to the cisplatin/infusional 5-FU combination. Regimens similar to those commonly used in head and neck cancer (100 mg/m^2 cisplatin with 4 or 5 days of infusional 5-FU at 1000 mg/m^2/day) have been tested at several centers as induction regimens, followed by either surgery or radiotherapy consolidation (Table 3.3). The frequency of pathological complete responses (CRs) has been less than in head and neck trials, but median survivals of 18–21 months have been the rule. Addition of radiotherapy has increased the percentage of pathological CRs at surgery, but not survival (Table 3.3).

Not all induction chemoradiotherapy studies in esophageal cancer have been as promising. When TAYLOR attempted to apply the integrated schedule of cisplatin/5-FU/radiotherapy which had been so successful in head and neck cancer (MURTHY et al. 1987), toxicity was more severe and tended to limit dosing. Although an overall 47% clinical CR rate was documented, median survival was 13 months and median time to recurrence was only 7 months (TAYLOR et al. 1986).

Protracted infusion schedules of 5-FU (PIF) have also been explored in esophageal carcinoma. PIF alone was studied by LOKICH et al. (1987) as the initial phase of a combined modality trial.

Table 3.3. Trials of cisplatin/infusional 5-FU as induction therapy in squamous carcinoma of the esophagus

Cisplatin dose	5-FU dose	Frequency	Patients	CR + PR	Resected	Path.CR	Survival	Reference
100 mg/m^2	1000 mg/m^2/day × 4	q 3 wk × 2	35	20 (57%)	27 (77%)	2 (6%)	20 mos.	HILGENBERG et al. 1988 CAREY et al. 1986
100 mg/m^2	1000 mg/m^2/day × 5	q 3 wk × 3	26	11 (42%)	14 (54%)	2 (8%)	18 mos.	KIES et al. 1987
20 mg/m^2 × 5	1000 mg/m^2/day × 5	q 3 wk × 2–6	25	18 (72%)	12 (48%) 8 (32%) RT	2 (8%)	21 mos.	AJANI et al. 1987
100 mg/m^2	1000 mg/m^2/day × 4	q 4 wk × 2 + RT 30 Gy	21	NS	15 (71%)	5 (24%)	18 mos.	LEICHMAN et al. 1984
75 mg/m^2	1000 mg/m^2/day × 4	q 4 wk × 2 + RT 30 Gy	106	NS	55 (52%)	18 (17%)	12 mos.	POPLIN et al. 1987

After 6 weeks of 5-FU at $300\,mg/m^2$/day, 11 of 13 patients were judged to have responded. With the excellent toxicity profile of PIF and the activity of cisplatin, it would seem appropriate to consider weekly low dose cisplatin in combination with PIF for esophageal cancer; however, results with this combination have not yet been reported.

3.1.1.3 Cisplatin/Infusional 5-FU in Non-Small Cell Lung Cancer

Protracted infusional 5-FU has also undergone little investigation in non-small cell lung cancer (NSCLC), but 5-day schedules have been studied in combination with cisplatin. Two phase 2 trials of the cisplatin/infusional 5-FU combination in NSCLC have been described. WEIDEN et al. (1985) and HEIM et al. (1986) both combined relatively high doses of cisplatin ($100\,mg/m^2$ and $120\,mg/m^2$ respectively) with 5-day infusions of 5-FU at 1000 and $900\,mg/m^2$/day. In the case of HEIM's trial, the cisplatin was also given as a 24-h infusion. Response

rates were 37% and 47% respectively. When the HEIM regimen was restudied in a small confirmatory MAOP trial, a similar response rate, 43%, was obtained (Table 3.4).

The addition of the 5-day infusional 5-FU schedule to the cisplatin/vinblastine combination has been investigated in a randomized prospective study by the Central Pennsylvania Oncology Group (CPOG). After stratification for performance status and histological type, 75 patients with stage IV NSCLC were randomized either to cisplatin $100\,mg/m^2$ on day 1 plus vinblastine $5\,mg/m^2$ on days 1 and 14, given in 28-day cycles, or to the same combination to which was added infusional 5-FU, $1\,g/m^2$/day $\times$ 5, on days 1–5 (SHAH et al. 1988). Patients receiving the 5-FU had a higher objective response rate [27% vs 18%, all partial responses (PRs)], duration of response (44 vs 16 weeks), and survival (28 vs 16 weeks). Because of the relatively small number of patients, none of the above differences reached statistical significance at the $P = 0.05$ level except in subgroup analysis of those patients with adenocarcinoma,

Table 3.4. Trials of cisplatin/infusional 5-FU in advanced/metastatic NSCLC

Cisplatin dose	5-FU dose	Frequency	CR + PR	CR	Patients	Reference
$100\,mg/m^2$	$1000\,mg/m^2$/day $\times$ 5	q 3/4/6 wk	37%	0	19	WEIDEN et al. 1985
$120\,mg/m^2$	$900\,mg/m^2$/day $\times$ 5	q 3 wk	47%	3%	32	HEIM et al. 1986
$120\,mg/m^2$	$900\,mg/m^2$/day $\times$ 5	q 3 wk	43%	3%	63	Mid-Atlantic Oncology Program (unpublished data)
$100\,mg/m^{2a}$	$1000\,mg/m^2$/day 5		33%	5%	21	COHEN et al. 1987

[a] Divided doses, schedule based on RBC deformability

Table 3.5. Pilot studies in NSCLC in which one or more additional drugs have been added to cisplatin/infusional 5-FU

Cisplatin	5-FU	Added drug(s)	CR + PR	CR	Patients	Reference
$100\,mg/m^2$	$30\,mg/m^2$/day $\times$ 3	VLB $5\,mg/m^2$ days 1,3	19%	NS	100+	PERRY et al. 1987[a]
$25\,mg/m^2 \times 4$	$800\,mg/m^2$/day $\times$ 4	MMC $8\,mg/m^2$ alt cycles	37%	0	30	HASKETH et al. 1988
$15\,mg/m^2 \times 5$	$600\,mg/m^2$/day $\times$ 5	MTX $60\,mg/m^2$ + LV day 1	30%	NS	33	TAKITA et al. 1987
$20\,mg/m^2 \times 5$	$800\,mg/m^2$/day $\times$ 5	MTX $200\,mg/m^2$ + LV days 15,22	67%	NS	21	WHEELER et al. 1986
$120\,mg/m^2$/24 h	$800\,mg/m^2$/day $\times$ 5	DCM $400\,mg/m^2$ 4 h before cisplatin	14%	7%	43	Mid-Atlantic Oncology Program (unpublished data)
$100\,mg/m^2$/24 h	$900\,mg/m^2$/day $\times$ 5	VP-16 $100\,mg/m^2$ p.o. $\times$ 3 prior to cisplatin		Too early	60+	Mid-Altantic Oncology Program (unpublished data)
$70\,mg/m^2$	$800\,mg/m^2$/day $\times$ 5	VP-16 $60\,mg/m^2 \times 5$	0	0	10	LEE et al. 1987

Abbreviations: DCM, dichloromethotrexate; MMC, mitomycin C; methotrexate; NS, not stated; VLB, vinblastine; VP-16, etoposide; LV, Leucovorin
[a] Randomized study against cisplatin/5-FU: no advantage for added vinblastine

who had a median survival of 36 vs 13 weeks $P =$ 0.01).

The combination of cisplatin with infusional 5-FU usually has minimal myelotoxicity, suggesting that a third drug might be added to increase cytotoxicity further. This has been attempted in pilot studies with a number of drugs (Table 3.5). None of these small trials has yet shown a result which is convincingly better than cisplatin/infusional 5-FU alone, and some have produced disappointingly low response rates. In one randomized study by the Cancer and Leukemia Group B (CALGB), cisplatin $(100 \, mg/m^2)$ plus 3 days of infusional 5-FU $(30 \, mg/kg/day)$ was compared with the same regimen to which was added vinblastine $3 \, mg/m^2$ on days 1 and 3; the group receiving vinblastine experienced greater toxicity but no significant benefit in response or survival (PERRY et al. 1987).

Both cisplatin and 5-FU have shown synergy with antifols in some systems. Thus, it is theoretically attractive to add an antifol to the cisplatin/ infusional 5-FU combination. This has been addressed in three phase II trials, with mixed success. Using relatively low doses of cisplatin/5-FU $(15 \, mg/m^2/day \times 5$ and $600 \, mg/m^2/day \times 5)$, TAKITA and colleagues (1987) added methotrexate, $60 \, mg/m^2$ on day 1, with leucovorin rescue, and obtained a 30% response rate in 33 patients. WHEELER and co-workers (1986) used a similar combination with higher doses of all three drugs $(20 \, mg/m^2 \times 5$ cisplatin, $800 \, mg/m^2/day \times 5$ 5-FU, $200 \, mg/m^2$ methotrexate on days 15 and 22) and obtained a 67% response rate in 21 patients. MAOP (unpublished data) administered dichloromethotrexate 4 h before a 5-day course consisting of $120 \, mg/m^2$ (24-h infusion) of cisplatin and $800 \, mg/m^2/day \times 5$ of 5-FU; response was only 14% in 43 patients although CRs were seen in 7%. All of these regimens were well tolerated.

One of the most interesting recent applications of short-term infusional 5-FU in NSCLC has been the use of cisplatin/5-day infusional 5-FU with concurrent radiotherapy as preoperative conditioning ("neoadjuvant") chemotherapy in stage III NSCLC, as developed at Rush-Presbyterian-St. Luke's Medical Center (TAYLOR et al. 1987, 1988b). Patients with stage III NSCLC without distant metastases were treated with four cycles of cisplatin $(60 \, mg/m^2$ day 1) and infusional 5-FU $(800 \, mg/m^2/day \times 5$, days 1–5) with concomitant radiotherapy $(2 \, Gy/day \times 5$, days 1–5). This is the same regimen used by the Rush-Presbyterian group in head and neck cancer. As in head and

neck cancer, it was found to be tolerable when repeated in 14-day cycles.

The objective of this therapy was to render the tumor resectable, and 61% of patients (39/64) were able to undergo exploration 4 weeks after the fourth cycle of chemoradiotherapy. Evaluation prior to surgery showed a response rate of 56% (36/64, 5 CRs, 31 PRs) by CT scan; only 3 of the 64 patients developed metastatic disease during preoperative therapy. A major reason for patients not undergoing exploration was patient refusal (11 of 50 deemed eligible). Most patients who did not undergo surgery received one or two additional cycles of chemoradiotherapy.

All but one of the patients explored underwent resection. Pathological evaluation of the resected specimens revealed 23% (9/39) without evidence of viable cancer, 21% (8) with microscopic tumor only, and 56% (22) with gross residual disease; 26% of the last group had microscopic involvement of resection margins. An interesting finding was a lack of correlation between complete response by CT scan and complete pathological response. Surgery was complicated by fibrosis and obliteration of tissue planes, but perioperative morbidity and fatality (5%) appeared acceptable.

Median survival among all patients was 15 months; 3-year survival was 22%. With median follow-up of 33 months, 43 patients had suffered recurrences and 33% of patients who underwent surgery were disease free (TAYLOR et al. 1988b).

A somewhat similar regimen has been reported by the Lung Cancer Study Group (LCSG) but with less frequent chemotherapy (two cycles, weeks 1 and 4) and less radiotherapy (30 Gy, not coordinated with the chemotherapy) (WEIDEN and PIANTADOSI 1988). A preliminary report showed survival to be shorter (median 10.5 months), but 13% of patients (23% of responders) were pathologically tumor-free at surgery. The CALGB is also studying a similar regimen employing two cycles of cisplatin/vinblastine/infusional 5-FU (3 days) with 30 Gy of radiation prior to surgery (STRAUSS et al. 1988a).

The Rush group is currently exploring the use of a regimen similar to their original cisplatin/ infusional 5-FU combination but to which etoposide has been added. This regimen, together with coordinated radiotherapy, 10 Gy per course, is repeated every 3 weeks for a total of four courses prior to surgery. Early results showed a 73% clinical response rate in the first 32 patients (BONOMI et al. 1988) and no viable tumor in nine of the first 19 surgical specimens (ROWLAND et al. 1988).

The results from Rush-Presbyterian (TAYLOR et al. 1988b; BONOMI et al. 1988) (as well as the HEIM and MAOP trials; HEIM et al. 1986) suggest that the most valuable applications of infusional chemotherapy in NSCLC may be to enhance the potentially curative results of surgery or radiotherapy. In the Heim and MAOP studies, patients with bulky stage III disease (T > 5 cm) received four cycles of cisplatin/5-FU, then went on to aggressive radiotherapy (60 Gy) to the thorax. In this subgroup of patients 3-year survival has also been in excess of 20%, even without surgery. CALGB has also now reported a prospective trial in which stage III patients were randomized to receive either radiotherapy (60 Gy) or radiotherapy preceded by a brief course of chemotherapy (vinblastine 5 mg/m^2 days 1–5, cisplatin 100 mg/ m^2 days 1 and 29). Survival favored the group receiving chemotherapy, with median survival of 16.5 vs 8.5 months ($P = 0.0028$, log rank test) (DILLMAN et al. 1988).

3.1.1.4 Cisplatin/Infusional 5-FU in Small Cell Lung Cancer

Small cell lung cancer (SCLC) is much more chemosensitive than NSCLC, with chemotherapeutic cures possible in a small fraction of patients. It is therefore surprising that in SCLC, where the potential impact of improvements in therapeutic index may be considerably greater than in NSCLC, infusional chemotherapy has been almost entirely overlooked.

5-Fluorouracil, by both bolus and infusional schedules, remains largely unexplored in SCLC. As part of a broad phase II protocol exploring 5-FU activity in resistant or refractory malignancies, MAOP is presently studying protracted infusional 5-FU in SCLC. The study is too immature to cite meaningful response rates, but major responses have been seen and infusional 5-FU appears to be active in SCLC.

The combination of cisplatin with shorter course (5 day) infusional 5-FU has been investigated in France by MORERE and colleagues (1988). They administered cisplatin (20 mg/m^2 × 5) with infusional 5-FU (600 mg/m^2/day × 5) to a mixed population of 20 patients (8 pretreated, 17 with extensive disease including 13 with central nervous system metastases). Overall response rate was

75%, with 30% complete responses. Interestingly, 9 of 13 patients with CNS metastases responded, including 4 CNS CRs (infusional 5-FU equilibrates across the blood–brain barrier).

3.1.1.5 Cisplatin/Infusional 5-FU in Breast Cancer

Infusional 5-FU has substantial activity in breast cancer, even in patients who have received bolus 5-FU as a part of earlier regimens. Protracted infusion schedules have been investigated as second- and third-line therapy for refractory breast cancer, with two small series reporting response rates of 25%–50% in heavily pretreated patients (HUAU et al. 1988; JABBOURY et al. 1988). STRAUSS et al. (1988b) have studied the addition of weekly low dose cisplatin to the protracted infusion schedule of 5-FU (PIF). Of 21 patients treated with PIF, ten also received weekly cisplatin, 20 mg/m^2. Objective response rates were 3/11 (27%) for PIF and 7/10 (70%) for PIF + weekly cisplatin. The activity of PIF in heavily pretreated breast cancer patients suggests that PIF should perhaps be incorporated into front-line combination chemotherapy for breast cancer. Such studies are underway but have not yet been reported.

3.1.1.6 Cisplatin/Infusional 5-FU in Gastric and Pancreatic Cancer

Cisplatin has activity in upper gastrointestinal cancer and has been used in combination with bolus 5-FU plus doxorubicin (FAP combination) in gastric and pancreatic cancer (MOERTEL et al. 1986). The combination of cisplatin with infusional schedules of 5-FU is under active investigation.

In gastric cancer, a small pilot study of cisplatin (100 mg/m^2) in combination with a 5-day infusion of 5-FU (100 mg/m^2/day) produced a 55% response rate (11% CRs) in 18 evaluable patients, with low toxicity (ROUNIEA et al. 1988). MAOP is currently investigating the combination of protracted infusional 5-FU (300 mg/m^2/day) with weekly low dose cisplatin (20 mg/m^2) or carboplatin (100 mg/m^2) in pancreatic cancer.

3.1.1.7 Cisplatin/Infusional 5-FU in Colorectal Cancer

In contrast with all of the tumor types considered above, cisplatin has no clearly recognized single-agent clinical activity in colorectal cancer. Nevertheless, some studies have suggested synergy with 5-FU, and trials have been conducted in colorectal cancer on this basis. In preclinical studies using human colorectal carcinoma cell lines, one study showed only additive activity (Bergerat et al. 1979), while another showed synergy at some drug ratios (5-FU excess) and antagonism at others (cisplatin excess) (Ortiz and Woolley 1987).

Clinical trials of cisplatin/5-FU in colorectal cancer have been conducted using bolus (Loehrer et al. 1988), 5-day infusion (Richards et al. 1988; Dy et al. 1986), and protracted infusion (Cantrell et al. 1987; Lokich et al. 1989b) schedules. Neither the bolus nor the 5-day schedule produced results likely to be superior to 5-FU alone on the same schedule. However, one phase II trial of protracted infusional 5-FU with weekly low dose cisplatin reported a 63% response rate among 32 patients (Cantrell et al. 1987). This led to a prospective randomized trial which was recently reported (Lokich et al. 1989b, 1990). Among 179 patients, both response rate (33% vs 35%) and preliminary survival showed no difference between PIF monotherapy and PIF plus weekly cisplatin. When weekly cisplatin was added to PIF in patients with metastatic colorectal cancer shown to progress while receiving PIF monotherapy occasional objective responses were observed, but the response rate was only 5% (Ahlgren et al. 1991).

3.1.2 Mitomycin C/Infusional 5-FU Regimens

Mitomycin C has substantial activity in many solid tumors. Its severe and cumulative marrow toxicities have limited its use in combination chemotherapy with other myelotoxic drugs. The relative freedom from myelotoxicity seen with infusional 5-FU, however, makes infusional 5-FU an attractive agent for combination therapy with mitomycin C. This combination has seen extensive use in squamous carcinoma of the anal canal and has also been explored in esophageal and breast cancer.

Standard primary treatment in most centers for squamous carcinoma of the anal canal now consists of radiotherapy in combination with one or two cycles of mitomycin C/infusional 5-FU (Table 3.6). Most patients avoid surgery but local excision or AP resection is used for those patients who do not achieve a biopsy-proven complete response. Five-year survival is of the order of 75%.

The same general approach has been studied in esophageal cancer at Fox Chase Cancer Center. Patients receive two 5-day cycles of infusional 5-FU ($1000 \, mg/m^2$/day) with one dose of mitomycin C ($10 \, mg/m^2$) on day 2. Radiotherapy totals 60 Gy. Of 30 stage I/II patients treated with curative intent, actuarial survival was 47% at 2 years and 32% at 5 years (Coia et al. 1987). Of 20 stage III/IV patients treated to 50 Gy for palliation, local control was maintained until death in 64%, with median survival of 8 months.

3.1.3 PALA/Infusional 5-FU Regimens

PALA (N-(phosphonacetyl)-L-aspartic acid) is an antimetabolite which blocks de novo pyrimidine synthesis. Although fairly toxic doses are required for PALA to exert direct cytotoxic effects, at much lower doses it is able to reduce substantially the intracellular pool of uracil nucleotides. This allows 5-FU to function more effectively as an inhibitor of thymidylate synthetase. Relatively effective blockade of uracil synthesis is maintained for a week after a single dose of $250 \, mg/m^2$ of PALA, permitting a relatively nontoxic dose to act synergistically with 5-FU. Ardalan and colleagues have investigated this combination in advanced pancreatic and colorectal cancer, using a weekly high dose infusion (up to $3400 \, mg/m^2$ over 24 h) of 5-FU (Ardalan et al. 1988). Response rate with PALA was 39% (11/28 patients;

Table 3.6. Trials of mitomycin C/infusional 5-FU/radiotherapy in squamous carcinoma of the anal canal

Mitomycin C dose	5-FU dose	Courses of 5-FU	RT	CR	Patients	Survival	Reference
$15 \, mg/m^2$	$1000 \, mg/m^2$/day × 4	2	30 Gy	84%	45	89% 50 mos	Leichman et al. 1985
$15 \, mg/m^2$	$750 \, mg/m^2$/day × 5	1	30 Gy	43%	30	75% 5 yrs	Michaelson et al. 1983
$10 \, mg/m^2$	$1000 \, mg/m^2$/day × 4	2	45 Gy	76%	33	NS	Sischy 1985
$10 \, mg/m^2$	$1000 \, mg/m^2$/day × 4	1	50 Gy	93%	30	70% 5 yrs	Cummings et al. 1984
$15 \, mg/m^2$	$1000 \, mg/m^2$/day × 4	2	30 Gy	84%	19	87% 40 mos	Meeker et al. 1986
$10 \, mg/m^2$	$1000 \, mg/m^2$/day × 4	2	50 Gy	86%	30	(immature)	Sischy et al. 1988

two CRs) versus 22% (4/19; no CRs) with 5-FU monotherapy. Based upon these results, MAOP has begun a phase III trial of protracted infusional 5-FU with or without weekly PALA.

3.2 Combination Chemotherapy Employing Infusional Bleomycin

Bleomycin shows a moderate degree of cytokinetic specificity, with maximum cell killing occurring during the G_2 phase (BARRANCO et al. 1971), but has a relatively short plasma half-life of 2–4 h (ALBERTS et al. 1978). Thus, the possibility of increasing cell kill in the G_2 phase has led to the investigation of infusional schedules of bleomycin. These schedules are made more attractive by both animal (SIKIC et al. 1978) and clinical (COOPER and HONG 1981) evidence suggesting that the pulmonary toxicity of bleomycin can be reduced by long-term infusion.

In addition, there is the suggestion that bleomycin may be an inhibitor of type 2 DNA polymerase, required for excision repair processes. If this were to form the basis for the synergy of bleomycin with cisplatin (OKUYAMA and MISHINA 1980), longer term infusional schedules of bleomycin should enhance the synergy by prolonging the duration of repair inhibition. This should permit more cisplatin adducts to be converted into DNA cross-links, a relatively slow process which is opposed by excision repairs (ROBERTS and THOMPSON 1979).

3.2.1 Cisplatin/Infusional Bleomycin in Squamous Carcinoma of the Head and Neck

The combination of cisplatin and infusional bleomycin has been investigated as induction therapy for squamous carcinoma of the head and neck by two cooperative groups. Both used a schedule of cisplatin 100 mg/m^2 followed on day 3 by a 15 U/m^2 bolus of bleomycin and then a 5-day infusion at 15 U/m^2/day. In the Radiation Therapy Oncology Group (RTOG) pilot study one cycle of chemotherapy was given prior to radiotherapy (GLICK et al. 1980). When evaluated after one cycle of therapy, the response rate was 48% (no CRs). The Head and Neck Contracts Program study was a randomized trial between surgery

followed by postoperative radiotherapy (standard therapy), standard therapy preceded by one cycle of induction chemotherapy, and induction therapy plus standard therapy plus six cycles of monthly cisplatin. One cycle of induction therapy resulted in a 37% response rate (3% CRs) among 104 patients. There was no significant impact on survival (Head and Neck Contracts Program 1987). Using a more intensive schedule (cisplatin 120 mg/m^2 days 1, 22; bleomycin 15 U/m^2/day days 3–9 after a 15 U bolus), PENNACHIO et al. (1982) reported an overall induction response rate of 70% (17% CRs) in a group of 41 stage IV unresectable patients. These patients then underwent resection (if possible) or received radiotherapy. Projected survival was 29 months, compared with 4.5 months for a comparable historical control group. This was not a prospectively randomized trial. In none of these trials was the scheduling optimized to exploit any putative synergy based on repair inhibition.

3.2.2 Cisplatin/Infusional Bleomycin in Non-Small Cell Lung Cancer

ISRAEL and colleagues (1987) studied the cisplatin/infusional bleomycin combination in NSCLC using a schedule designed to exploit possible repair inhibition activity of the bleomycin. In their studies, cisplatin was given at 20 mg/m^2/day for each of 5 consecutive days while bleomycin was administered by continuous infusion at a dose rate of 5 units/day for 5 days. Cycles were repeated every 21 days. This combination was well tolerated, with toxicity primarily limited to pulmonary compromise. An average of five cycles could be given before pulmonary toxicity was observed; pulmonary toxicity was reported in 51/713 patients, with four deaths due to pulmonary fibrosis.

Interpretation of ISRAEL et al.'s results is complicated by the wide diversity of patients treated (neoadjuvant, adjuvant, metastatic, locally advanced) and by the fact that in many cases additional drugs (mitomycin C, vindesine, etoposide, vincristine, or 5-FU) were added. However, when only the 215 patients with measurable disease treated with cisplatin/infusional bleomycin alone are evaluated there are adequate data to suggest that this is an active combination. These results are summarized in Table 3.7. The overall response rate was reported as 73% (15% CRs) in 215 pa-

Table 3.7. Cisplatin/infusional bleomycin in advanced NSCLC (summarized from ISRAEL et al. 1987)

Patient group	Response rate		Patients
	CR + PR	CR	
Total	73%	15%	215
Neoadjuvant	79%	12%	17
Bulky localized (unresectable)	73%	16%	188
Metastatic	60%	0	10

tients, but the series was heavily weighted (91%) with early and nonmetastatic lesions, which would be expected to respond better. The results with this regimen need confirmation in a metastatic population.

3.3 Combinations Employing Infusional Etoposide

The epipodophyllotoxins have moderate kinetic specificity, with maximum cell killing occurring in the G_2 phase. This lends a theoretical rationale to the possible use of infusional schedules. However, the terminal plasma half-life of etoposide, 15 h (ALLEN and CREAVER 1975), is considerably longer than that of 5-FU or even bleomycin. This suggests that much of the advantage of infusional schedules might be realized with a course of daily or twice daily bolus doses, and sequential daily bolus schedules do appear to be more effective than the same dose in a single bolus, in both animal (STAHELIN 1973) and clinical (CAVALLI et al. 1978) studies. Etoposide acts by stabilizing strand breaks induced by topoisomerase 2; if this action were to interfere with DNA repair, similar arguments could also be advanced for infusional schedules of etoposide enhancing synergy with alkylating agents, as led to ISRAEL et al.'s work cited above with cisplatin/bleomycin. However, in at least one system, excision repair appears to proceed without inhibition by etoposide (DOWNES et al. 1987). An alternative mechanism for synergy might involve cisplatin cross-linking tumor DNA while it is in a partially relaxed configuration due to the etoposide-induced strand break. This mechanism should also be enhanced by an infusional schedule of etoposide.

KROOK and colleagues reported a small pilot trial in which a 3-day infusion of etoposide (65–

130 mg/m^2/day) was combined with daily bolus cisplatin (30 mg/m^2 × 3) or infusional cisplatin (45 mg/m^2/day × 2). Among 16 NSCLC patients treated, 8 (50%) achieved an objective response (KROOK et al. 1987). Early results suggested a higher response rate with the infusional cisplatin (five of seven patients) than with the bolus schedule (three of nine). Based upon these early data, the North Central Cancer Treatment Group (NCCTG) performed a randomized trial in extensive NSCLC comparing cisplatin/etoposide therapy given by bolus with the same drugs both given by infusion; there was no difference in response rate but the infusional schedule was more toxic (GOLDBERG et al. 1990).

In SCLC, REMICK and colleagues (1987) have explored a 5-day infusion schedule of etoposide (50 mg/m^2/day) in combination with cisplatin (75 mg/m^2/day on day 6) and hexamethylmelamine (150 mg/m^2 orally for 10 days beginning day 8). Treatments were repeated on a 21-day cycle. Among 25 extensive disease patients without prior chemotherapy, there were 19 (76%) responses, including 12% CRs. Among 23 previously treated patients with extensive disease, a 39% response rate (all PRs) was seen.

3.4 Combinations Employing Infusional Vincas

The vinca alkaloids are cycle specific drugs with activity restricted to the M phase. In addition, they have relatively short plasma half-lives, making infusional schedules theoretically advantageous. The majority of clinical investigations with infusional vincas have been with vinblastine. Vinblastine was investigated by YAP and colleagues in refractory breast cancer using a 5-day infusion schedule at 1.4–2.0 mg/m^2/day (YAP et al. 1980). Myelosuppression was substantial at the higher doses, but the 36% response rate reported (25/70, five CRs) was considerably higher than historical data for vinblastine monotherapy (FRASCHINI et al. 1982). Activity is also reported in renal carcinoma (KUEBLER et al. 1984).

Combinations employing infusional vincas have been investigated by two groups in NSCLC. HUBERMAN and colleagues (1986) studied a 5-day infusion of vinblastine, 1.5 mg/m^2/day, combined with cisplatin 60 mg/m^2 on day 5. A 29% response rate (9/31 patients, two CRs) was reported with considerable toxicity. The authors concluded that the infusional schedule had no advantage over bolus administration.

Using the same schedule of vinblastine infusion with a higher cisplatin dose (40 mg/m^2 daily × 5), BLUMENREICH and colleagues (1987) treated 47 patients with locally advanced or metastatic NSCLC and obtained an objective response rate of 28% (13/47, no CRs). They also concluded that the regimen offered no advantage in survival or quality of life.

3.5 Conclusions and Direction of Continuing Research

Infusional chemotherapy offers the possibility of improving the therapeutic index of a number of available agents. Combination regimens based on infusional schedules can exploit this improved index and can also exploit mechanisms of synergy which are dependent on prolonged drug exposure. The potential is considerable and the field is in its infancy. Protracted infusional schedules in particular require much more investigation, and may reward it in a major way.

References

Adelstein DJ, Sharan VM, Earle AS et al. (1986) Chemo-radiotherapy as initial management in patients with squamous cell carcinoma of the head and neck. Cancer Treat Rep 70: 761–767

Adelstein DJ, Sharan VM, Earle AS et al. (1988) Simultaneous radiotherapy and chemotherapy with 5-fluorouracil and cisplatin for locally confined squamous cell head and neck cancer. NCI Monogr 6: 347–351

Ahlgren JD, Trocki O, Gullo JJ et al. (1991) Continuous infusion 5-FU with weekly low-dose cisplatin as second-line therapy in patients with metastatic colorectal cancer who have failed 5-FU monotherapy. Cancer Investigation, 1990, in press

Ajani J, McMurtrey M, Rich T et al. (1987) Combined modality therapy with effective prolonged systemic component for the locally advanced squamous cell carcinoma of the esophagus (SCCE). Proc ASCO 6: 82

Alberts DS, Chen HSG, Liu R et al. (1978) Bleomycin pharmacokinetics in man. I. Intravenous administration. Cancer Chemother Pharmacol 1: 177–181

Allen LM, Creaver PJ (1975) Comparison of the human pharmacokinetics of VM-26 and VP-16, two antineoplastic epipodophyllotoxin glucopyranoside derivatives. Eur J Cancer 11: 697–707

Amrein PC, Weitzman SA (1985) Treatment of squamous-cell carcinoma of the head and neck with cisplatin and 5-fluorouracil. J Clin Oncol 3:1632–1639

Ardalan B, Singh G, Silberman H (1988) A randomized phase I and II study of short-term infusion of high-dose fluorouracil with or without N-(phosphonacetyl)-L-aspartic acid in patients with advanced pancreatic and colorectal cancers. J Clin Oncol 6: 1053–1058

Barranco SC, Humphrey RM (1971) The effects of bleomycin on survival and cell progression in Chinese hamster cells in vitro. Cancer Res 31: 1218–1223

Bergerat JP, Green C, Drewinko B (1979) Combination chemotherapy in vitro. IV. Response of human colon carcinoma cells to combinations using cis-diamminedichloroplatinum. Cancer Biochem Biophys 3: 173–180

Blumenreich MS, Woodcock TM, Gentile PS et al. (1987) High-dose cisplatin and vinblastine infusion with or without radiation therapy in patients with advanced non-small cell lung cancer. J Clin Oncol 5: 1725–1730

Bonomi P, Rowland KM Jr, Taylor SG IV et al. (1988) Phase II trial of therapy with etoposide, 5-fluorouracil by continuous infusion, cisplatin and simultaneous split-course radiation in stage III non-small cell bronchogenic carcinoma. NCI Monogr 6: 331–334

Cantrell JE, Hart RD, Taylor RF, Harvey JC (1987) Pilot trial of prolonged continuous infusion 5-fluorouracil and weekly cisplatin in advanced colorectal cancer. Cancer Treat Rep 71: 615–618

Carey RW, Hilgenberg AD, Wilkns EW et al. (1986) Prospective chemotherapy followed by surgery with possible postoperative radiotherapy in squamous cell carcinoma of the esophagus: evaluation of the chemotherapy component. J Clin Oncol 4: 697–701

Cavalli F, Sonntag RW, Jungi F et al. (1978) VP-16-213 monotherapy for remission induction in small cell lung cancer: a randomized trial using three dosage schedules. Cancer Treat Rep 62: 473–475

Choksi AJ, Hong WK, Dimery IW et al. (1988) Continuous cisplatin (24 hour) and 5-fluorouracil (120 hour) infusion in recurrent head and neck squamous cell carcinoma. Cancer 61: 909–912

Cohen MH, Krasnow SH, Anderson AJ et al. (1987) Modified continuous infusion 5 flurouracil-platinum (CIF-P) in non-small cell lung cancer (NSCLC) patients. Proc ASCO 6: 185

Coia LR, Engstrom PF, Paul A (1987) Nonsurgical management of esophageal cancer: report of a study of combined radiotherapy and chemotherapy. J Clin Oncol 5: 1783–1790

Cooper KR, Hong WK (1981) Prospective study of the pulmonary toxicity of continuously infused bleomycin. Cancer Treat Rep 65: 419–425

Cummings B, Keane T, Harwood A et al. (1984) Results and toxicity of the treatment of anal canal carcinoma by radiation therapy or radiation and chemotherapy. Cancer 54: 2062–2068

Dasmahapatra KS, Citrin P, Hill GJ et al. (1985) A prospective evaluation of 5-fluorouracil plus cisplatin in advanced squamous-cell cancer of the head and neck. J Clin Oncol 3: 1486–1489

Dillman RO, Seagren SL, Propert K et al. (1988) Proto-chemotherapy improves survival in regional non-small cell lung cancer (NSCLC). Proc ASCO 7: 195

Dionet C, Verrelle P (1984) Curability of mouse L1210 leukemia by combination of 5-fluorouracil, cis-diamminedichloroplatinum (II) and low doses of x-rays. Cancer Rep 44: 652–656

Downes CS, Mullinger EM, Johnson RT (1987) Action of etoposide (VP-16-213) on human cells: no evidence for topoisomerase II involvement in excision repair of u.v.-induced DNA damage, nor for mitrochondrial hypersensitivity in ataxia telangiectasia. Carcinogenesis 8: 613–618

Dy C, Gil A, Algana SA, et al. (1986) Combination chemotherapy of cisplatin and 5-FU in advanced colorectal carcinoma. Cancer Treat Rep 70: 465–468

Fraschini G, Yap HY, Barnes BC et al. (1982) Continuous five-day infusion of vinblastine for refractory metastatic breast cancer. Proc ASCO 1: 78

Glick JH, Marcial V, Richter M, Velez-Garcia E (1980) The adjuvant treatment of inoperable stage III and IV epidermoid carcinoma of the head and neck with platinum and bleomycin infusions prior to definitive radiotherapy: an RTOG pilot study. Cancer 46: 1919–1924

Goldberg RM, Jett JR, Therneau TM et al. (1990) Bolus versus infusin regimens of etoposide and cisplatin in treatment of non-small cell lung cancer: a study of the North Central Cancer Treatment Group. J Natl Cancer Dust 82: 1899–1903

Haas C, Byhardt R, Cox J et al. (1985) Randomized study of 5-fluorouracil (F) and cis-platinum (P) as initial therapy of locally advanced carcinoma of the head and neck (LASCHN). Proc ASCO 4: 143

Hasketh PJ, Cooley TP, Finkel HE et al. (1988) Treatment of advanced non-small cell lung cancer with cisplatin, 5-fluorouracil, and mitomycin-C. Cancer 62: 1466–1470

Head and Neck Contracts Program (1987) Adjuvant chemotherapy for advanced head and neck squamous carcinoma. Cancer 60: 301–311

Heim W, Brereton H, Shebaugh D (1986) Infusional high-dose cisplatinum and 5 fluorouracil in advanced non-small cell lung cancer: a Mid-Atlantic Oncology Program pilot study. Proc ASCO 5: 174

Hilgenberg AD, Carey RW, Wilkens EW Jr et al. (1988) Preoperative chemotherapy, surgical resection, and selective postoperative therapy for squamous cell carcinoma of the esophagus. Ann Thorac Surg 45: 357–363

Huau S, Singhakowinta A, Saual B, Pazdur R (1988) Efficacy of continuous infusion low-dose 5-FU (CILD-FU) in previously treated metastatic breast cancer. Proc ASCO 7: 37

Huberman M, Lokich J, Green R et al. (1986) Vinblastine plus cisplatin in advanced non-small cell lung cancer: lack of advantage for vinblastine infusion schedule. Cancer Treat Rep 70: 287

Israel L, Bream JL, Morere JF (1987) Lung cancer. In: Lokich JJ (ed) Cancer chemotherapy by infusion, 1st edn. Precept, Chicago, pp 338–352

Jabboury K, Holmes F, Theriault R, Hortobagyi G (1988) Fluorouracil rechallenge by protracted continuous infusion in refractory breast cancer. Proc ASCO 7: 39

Jacobs C, Goffinet DR, Goffinet L et al. (1987) Chemotherapy as a substitute for surgery in the treatment of advanced resectable head and neck cancer. Cancer 60: 1178–1183

Jacobs C, Lyman G, Velez-Garcia E et al. (1988) Comparison of infusional 5 fluorouracil (5FU) and cisplatin (CDDP) in combination and as single agents for recurrent and metastatic head and neck cancer. Proc ASCO 7: 154

Kies MS, Lester EP, Gordon LI et al. (1985) Cis-platin and infusion 5-fluorouracil (5-FU) in stage III and IV

squamous cancer of the head and neck. Proc ASCO 4: 139

Kies MS, Rosen ST, Tsang T-K et al. (1987) Cisplatin and 5-fluorouracil in the primary management of squamous esophageal cancer. Cancer 60: 2156–2160

Kish J, Drelichman A, Jacobs J et al. (1982) Clinical trial of cisplatin and 5-FU infusion as initial treatment for advanced squamous cell carcinoma of the head and neck. Cancer Treat Rep 66: 471–474

Kish JA, Weaver A, Jacobs J et al. (1984) Cisplatin and 5-fluorouracil infusion in patients with recurrent and disseminated epidermoid cancer of the head and neck. Cancer 53: 1819–1824

Kish JA, Ensley JF, Jacobs J et al. (1985) A randomized trial of cisplatin (CACP) + 5-fluorouracil (5-FU) infusion and CACP + 5-FU bolus for recurrent and advanced squamous cell carcinoma of the head and neck. Cancer 56: 2740–2744

Krook J, Jett J, Little C (1987) A pilot study of infusion VP-16 followed by cisplatin (CDDP) in lung cancer. Proc ASCO 6: 182

Kuebler JP, Hogan TF, Trump DL et al. (1984) Phase II study of continuous five-day vinblastine infusion in renal adenocarcinoma. Cancer Treat Rep 68: 925–926

Lee JS, Dhingra HM, Chiuten DF et al. (1987) A pilot study of etoposide (E), cisplatin (P) and 5-FU (F) continuous infusion (CI) for extensive non-small cell lung cancer (E-NSCLC). Proc ASCO 6: 173

Leichman L, Steiger Z, Seydel HG et al. (1984) Preoperative chemotherapy and radiation therapy for patients with cancer of the esophagus: a potentially curative approach. J Clin Oncol 2: 75–79

Leichman L, Nigro N, Vaitkevicius VK et al. (1985) Cancer of the anal canal: model for preoperative combined modality therapy. Am J Med 78: 211–215

Loehrer PJ, Turner S, Kubilis P et al. (1988) A prospective randomized trial of fluorouracil versus fluorouracil plus cisplatin in the treatment of metastatic colorectal cancer. A Hoosier Oncology Group trial. J Clin Oncol 6: 642–648

Lokich JJ, Shea M, Chaffey J (1987) Sequential infusion of 5-fluorouracil followed by concomitant radiation for tumors of the esophagus and gastroesophageal junction. Cancer 60: 275–279

Lokich JJ, Ahlgren JD, Gullo JJ et al. (1989a) A prospective randomized comparison of continuous-infusion fluorouracil with a conventional bolus schedule in metastatic colorectal carcinoma: a Mid-Atlanti Oncology Program Study. J Clin Oncol 7: 425–432

Lokich JJ, Cantrell J, Ahlgren J, Phillips J (1989b) A phase III trial of protracted infusional 5-FU (PIF) vs PIF plus weekly bolus cisplatin (CDDP) in advanced measurable colon cancer (MAOP protocol 5286). Proc ASCO 8: 104

Lokich JJ, Cehlgren JD, Cantrell J, Gullo JJ, Fryer JG (1991) A prospective randomized comparison of protracted infusional 5-fluorouracil with or without weekly bolus cisplatin in metastatic colorectal carcinoma: a Mid-Atlantic Oncology Program Study. Cancer (in press)

Macmillan WE, Wobury WH, Welling PG (1978) Pharmacokinetics of 5-fluorouracil in humans. Cancer Res 38: 3479–3482

Meeker WR, Sickle-Santanello BJ, Philpott G et al. (1986) Combined chemotherapy, radiation and surgery for epithelial cancer of the anal canal. Cancer 57: 522–529

Michaelson R, Magill GB, Quan SHQ et al. (1983) Preoperative chemotherapy and radiation therapy in the management of anal epidermoid cancer. Cancer 51: 390–395

Moertel C, Rubin J, O'Connell M et al. (1986) A phase II study of combined 5-fluorouracil, doxorubicin and cisplatin in the treatment of advanced upper gastrointestinal adenocarcinomas. J Clin Oncol 4: 1053–1057

Morere JF, Tcherakian F, Breau JL et al. (1988) Successful chemotherapy with cisplatinum (DDP) and 5-fluorouracil (5-FU) in small cell lung cancer. Proc ASCO 7: 210

Murthy AK, Taylor SG IV, Showel J et al. (1987) Treatment of advanced head and neck cancer with concomitant radiation and chemotherapy. Int J Radiat Oncol Biol Phys 13: 1807–1813

Okuyama S, Mishina H (1980) Consecutive therapy of cancer aimed at perpetuation of repairable damage: a hypothesis unifying radiotherapy and chemotherapy. J Clin Hematol Oncol 10: 83–93

Ortiz J, Wooley PV (1987) A study of the synergistic cytotoxic effects of 5-fluorouracil and cisplatin against colon carcinoma cells using median effect analysis. Proc AACR 28: 414

Paredes J, Hong WK, Felder TB et al. (1988) Prospective randomized trial of high-dose cisplatin and fluorouracil infusion with or without sodium diethyldithiocarbanate in recurrent and/or metastatic squamous cell carcinoma of the head and neck. J Clin Oncol 6: 955–962

Pennachio JL, Hong WK, Shapshay S et al. (1982) Combination of cisplatinum and bleomycin prior to surgery and/or radiotherapy compared with radiotherapy alone for the treatment of advanced squamous cell carcinoma of the head and neck. Cancer 50: 2795–2801

Perry D, Richard F II, Prospect K et al. (1987) 5-FU and cisplatin (DDP) vs 5-FU, DDP and vinblastine (VBL) in advanced non-small cell lung cancer (NSCLC). Proc ASCO 6: 168

Poplin E, Fleming T, Leichman L et al. (1987) Combined therapies for squamous cell carcinoma of the esophagus, a Southwest Oncology Group study (SWOG-8037). J Clin Oncol 5: 622–628

Remick SC, Neville AJ, Willson JKV (1987) Phase II trial evaluating continuous infusion of etoposide, cisplatin, and hexamethylmelamine in extensive disease small cell carcinoma of the lung. Cancer Treat Rep 71: 575–580

Richards F II, Beck J, Muss H et al. (1988) Continuous infusion 5-fluorouracil (5-FU) with bolus cisplatin (P) in the treatment of metastatic colorectal cancer. Proc ASCO 7: 96

Roberts JJ, Thompson AJ (1979) The mechanism of antitumor platinum compounds. Prog Nucleic Acid Res Mol Biol 22: 71–133

Rooney M, Kish J, Jacobs J et al. (1985) Improved complete response rate and survival in advanced head and neck cancer after three course induction therapy with 120-hours 5-FU infusion and cisplatin. Cancer 55: 1123–1128

Rouniea PH, Oliveira J, Droz JP et al. (1988) Cisplatin (P) + five days continuous infusion 5-FU (c.i. 5FU) in advanced gastric cancer: preliminary results of a phase II trial. Proc ASCO 7: 106

Rowland KM, Taylor SG IV, O'Donnell MR et al. (1984) Cisplatin/5-fluorouracil infusion chemotherapy in advanced recurrent cancer of the head and neck. Proc ASCO 3: 184

Rowland K, Bonomi P, Taylor SG IV et al. (1988) Phase II trial of etoposide, cisplatin, 5-FU and concurrent split-course radiation in stages 3A and 3B non-small cell lung cancer (NSCLC). Proc ASCO 7: 203

Schabel FM Jr, Trader MW, Laster WR et al. (1979) cis-Dichlorodiammineplatinum (II): combination chemotherapy and cross-resistance studies with tumors of mice. Cancer Treat Rep 63: 1459–1473

Shackney SE (1985) Cell kinetics and cancer chemotherapy. In Calabrisi P, Schein PS, Rosenberg SA (eds) Medical oncology. MacMillan, New York, pp 41–60

Shah S, Harvey H, Lipton A et al. (1988) A randomized study of vinblastine and cisplatinum (VBL + CDDP) vs vinblastine, cisplatinum and 5-FU five day continuous infusion in advanced non-small lung cancer (NSCLC). Proc ASCO 7: 211

Sikic B, Collins JM, Mimnaugh EG, Gram TE (1978) Improved therapeutic index of bleomycin when administered by continuous infusion in mice. Cancer Treat Rep 62: 2011–2017

Sischy B (1985) The use of radiation therapy combined with chemotherapy in the management of squamous cell carcinoma of the anus and marginally resectable adenocarcinoma of the rectum. Int J Radiat Oncol Biol Phys 11: 1587–1593

Sischy B, Lefkopoulou M, Mittleman A et al. (1988) Interim report of EST 7283: a phase II study to evaluate the effectiveness of 5-FU and mitomycin-C combined with irradiation in the management of carcinoma of the anal canal. Proc ASCO 7: 107

Stahelin H (1973) Activity of new glycosidic lignan derivative (VP-16-213) related to podophyllotoxin in experimental tumors. Eur J Cancer 9: 215–221

Strauss G, Sherman D, Mathison D et al. (1988a) Concurrent chemotherapy (CT) and radiotherapy (RT) followed by surgery (S) in marginally resectable stage IIIA non-small cell carcinoma of the lung (NSCLC): a Cancer and Leukemia Group B Study. Proc ASCO 7: 203

Strauss G, Schwartz J, Nickerson J, Lokich J (1988b) Continuous infusion (CI) 5-fluorouracil (5-FU) with or without cisplatin as third line therapy for metastatic breast cancer. Proc ASCO 7: 39

Takita H, Regal AM, Antowiak JG (1987) Continuous five-day infusion of cis-platinum and 5-FU with methotrexate day one, in non-small cell lung carcinoma. Proc ASCO 6: 178

Tannock IF, Browman G (1986) Lack of evidence for a role of chemotherapy in the routine management of locally advanced head and neck cancer. J Clin Oncol 4: 1121–1126

Taylor SG IV, Murthy AK, Showel JJ et al. (1985) Improved control in advanced head and neck cancer with simultaneous radiation and cisplatin/5-FU chemotherapy. Cancer Treat Rep 69: 933–939

Taylor SG IV, Bonomi PD, Kiel KD et al. (1986) Failure of simultaneous cisplatin/5-FU infusion chemotherapy and radiation to improve control of esophageal cancer. Proc ASCO 5: 88

Taylor SG IV, Trybula M, Bonomi PD et al. (1987) Simultaneous cisplatin fluorouracil infusion and radiation followed by surgical resection in regionally localized stage III non-small cell lung cancer. Ann Thorac Surg 43: 87–91

Taylor SG IV, Murthy AK, Showel J et al. (1988a) Concomitant therapy with infusion of cisplatin and 5-fluorouracil plus radiation in head and neck cancer. NCI Monogr 6: 343–345

Taylor SG IV, Murthy AK, Bonomi P et al. (1988b) Concomitant therapy with infusional cisplatin and 5-fluorouracil plus radiation in stage III non-small cell lung cancer. NCI Monogr 6: 327–329

Weiden P, Piantadosi S (1988) Preoperative chemo-radiotherapy in stage III non-small cell lung cancer (NSCLC): a phase II study of the Lung Cancer Study Group (LCSG). Proc ASCO 7: 197

Weiden PL, Einstein AB, Rudolph RH (1985) Cisplatin bolus and 5-FU infusion chemotherapy for non-small cell lung cancer. Cancer Treat Rep 69: 1253–1255

Wheeler C, Ervin T, Come S et al. (1986) Platinum, 5-FU and methotrexate (PFM): an active regimen in non-small cell lung cancer (NSCLC). Proc ASCO 5: 181

Yap HY, Blumenschein BR, Keating MJ et al. (1980) Vinblastine given as a continuous 5-day infusion in the treatment of refractory advanced breast cancer. Cancer Treat Rep 64: 279–283

4 Admixtures of Chemotherapy Agents by Continuous Infusion

Jacob J. Lokich

CONTENTS

4.1 Introduction

The application of multiple drugs or combination chemotherapy for the treatment of cancer has become standard practice since its introduction in the 1960s for the treatment of first testicular cancer and subsequently leukemias and Hodgkin's disease. Today chemotherapy for malignancies virtually always entails the application of multiple agents, either simultaneously or in some planned sequence. The rationale for combination chemotherapy is based upon the concept of affecting multiple metabolic sites within the tumor cell or multiple points during the tumor cell cycle. At a practical level, the use of non-cross-resistant agents without overlapping toxicity maximizes the effectiveness of such combinations. Recent conceptual advances in the application of cancer chemotherapy have introduced the concept of alternating non-cross-resistant agents applied intensively on a weekly basis. Another conceptual development has been the application of biochemical modulation utilizing a noncytotoxic enhancing agent in conjunction with a primary cytotoxic drug.

Another major development in cancer chemotherapy has been the recognition of the importance of the drug schedule in maximizing the effectiveness of antineoplastic agents, particularly those agents which are schedule dependent, such as the antimetabolite class of compounds. The introduction of ambulatory delivery systems has made it feasible for schedule-dependent agents to be administered conveniently. This concept of schedule dependency has been translated into the use of infusional schedules for a whole host of drugs. The infusional schedule administers chemotherapeutic agents for 24-h periods for a variety of durations depending on the agent and the dose rate.

Integrating the concepts of multidrug therapy and infusional delivery systems is difficult from a technological standpoint. In many combination chemotherapy programs one of the agents is administered as an infusion while the second or third agent is administered on a bolus schedule. Thus, for example, in the case of the common combination of 5-fluorouracil (5-FU) and cisplatin, the former agent is administered as a 5-day infusion and the latter as a daily bolus. A second method for combination chemotherapy by infusion would be to administer the agents simultaneously through multiple access sites utilizing multiple infusion devices. This proposal has obvious limitations in terms of patient comfort and convenience. A third method would be to administer multiple agents in sequence over the 24-h period, perhaps, for example, changing the agent every 8 h. The most convenient and practical method of simultaneous infusional delivery for multiple agents is the creation of admixtures or solutions which contain the component drugs of a combination in a single reservoir for delivery. The present report reviews the phase I studies from The Cancer Center, which has established the compatibility of a number of classes of agents. Multiagent admixtures of the

Jacob J. Lokich, MD, Chief of Neoplastic Disease, New England Baptist Hospital, Medical Director, Boston Cancer Center, 125 Parker Hill Avenue, Boston, MA 02120, USA

fluoropyrimidines and the anthracyclines, and the special combination of etoposide and cisplatin, are reviewed.

4.2 Preclinical Pharmacy Studies of Admixtures

The miscibility of two or more neoplastic agents depends upon the stability of the reconstituted agent and the compatibility of the agents with each other.

Stability is an essential component in order that the agent or agents be capable of administration in an ambulatory setting for reasonable periods of time depending upon the planned duration of the infusions. Stability studies are carried out at room temperature and in containers or drug reservoirs employed for the specific infusion device to be used. For the studies reported here, stability data were accumulated for the individual agents in polyvinyl plastic bags with a 60-cc capacity. The criterion for optimal stability was 90% retention of the parent compound or a less than 10% loss over a 7-day period. Drug assays were carried out using high pressure liquid chromatography.

Compatibility studies are carried out utilizing the same conditions of room temperature and the polyvinyl plastic reservoir. A major determinant of compatibility may relate to the pH of the solution and the diluent necessary for the individual drugs. The fact that 5-FU has a pH of 9.5 and limited solubility makes it incompatible with drugs such as doxorubicin and cisplatin. Therefore, admixtures of the fluoropyrimidines preferentially use floxuridine or FUdR, which maintains a pH of 7.5 and is much more soluble than 5-FU. Solubility is another important characteristic dictating whether or not an agent is available for practical purposes to be delivered on infusion schedules. Etoposide or VP-16-213 is of particular importance in this regard. Etoposide solubility is limited to a concentration of 0.4 mg/cc when reconstituted. For the optimal dose of administration on an infusion schedule, for example, of 30 mg/m²/day for a 5-day infusion or a total dose of 45 mg/day, the minimum volume of infusion per day would be greater than 110 cc. Because of the reservoir volume in most delivery systems, the delivery of etoposide on the proposed dose rate schedule would necessitate patient exchange of the cassette reservoir at least daily, increasing the complexity

of an ambulatory system for this agent. As a consequence, the majority of infusion programs utilizing etoposide have been short-term infusions in hospitalized patients.

4.3 Principles of Phase I Trial Studies of Admixtures

Phase I studies are more complicated for infusion schedules in general because of the difficulty in establishing a starting dose based upon animal trials. The execution of phase I trials for admixtures is particularly complex. In the single agent phase I infusional studies performed by LOKICH (1986) utilizing a protracted infusion for 28 days or more, the cumulative doses delivered were variable depending upon the agent. Thus, for example, the cumulative dose of 5-FU delivered at a dose rate of 300 mg/m²/day is four times that which can be delivered on a standard bolus schedule of this agent. In contrast, for FUdR and for methotrexate, the optimal dose rate for infusion is markedly diminished to one-tenth that which is tolerated on a bolus schedule. For the vast majority of other antineoplastic agents the cumulative dose delivered on an infusion schedule is comparable to that delivered on a bolus schedule. It has been suggested that for phase I studies of infusional delivery a maximum cumulative dose of 25% of the usual bolus dose be employed as the starting dose for initial patient entries. The general rules for phase I studies of admixtures of two or more agents require starting doses for both agents which are 50% or more below the starting dose rate for infusion of the individual agents. The dose duration selection should similarly be factored into the equation in determining the starting dose rate. Finally, the execution of a phase I trial utilizing admixtures of two or more cytotoxic agents should fix the dose rate of all but one of the agents and escalate that one agent until the identification of dose-limiting toxicity is achieved. Subsequent patient entries should involve escalation of the dose rate for the previously fixed agent(s) and the admixed drug should then return to the baseline and be escalated to the point of dose-limiting toxicity. The optimal dose rate for an admixture will be established when (a) the maximal dose of each of the component drugs is delivered with (b) dose-limiting toxicity observed in 50% or less of patients without life-threatening toxicity.

The duration of the infusion is a critical component in phase I trials, as indicated above. In addition, however, the duration of infusion has practical as well as biological implications. Open-ended infusions for 28 or more days are inconvenient for patient tolerance and increase the risk for the development of hand-foot syndrome. In addition, continuous exposure to a cytotoxic agent may result in the emergence of resistant tumor cell lines. For these reasons, the durations of infusion for ambulatory programs and phase I trials from The Cancer Center have focused on 14-day periods. For programs involving etoposide, in particular, the infusional periods have ranged from 72 to 120 h.

4.4 Fluoropyrimidine-Based Admixture Infusions

5-Fluorouracil has been the standard agent for the treatment of gastrointestinal cancers in particular for more than 20 years. Recent studies utilizing prospective randomized designed trials have confirmed that the infusional schedule for this agent is the optimal mode of delivery (SEIFERT et al. 1975; KISH et al. 1984; LOKICH et al. 1989b). Infusional 5-FU is commonly employed with additional agents administered as a bolus in the treatment of head and neck cancer, esophageal cancer, and anal cancer.

The most common drugs employed in conjunction with 5-FU include cisplatin, methotrexate, mitomycin C, and doxorubicin. Of this group, only methotrexate is compatible with 5-FU in a single solution. Leucovorin is another noncytotoxic drug utilized for biochemical modulation of 5-FU and it too is compatible with 5-FU. FUdR may be substituted for 5FU in the combination to create an acceptably compatible admixture for infusional delivery.

A summary listing of the clinical trials carried out using admixture infusions of the fluoropyrimidines is provided in Table 4.1 (LOKICH et al. 1985, 1988; ANDERSON et al. 1989a, c). The cited studies are all phase I trials which established the optimally tolerated dose rates for the admixture infusions. Clinical phase II studies to establish the therapeutic effect of these combinations have not been reported. The combination of 5-FU and methotrexate has been studied based on In vitro studies demonstrating that incorporation of 5-FU

Table 4.1. Fluoropyrimidine-based admixtures

	Trials	Optimal dose rates (mg/m²/day)	Reference
Fluorouracil +		300	LOKICH
Methotrexate	Phase I	0.75	et al. 1985
Leucovorin	Phase I	5[a]	ANDERSON et al. 1989c
Floxuridine	Phase I	0.1	ANDERSON et al. 1989a
Floxuridine + (FUdR)		15	
Cisplatin	Phase I	7.5	LOKICH et al. 1988
Leucovorin	Phase I	5	ANDERSON et al. 1989c

[a] 5-FU dose reduced to 200

into RNA is facilitated by methotrexate. The phase I study of the continuous infusion of the admixture of 5-FU and methotrexate was carried out in 29 patients employing two schedules. Dose-limiting toxicity was related predominantly to the methotrexate component, with thrombocytopenia, stomatitis, and chemical hepatitis being observed at the highest dose rates. For a 14-day infusion, the optimal dose rates were 300 mg/m²/day for 5-FU and 0.75 mg/m²/day for methotrexate. Six responses were observed in 19 patients with colon cancer and an additional five patients had an antitumor effect demonstrated by a decrease in carcinoantibiotic antigen levels. Definitive phase II trials have not been reported.

5-Fluorouracil has been combined with leucovorin in a variety of clinical trials utilizing a variety of doses and schedules for both the 5-FU and leucovorin. The combination of these two agents results in a biochemical modulation based upon stabilization of the thymidylate synthetase and FdUMP complex. A phase I trial of the simultaneous delivery of 5-FU or 5-FUdR admixed with leucovorin in a 14-day infusion has been reported (ANDERSON et al. 1989c). For 5-FU and leucovorin the optimal dose rate of delivery was 200 mg/m²/day and 5 mg/m²/day respectively. Dose-limiting toxicity was stomatitis. Using the infusion schedule for leucovorin resulted in biochemical modulation, at least in terms of toxicity, and two points may be emphasized. First, modulation is achieved with an extraordinarily low dose of leucovorin. Secondly, the evidence of modulation is based upon a substantial reduction in the optimally tolerated dose rate for 5-FU. The addition of leucovorin at the very low dose reduces the dose rate for 5-FU from 350 mg/m^2/day to a maximum of 200 mg/m^2/day.

For the FUdR plus leucovorin infusion the optimal dose rates for the two agents were 0.075 mg/kg/day and again 5 mg/m^2/day. Dose rate limiting toxicity for FUdR plus leucovorin was diarrhea related to the appearance of regional enteritis. Evidence for leucovorin-induced biochemical modulation was again provided by the fact that the optimally tolerated dose of FUdR was reduced by 60%.

5-Fluorouracil and FUdR are distinctive fluoropyrimidines, differing chemically and in terms of their specific mechanism of action intracellularly. They are also distinctive clinically, at least as regards manifested dose rate limiting toxicity, and although comparative trials are sparse and in fact date back to the 1960s, there is some evidence of differences in therapeutic efficacy. A phase I study of the admixture of the two fluoropyrimidines has been reported (ANDERSON et al. 1989a). In that study, the optimal dose rate of the individual fluoropyrimidines was for the most part maintained. Thus, the dose rate for 5-FU for a 14-day infusion is 350 mg/m^2/day and for FUdR, 0.125 mg/kg/day, with only the latter drug being reduced in the admixture setting (to 0.1 mg/kg/day).

5-Fluorouracil combined with cisplatin has been applied successfully to a number of tumors, including head and neck cancer, lung cancer, and other tumors. Studies of the compatibility of 5-FU and cisplatin, however, demonstrated that because of the high pH of 5-FU, cisplatin was not stable. FUdR, on the other hand, with a pH of 7.5, is compatible with cisplatin and stability is maintained for at least 7 days at room temperature. On this basis, a phase I study was carried out (LOKICH et al. 1988). The admixture was administered for a period of 14 consecutive days and in the phase I study the optimal dose rates were 0.075 mg/kg/day for FUdR and 7.5 mg/m^2/day for cisplatin. Dose rate limiting toxicity was again related to the FUdR, as manifested by enteritis. It is apparent that cisplatin infusion does result in modulation of the maximum dose rate of FUdR.

4.5 Anthracycline-Based Admixture Infusions

The optimal dose rate for infusion of doxorubicin has been established both for short-term infusions

Table 4.2. Doxorubicin-based admixtures

Agent	Trials	Optimal dose rates (mg/m^2/day)	Reference
Cyclophosphamide	Phase I	50	LOKICH et al. 1986
Vinblastine	Phase I	0.5	LOKICH et al. 1986
Vincristine	Phase II	0.5	BARGOLIE et al. 1984
Dacarbazine	Phase II	100	LEGHA et al. 1982
Bleomycin	Phase I-II	1.0	ROSENTHAL 1988

of 96 h and for protracted infusions for 28 days or more. On the infusion schedule the acute toxicity profile is altered, with a lesser incidence of nausea but a frequent incidence of dose rate limiting stomatitis. In addition, particularly with protracted infusion, the hand-foot syndrome has been observed. A summary of the doxorubicin combinations in which admixtures have been employed is detailed in Table 4.2. These studies for the most part represent phase II type studies in which a fixed dose of the admixed agents is established. The durations of infusion are variable as well.

Doxorubicin admixed with cyclophosphamide was studied in a protracted infusion system (LOKICH et al. 1986). The dose rate for doxorubicin was fixed at 3 mg/m^2/day and cyclophosphamide was added at 50 mg/m^2/day. The median duration of infusion was 20 days, with a range of 7–56 days. Dose rate limiting toxicity was leukopenia. Responses were observed in three patients with advanced measurable breast cancer.

The combination of doxorubicin and periwinkle alkaloids, specifically vinblastine or vincristine, has been reported in two studies. Doxorubicin admixed with vinblastine, the latter administered at a dose rate of 0.5 mg/m^2/day, was studied in 32 patients, again with open-ended infusion. The median duration of infusion was 18 days, with a range of 5–48 days. Dose rate limiting toxicity was leukopenia. Subsequently this two drug regimen, as well as the combination of doxorubicin and cyclophosphamide, has been studied in fixed duration infusions of 14 days repeated at 28-day intervals.

Doxorubicin admixed with vincristine has been studied in a phase II program for multiple myeloma refractory to alkalating agent therapy (BARGOLIE et al. 1984). The dose rates of the two agents, at 15 mg/m^2/day and 1 mg/m^2/day with a fixed duration of 4 days, resulted in the expected toxicity of stomatitis and bone marrow suppression. The clinical effect of this regimen, however, was remarkable for such refractory patients.

A similar program combining doxorubicin and dacarbazine as an admixture for a fixed 96-h infusion has been studied by the SWOG. Studies have demonstrated a similar dose rate limiting toxicity to other 96-h infusion studies of doxorubicin. Clinical effectiveness is retained on the infusion schedule. Controversy still exists as to whether DTIC adds to the clinical effectiveness of the infusion (LEGHA et al. 1982).

Doxorubicin and bleomycin are presently being studied in conjunction with radiation therapy. The admixture of doxorubicin and bleomycin is apparently stable and a phase I trial is in progress (ROSENTHAL 1988)

There are other potential admixture possibilities for the anthracyclines which have not been explored because of established incompatibilities. Because of its pH at 9.5, 5-FU is not compatible with doxorubicin. Similarly, cisplatin is not compatible with doxorubicin beyond 3 days, at which time there is a change in the HPLC chromatogram. The possibility exists that newer analogs of platinum display compatibility with one or more of the anthracyclines, and this awaits further investigation.

With regard to other anthracyclines, only daunorubicin has been studied on an infusion schedule in an admixture with cytarabine and a third agent, etoposide (SEARGENT et al. 1987) The in vitro stability and compatibility of this three drug regimen was established again using HPLC methodology and monitoring the levels over a 72-h period. However, clinical studies using the three drug regimen as an admixture infusion have not been reported.

4.6 Etoposide-Cisplatin Admixture Infusion

Etoposide or VP-16-213 and cisplatin are two agents for which infusional schedules have been developed predominantly focusing on 5-day durations. The optimal dose rate for etoposide has been defined by two phase I studies as a dose rate of 60–100 mg/m^2/day for a cumulative 5-day dose of 300–500 mg/m^2/day. Cisplatin in phase I trials achieves an optimal dose of 20 mg/m^2/day for 5 days, with the result that the cumulative dose

by infusion is comparable to the bolus dose. There are both experimental and pharmacological reasons for the infusion schedule for each of the agents and clinical activity for the infusional schedule has been established in a variety of tumor categories.

Combination chemotherapy employing a two drug regimen of etoposide and cisplatin in both experimental systems and clinical trials has demonstrated synergism for the combination. Since the stability of an admixture of the two drugs was established, three categories of admixture infusions have been studied; (a) 72-h infusion, (b) 120-h continuous infusion, and (c) 14-day infusion. For the 3-day infusion, etoposide and cisplatin were mixed in 2–3 liters of normal saline in a phase I clinical design with escalation of etoposide from 50 to 100 mg/m^2/day and of cisplatin from 20 to 40 mg/m^2/day. At the maximum dose of etoposide, 6 of 17 courses were associated with life-threatening leukopenia and four patients died of sepsis. The optimal dose rate for the two drug admixture over a 3-day period was defined by an etoposide dose of 75 mg/m^2/day and a cisplatin dose of 30 mg/m^2/day (ANDERSON et al. 1989b).

An extension of the phase I trial was carried out in a total of 94 patients of which 77 or 82% were evaluable (CREAGAN et al. 1988). Tumor responses were observed in four of four patients with previously untreated gastric or gastroesophageal junction cancer and two of two patients with endometrial cancer. In addition, 8 of 12 patients with measurable non-small cell lung cancer responded to therapy. Therefore, clinical activity for the two drugs administered as an admixture infusion is established.

The 5-day infusional delivery of an admixture of etoposide and cisplatin identified the optimal dose rates as 30 mg/m^2/day and 20 mg/m^2/day respectively (LOKICH et al. 1989c). Dose rate limiting toxicity again is hematological and the clinical activity of the program was established in three of three patients with gastric cancer. The optimal dose rates of delivery resulted in a cumulative dose of 150 mg/m^2 etoposide and 100 mg/m^2 cisplatin. Thus, comparing the single agent etoposide for 5 days with the combination of etoposide and platinum, there is a decrease in the maximum cumulative dose by approximately 50% from 300 mg/m^2 cumulative to 150 mg/m^2. For the 3-day infusion of etoposide mixed with cisplatin, the cumulative etoposide dose is somewhat intermediate at 225 mg/m^2.

The more protracted infusions, specifically for

14 days, have been studied by 2 groups (LOKICH et al., unpublished observations). The practical delivery of infusional etoposide in an ambulatory setting, however, is limited because of the limited solubility of the agent requiring large volumes. Thus the daily dose to be delivered would require something over 150 cc of fluid, which is at the maximum level for most of the portable infusion pumps and would necessitate either daily exchanges of the drug infusion reservoir or the capacity for carrying large volumes of a liter or more at a time, making the ambulatory system awkward.

4.7 Cyclophosphamide, Methotrexate, and 5-Fluorouracil Admixture Infusions

Because of its ubiquitous use in chemotherapy for breast cancer in both the adjuvant and advanced disease settings, cyclophosphamide, methotrexate, and 5-FU (CMF) may well be the most common chemotherapy regimen utilized in the treatment of cancer. Each of the component drugs has been studied in phase I trials to establish the optimal dose rate of delivery, although only 5-FU has been established to have activity on an infusion schedule and, in fact, in comparative trials against the bolus is clearly superior on the infusion schedule.

The use of an admixture infusion for the administration of CMF has been reported in a phase I trial utilizing a 14-day duration for the infusion (LOKICH et al. 1989a). The 14-day period has been selected on the basis of patient convenience and to avoid the development of the hand-foot syndrome. However, another important part of the rationale for this duration of infusion is based upon planned trials to compare a 14-day infusion with the usual 14-day bolus administration of CMF.

In the phase I trial the optimal dose rates of 5-FU and methotrexate were fixed at 300 mg/m^2/day and 0.75 mg/m^2/day respectively, and the cyclophosphamide dose was escalated from 25 to 100 mg/m^2/day. The trial basically demonstrated that the cumulative dose delivered for the cyclophosphamide and 5-FU components is increased while the methotrexate dose is markedly decreased on an infusion schedule. Clinical activity for the admixture infusion was also demonstrated in the phase I study.

An ongoing phase II study in previously untreated patients with advanced measurable breast cancer is in progress.

4.8 Summary

The administration of cancer chemotherapy by infusional systems for 24 h a day for a variety of durations is becoming increasingly common clinical practice. The use of multiple agents administered simultaneously on the basis of multiple cytotoxic lethal injury or on the basis of biochemical modulation is similarly commonplace and in fact represents the standard practice in the use of cancer chemotherapy. Finally, ambulatory therapy is a practical consideration in virtually all approaches to treatment of the cancer patient. Combination chemotherapy utilizing admixtures of drugs that are compatible and stable is an innovative and creative means of addressing combination chemotherapy. For the most part, clinical trials to date have reported phase I data to establish the optimum dose rates of delivery of the component drugs. The majority of the reports have involved fluoropyrimidine-based admixtures and anthracycline- or doxorubicin-based combinations. These studies reflect the fact that these agents have been the most studied with infusional delivery systems.

The synergistic combination of cisplatin and etoposide is receiving increasing attention in expanded phase II trials. The limitations for the combination in an ambulatory setting based upon the poor solubility of etoposide may result in either a search for other analogues with greater solubility or the development of more optimal delivery systems.

Admixtures will continue to be explored as a means of delivery of multiple agents on an infusion schedule simultaneously.

References

Anderson N, Lokich J, Bern M et al. (1989a) Combined 5-fluorouracil administered as a 14-day infusion. Cancer 63: 825–827

Anderson N, Wallach S, Lokich J et al. (1989b) VP16-213 + cisplatinum: 72 hour continuous admixed infusion in 94 patients. ASCO Abs.

Anderson N, Lokich J, Bern M et al. (1989c) A Phase I clinical trial of combined fluoropyrimidines with leucovorin in a 14-day infusion. Cancer 6: 233–237

Bargolie B, Smith L, Alexamann R (1984) Effective treatment of advanced multiple myeloma refractory to alkylating agents. N Engl J Med 310: 1353–1356

Creagan E, Richardson R, Kovach J (1988) Pilot study of a continuous five-day intravenous infusion of etoposide concomitant with cisplatin in selected patients with advanced cancer. J Clin Oncol 6: 1197–1201

Kish J, Eusley J, Weaver A et al. (1984) Superior response rate with 96 hours 5FU infusion vs 5FU bolus. PASCO Abs. C-695

Legha SS, Benjamin RS, MacKay B et al. (1982) Role of Adriamycin in breast cancer and sarcomas. In: Muggia FM, Young CW, Carter SK (eds) Anthracycline antibiotics in cancer therapy. Nijhoff, The Hague, pp 432–434

Lokich J (1986) Protracted infusional chemotherapy. In: Lokich J (ed) Cancer chemotherapy by infusion. Precept, Chicago, pp 243–264

Lokich J, Phillips D, Green R et al. (1985) 5-Fluorouracil and methotrexate administered simultaneously as a continuous infusion. Cancer 56: 2395–2398

Lokich J, Zipoli T, Moore C et al. (1986) Doxorubicin/vinblastine and doxorubicin/cyclophosphamide combination chemotherapy by continuous infusion. Cancer 58: 1020–1023

Lokich J, Anderson N, Bern M et al. (1988) Combined floxuridine and cisplatin in a fourteen day infusion. Cancer 62: 2309–2312

Lokich J et al. (1989a) Cyclophesphamide, methotrexate, and 5-fluorouracil in a three-drug admixture. Cancer 1989: 63: 822–824

Lokich J, Ahlgren J, Gullo J et al. (1989b) A prospective randomized comparison of continuous infusion fluorouracil with a conventional bolus schedule in metastatic colorectal carcinoma: a Mid-Atlantic Oncology Program Study. J Clin Oncol 7: 425–432

Lokich J, Anderson N, Bern M et al. (1989c) Etoposide admixed with cisplatin. Cancer 63: 818–821

Rosenthal J, Adriamycin and bleomycin combination admixture administered by continuous IV infusion alone and concomitantly with radiation therapy. (Protocol activated at Downstate 1988).

Seargeant L, Kobrinsky N, Sus C et al. (1987) In vitro stability and compatability of daunorubicin, cytarabine and etoposide. Cancer Treat Rep 71: 1189–1192

Seifert P, Baker LH, Reed ML et al. (1975) Comparison of continuously infused 5-fluorouracil with bolus injection in treatment of patients with colorectal cancer. Cancer 36: 123–128

5 Time-Specified Delivery of Chemotherapy by Implantable Programmable Pumps – Preliminary Data on 5-Fluoro-2'-deoxyuridine

Reinhard von Roemeling, Rosellen Lanning, Henry Wagner, Jr., Ronald DeConti, Lawrence E. Scheving, and William Hrushesky

CONTENTS

Introduction

Chemotherapy is curative in selected widespread malignancies, including childhood leukemia, testicular cancer, and malignant lymphomas. However, the most commonly occurring malignant diseases, including lung, gastrointestinal, and renal cell cancer, respond poorly or not at all even to aggressive cytotoxic therapy. The treatment goal for these metastatic tumors is palliation, not cure. As chemotherapy may not even prolong survival significantly, its application needs to be critically reviewed as to how it affects the patient's quality of life.

The intrinsic or acquired resistance of tumor cells against chemotherapy with fluoropyrimidines may be overcome in some cases by increased drug doses (Hryniuk et al. 1987), pharmacological manipulations (Pinedo and Peters 1988), or prolonged exposure of slowly dividing cells to cytotoxic agents (Vogelzang 1984; Lokich et al. 1989). These strategies are frequently limited by toxicity (Petrelli et al. 1988; Anderson et al. 1989).

Preclinical experiments, which have been performed during the past two decades, have reproducibly demonstrated that the toxicity and antitumor activity of at least 20 of the most commonly used cytotoxic drugs depend upon the time of day when the treatment is given (Levi et al. 1988). Underlying mechanisms of circadian-dependent pharmacodynamics are complex and involve rhythmic changes in cell cytokinetics of both normal and malignant tissues, drug pharmacokinetics, immune functions, and hormonc modulations. The therapeutic index can be raised if normal host tissues and tumor cells differ in the circadian patterns of their susceptibility rhythms to cytotoxic drugs, which should be administered at times of low host and high tumor toxicity.

The first clinical treatment schedules derived from these principles have been introduced during the past 5 years (Hrushesky 1985). A major obstacle has always been the logistical aspects of how to give treatment at specified times of the day that may not readily fit within common clinic or hospital routines. Since programmable pumps have been developed, even complex treatments may be given automatically and at the patient's home with a minimum of inconvenience or compromised quality of life.

Reinhard von Roemeling, MD, Assistant Professor, Division of Medical Oncology
Henry Wagner, Jr., MD, Assistant Professor, Division of Radiotherapy
Ronald DeConti, MD, William Hrushesky, MD, Professors, Division of Medical Oncology, Albany Medical College and Veterans Administration Center, 47 New Scotland Ave., A-52, Albany, NY 12208, USA

Rosellen Lanning, RN, OCN, Medtronic, Inc., 7000 Central Ave. NE, Minneapolis, MN 55432, USA

Lawrence E. Scheving, MD, Professor, Department of Anatomy, University of Arkansas for Medical Sciences, Little Rock, AR 77205, USA

5.2 Time-Specified Infusion Pattern of FUdR

5-Fluoro-2'-deoxyuridine (FUdR) is a nucleotide antimetabolite closely related to and interconvertible with 5-fluorouracil (5-FU). It interferes with DNA synthesis of actively dividing cells. Its half-life is short (about 10–15 min) following bolus i.v. injection (CHABNER 1982; PINEDO and PETERS 1988). In the mid 1960s, FUdR was compared to 5-FU in patients with metastatic colorectal cancer and found to be more toxic (REITEMEIER et al. 1965). While it was hardly used for some time, its renaissance began in the early 1980s, after ENSMINGER and colleagues had described response rates for hepatic arterial FUdR infusion four times as high as those achieved with intravenous 5-FU or FUdR treatment in patients with metastatic colorectal cancer confined to the liver (ENSMINGER et al. 1978). However, it was soon discovered that hepatic arterial infusion of FUdR over prolonged times (e.g., over 14 days, repeated every 4 weeks) resulted in severe liver toxicity as well as frequent gastric and intestinal complications (HOHN et al. 1986; KEMENY et al. 1987). Furthermore, it was technically difficult to perform such locoregional therapy (OBERMAN 1983). When intravenous infusions were tested in patients with widespread gastrointestinal carcinomas, constant-rate long-term FUdR delivery was limited by severe diarrhea before tumor-effective dose levels were reached (KEMENY et al. 1987; LOKICH et al. 1983).

These problems were severe enough to discourage its further use, had there been only a good treatment alternative for these unfortunate patients other than symptomatic care. Fluoropyrimidines are still the most active drugs for many adenocarcinomas 30 years after their development. Recent pharmacological manipulations of their transport and intracellular action has renewed hope for achieving greater antitumor activity, but has also been accompanied by severe toxicity problems (PINEDO and PETERS 1988; PETRELLI et al. 1988; ANDERSON et al. 1989).

Preclinical investigations using FUdR bolus injections and infusions in rodents with or without transplantable tumors have demonstrated that the drug is not only far better tolerated if given late in the activity span or in the early rest span of the recipient, but that tumor growth inhibition is also significantly greater during this circadian time span (ROEMELING et al. 1987a; ROEMELING and HRUSHESKY 1990). Findings from these studies were extrapolated for clinical trials using a circadian time-specified infusion pattern of FUdR. The daily dose was arbitrarily divided into four portions of 15%, 2%, 15%, and 68%. The largest fraction was given late in the day (from 1500 to 2100 hours). This infusion cycle was repeated daily for 14 days, followed by a 2-week treatment-free interval. Such treatments were given every 2 weeks on an outpatient basis using an automatic drug delivery device. This variable rate infusion was compared with constant rate infusion of FUdR (Fig. 5.1).

Fig. 5.1. Continuous infusion patterns for FUdR chemotherapy: the areas under the curves for each pattern are equivalent. To achieve a quasi-sinusoidal pattern in the time-modified schedule, the daily dose was divided into four portions of 6 h duration (15%, 68%, 15%, and 2%). The peak drug delivery was given between 1500 and 2100 hours

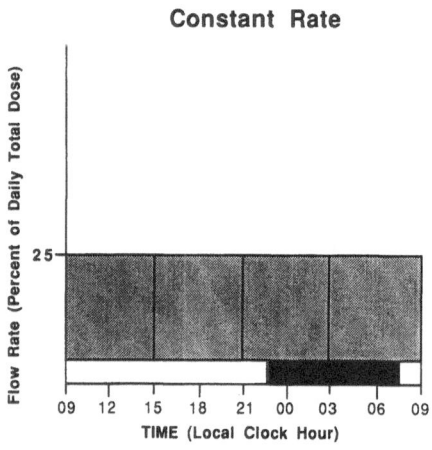

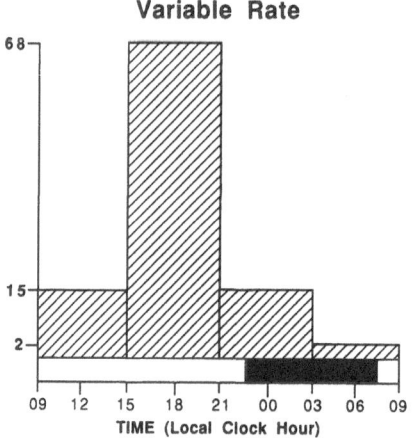

5.3 Automatic Drug Delivery

The Synchromed™ system (Medtronic, Inc., Minneapolis, Minnesota 55432) is the first and currently only available implantable, programmable drug administration system. This system offers a pump that can be noninvasively programmed. The pump contains a collapsible 18 cc drug reservoir. A peristaltic roller pump, driven by a long-lasting lithium thionyl battery module, delivers the drug. The rate of delivery is controlled by an inbuilt microcomputer. The infusion rate may vary between 0.009 and 0.9 cc/h. Program options include time-qualified bolus injections, continuous infusion at a constant flow rate, or a combination of both modes so that virtually any temporal infusion pattern can be achieved. The bolus-delay mode allows a series of exactly timed bolus injections. Complex delivery cycles can be created consisting of continuous infusion with multiple increases and decreases of the flow rate over time (ten steps per cycle; maximum cycle length = 100 h). Problems with the infusion system are rare and have been described in detail (VOGELZANG et al. 1985; ROEMELING and HRUSHESKY 1988 and 1989).

In our studies, the pump was subcutaneously implanted in the subclavian fossa for systemic drug delivery. This procedure was generally done with local anethesia on an outpatient basis, and treatment was started on the day of implantation. Prior to hepatic arterial infusion, a laparotomy was performed to place and pump catheter. The pump itself was implanted subcutaneously in the abdominal wall. Collateral blood vessels between the hepatic artery arising distal from the point of the catheter tip and the gastric/duodenal/pancreatic region were ligated to avoid extrahepatic FUdR perfusion. A cholecystectomy was performed to prevent drug-induced chronic cholecystitis. FUdR infusion was usually started on day 6 following the operation.

The treatment was offered on an outpatient basis. The patients returned to our or the referring physician's clinic every 2 weeks for pump refills. During therapy-free intervals, the pump was filled with sterile water (containing 1000 units/cc of heparin). Patients were seen by us at least every 6 weeks (normally every 4 weeks) for pump reprogramming procedures. Toxicity evaluations were done every 2 weeks by us or referring physicians. Tumor response evaluations were performed every 2 months. Standard criteria for toxicity and response evaluation were used according to the Eastern Cooperative Oncology Group guidelines (OKEN et al. 1982).

5.4 FUdR Toxicity Evaluations

Three phase I-II studies with FUdR by infusion have been performed at the University of Minnesota Hospital in Minneapolis (ROEMELING and HRUSHESKY 1988; ROEMELING and HRUSHESKY 1989).

1. Randomized Toxicity Comparison. In this study, 30 patients were randomized to receive intravenous FUdR infusion at a constant rate or a variable rate at 0.15 mg/kg/day × 14 days every 4 weeks. No dose escalations were permitted. The treatment continued until progression or until toxicity. At equal dose intensity there was a large difference in the incidence and severity of gastrointestinal toxicity with dose-limiting diarrhea. Forty-three percent of those on constant rate infusion had diarrhea of mild to severe grade versus 6% of the patients on the variable rate whose toxicity was only mild. Prolonged hospitalizations with rehydration were required for recovery from severe diarrhea in a fifth of the patients treated on flat infusion and in none of the patients using time-modified infusion (Fig. 5.2). Other toxicities were not seen, including hematological, hepatic, renal, neurological, and skin toxicity. Data from this study suggest that time modification of the infusion pattern reduces toxicity significantly. No loss of antitumor activity occurred with the less toxic variable rate infusion.

Six of the patients who started their therapy on constant rate infusion were treated until toxicity. After recovery, these patients were crossed over to time-modified infusion at the same dose intensity. This procedure reduced the rate and severity of diarrhea significantly. Nausea and vomiting were also less frequently observed.

2. Dose Escalation Study. Because of the mild toxicity associated with time-modified infusion, additional patients were accrued to a total of 39 cases. FUdR doses were escalated each month by 0.025 mg/kg/day as permitted by gastrointestinal toxicity described in our first study. Seventy-one percent of the patients did not have toxicity at the starting dose of 0.15 mg/kg/day. Fifty percent

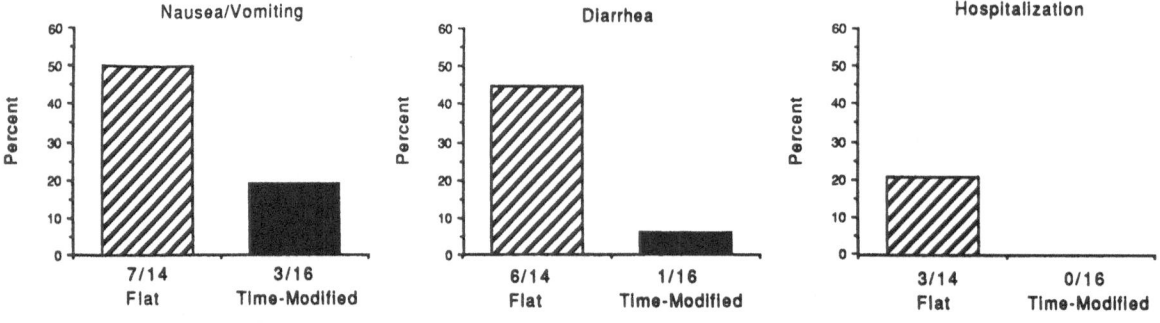

Fig. 5.2. Toxicity of intravenous FUdR infusion at equal dose intensity was found to vary depending upon infusion shape: the incidence and severity of nausea, vomiting, and diarrhea and the necessity of hospital admission for toxicity treatment were significantly lower after variable rate infusion as compared with constant rate infusion of equal dose intensity

reached the second escalation step and 26% were available for further escalation. The average tolerated dose was 0.2 mg/kg/day × 14 days. This compares to an average tolerated dose of 0.125 mg/kg/day for constant rate infusion. The maximum tolerated dose varied between individuals at a range between 0.15 mg/kg/day and 0.35 mg/kg/day. However, the overall toxicity of variable rate infusion remained below that of constant rate infusion even after dose escalation.

3. Hepatic Arterial Infusion. Fifty patients had metastatic colorectal cancer confined to the liver and received hepatic arterial FUdR infusions at 0.25 mg/kg/day × 14 days every 4 weeks. The infusion shape was either flat or time-modified, as described in Fig. 5.1. Hepatic toxicity, defined as a twofold rise in alkaline phosphatase or a serum bilirubin rise over 3 mg/dl in the absence of tumor progression, was dose limiting. Such an alkaline phosphatase rise was seen in 31% of patients following flat infusion versus 33% of patients after variable rate infusion. Over nine courses of treatment, the patients with variable rate infusion tolerated almost twice the dose intensity of FUdR (0.79 ± 0.06 mg/kg/week vs 0.46 ± 0.03 mg/kg/week). Sixteen percent versus 46% of the patients did not experience hepatic toxicity after flat versus variable rate infusion, respectively, despite higher dose intensity given to the latter group ($\chi^2 = 4.99$, $P = 0.03$). Survival did not differ significantly in the two groups (ROEMELING et al. 1987b; WESEN et al. 1989).

5.5 Response of Metastatic Renal Cell Cancer of FUdR

Sixty-eight consecutive patients were treated with infusional FUdR by implantable pump at the University of Minnesota between March 1985 and November 1988. Their characteristics have been described elsewhere (HRUSHESKY et al. 1989a, b). Briefly, 17 females and 51 males with a median age of 55 years suffered from progressive, measurable, metastatic renal cell cancer. Forty percent had failed prior systemic therapy. Ninety-eight percent had undergone nephrectomy prior to FUdR therapy. Sixty-one patients had widespread disease and were treated with intravenous FUdR infusion. In seven cases, metastatic disease was confined to the liver and treated with hepatic arterial FUdR infusion (at 0.25 mg/kg/day × 14 days every 4 weeks).

The median treatment duration for *intravenous* FUdR infusion was 6 months (range 2–30 months). In 56 evaluable patients, the following responses were documented: four complete responses (CRs), seven partial responses (PRs) (CRs + PRs = 19.6%), and four minor responses (MRs). The median duration of major responses was 9.4 months. Two patients, who achieved a partial response with systemic FUdR, underwent thoracotomy and resection of residual lung nodules. In 26 patients the previously progressive disease stabilized during therapy for a median of 6 months. Fifteen patients had tumor progression on therapy.

The median treatment duration for *hepatic arterial* FUdR infusion was 4 months (range 2–13 months) in a small group of seven patients with metastatic renal cell carcinoma confined to the liver. One complete response (after constant rate infusion) and three partial responses (one after constant rate and two after variable rate) were

Table 5.1. Comparison of two treatment schedules for the delivery of FUdR

Treatment period	No. of patients	No. of Rx periods	Dose intensity (mg/kg/week)	Nausea/ vomiting (grade 1)	Diarrhea (grade 1)	Hospitalization
qod × 28 days	7	21	0.742 ± 0.04	29%	0%	0%
qd × 14 days	7	20	0.581 ± 0.03	14%	29%	0%

seen in seven patients (objective response rate 57.2%). One patient had stable disease (SD), and two failed therapy.

Overall, complete, partial, and minor responses were seen in 30.2% of 63 evaluable patients receiving i.v. or i.a. FUdR infusion. Median survival of all 68 patients was 15 months (range of 3 to 37 months). These data demonstrate that FUdR infusion is among the most active systemic treatments available for this highly refractory disease. Its special value lies in its minimal interference with patients' quality of life, as it represents a low toxicity, outpatient regimen.

5.6 Feasibility Study of Long-Term Intermittent FUdR Infusion

We tested the implantable Synchromed pump for automatic, ambulatory intermittent drug delivery of FUdR over prolonged treatment durations. The goal was to maintain previously induced tumor remissions with a treatment schedule that offered maximal convenience and minimal toxicity. We chose the infusion pattern with the presumed best therapeutic index to be tested as a long-term maintenance regimen with minimum toxicity, reduced frequency of pump refill and programming procedures, and consequently fewer clinic visits.

Nine patients (six males, three females; median age 70 years) were treated with long-term FUdR infusion. They suffered from histologically proven metastatic malignancies (seven kidney cancers, two pancreatic cancers). FUdR was automatically delivered every other day (qod). The infusion pattern on treatment days was identical with the variable rate pattern described in Fig. 5.1. On off-days, the pump was delivering constant rate infusion at a minimum rate (e.g., 0.01 cc/day). All but one patient had previously received monthly FUdR infusions over 14 days, followed by a 2-week rest period. They had responded to this treatment (1 CR, 4 PRs, 1 MR, and 2 SD). The treatment was discontinued upon tumor progression.

Uninterrupted qod FUdR infusion was given for a mean of 178 ± 50 days. The mean dose on treatment days was 0.275 ± 0.03 mg/kg; the highest dose was 0.4 mg/kg. The mean dose intensity was 0.742 ± 0.041 mg/kg/week. Toxicity was mild and consisted of grade 1 nausea or diarrhea with no other toxicities. We compared this with the toxicity of 14-day FUdR infusions with an identical infusion pattern in the same patients (Table 5.1).

The frequency of toxicity was not significantly different (chi-square analysis), although dose intensity was 28% higher for the qod schedule ($t = 3.0$, $P < 0.01$). However, the qod infusion did not cause diarrhea.

All pumps worked reliably and accurately as determined by comparison of calculated and actually obtained residual volumes during pump refills. No catheter clotting problems occurred in spite of the low flow rate on off-days (the FUdR stock solution in the pump had a heparin concentration of 1000 units/cc). The pumps were refilled and reprogrammed every 2–8 weeks (average 33 ± 3 days). This long-term infusion of FUdR of intermittent sine-wave pattern has minimal toxicity and can be conveniently and cost-effectively offered to ambulatory patients (Lanning et al. 1989).

5.7 Cost-effectiveness

Our recent cost comparisons between implanted and portable drug delivery systems revealed that fluoropyrimidine infusion using a rented wearable device (with management and follow-up through a national home-care corporation) may be equally or more expensive depending upon the treatment duration. In addition, external pumps generally lack the programming capabilities of the Synchromed device. The implantable device is not reusable and increases the start-up cost of therapy; however, follow-up and maintenance procedures are simplified, and the therapy is more convenient. Both internal and external pump require central venous (or arterial) catheters, which are usually implanted and secured surgically. The break-even point for treatment cost with *intravenous* infusion (not considering treatment-related toxicity and subsequent expenses) using implanted or external devices will be reached at 3–6 months of treatment. For longer treatment durations, the implantable device is the more cost-effective and more convenient solution (LANNING et al. 1989). Similar experience has been reported for intrahepatic *arterial* chemotherapy infusion (PATT et al. 1987).

5.8 Infusion of Fluoropyrimidines as Radiosensitizers: Importance of Treatment Schedules

For three decades, but especially during the past few years, concurrent administration of 5-FU in conjunction with radiation therapy has been very popular, especially for treatment of gastrointestinal tumors and squamous cell carcinomas of the cervix or head and neck.

Studies using in vitro systems or animal tumor models have reported a variety of effects with these combinations. In some settings cell killing was additive; in others greater than additive killing was observed. The role of schedules of radiation and 5-FU chemotherapy combination varied from system to system (VIETTI et al. 1971; NAKAJIMA et al. 1979; VON DER MAASE 1987). The best in vitro data on scheduling of radiation and 5-FU administration indicate that enhanced toxicity is seen when 5-FU is given subsequent to radiation. This interval may be several hours without apparent abrogation of this effect. These findings suggest that inhibition of radiation-induced damage repair that occurs rapidly within 1 h is not the underlying mechanism of radiosensitization with 5-FU. The administration of 5-FU over a period of at least 48 h was needed to produce maximum effects (BYFIELD et al. 1982, 1985; WEINBERG and RAUTH 1987). The bulk of *animal data*, in which it has been possible to separately assess the sensitization (or dose modification) in tumor and normal tissue, has demonstrated minimal therapeutic gain. While there was clear evidence for dose modification, *differential* dose modification for tumor and nor-

mal tissue, a requisite for therapeutic gain, was not obtained generally. Even enhancement of permanent normal tissue damage was noted in some models (VON DER MAASE 1987; NIELSEN et al. 1988).

Despite the extensive *clinical experience* with the concurrent use of radiation therapy and 5-FU, there are few studies in which the use of such a combination has been unequivocally shown to be superior to treatment with radiation alone or to sequential treatment with 5-FU and radiation in which any interactions would be minimized. There is even less information available on FUdR combined with radiation. Thus, although the clinical impression is that these combinations are beneficial, it is far from clear what the magnitude and the mechanisms of such benefit might be. Some effects may not require any direct interaction between drug and radiation in enhancing cytotoxicity to tumor or protecting normal tissue. A specified sequence and interval between drug and radiation administration may be less important for such spatial cooperation and additive but independent cytotoxicity (STEEL and PECKHAM 1979). In contrast to STEEL (1988, 1989), however, we recommend further investigations with concurrent chemotherapy and radiation with careful consideration of treatment timepoints, sequence, and intervals rather than separation in time of both treatment modalities.

The effects of 5-FU and FUdR alone on normal tissue toxicity are substantially modified by circadian shaping of the infusion rate without diminishing antitumor response (LEVI et al. 1989; HRUSHESKY et al. 1989b). It is important to emphasize that 5-Fu and FudR have quantitatively different pharmacokinetics and pharmacodynamics and therefore different toxicity profiles. The dose-limiting toxicity may change with the administration schedule, as tissue response is a function of dose, route, delivery mode, and treatment duration. Consequently, the circadian toxicity profiles of both drugs may differ substantially and have to be determined separately for each drug at a defined delivery schedule (GONZALES et al. 1989). 5-FU is usually best tolerated during the late rest span of the recipients; FUdR is least toxic during the late activity or early rest span. Differences in the maximal tolerated doses (MTD), given during the circadian stages of best versus worst tolerance, may exceed 50% of the mean MTD.

In a next step, it is important to determine

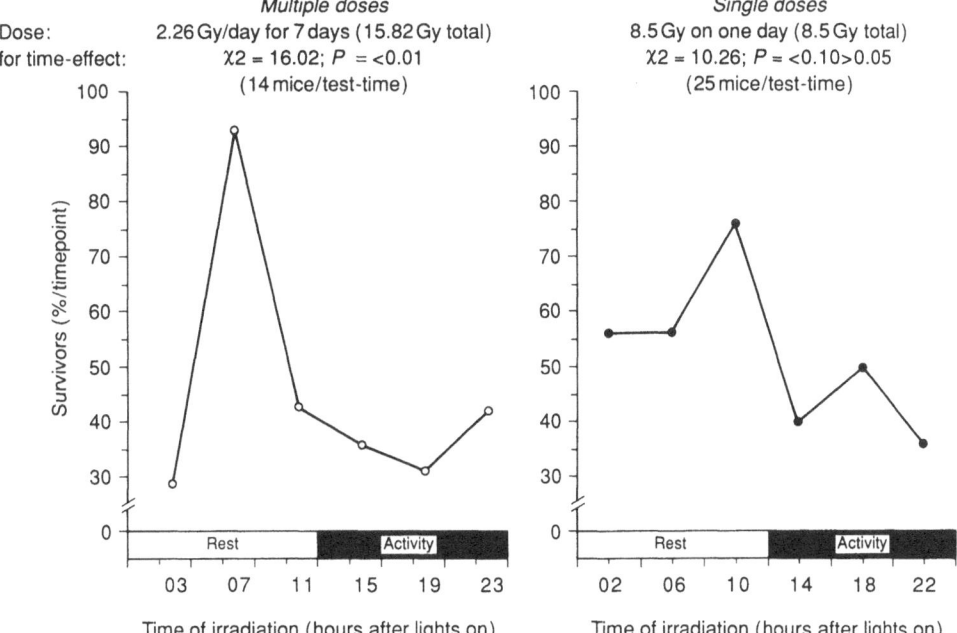

Fig. 5.3. Subgroups of mice standardized to 12:12 hours light on: off were irradiated at six different circadian stages and followed for suvival. Lethal toxicity varied significantly depending upon the circadian stage of treatment for both single-dose and multiple-dose exposures

whether there is a similar time dependence for the enhancement seen with radiation and 5-FU and FUdR. If this is the case, dose-limiting toxicity seen in tissues such as oropharyngeal or gastrointestinal mucosa might be diminished, allowing for greater treatment intensity of both radiation and chemotherapy. The availability of programmable infusion devices and the demonstration of feasibility of automatic time-specified treatment will facilitate the investigation of such hypotheses.

5.9 Circadian Susceptibility to Radiation

Much controversy was generated in the early 1960s over whether or not there was a circadian dependence of toxicity from ionizing radiation. More recent experiments with properly standardized animals and an increased number of sampling times have documented definite circadian radiosensitivity cycles. For practical reasons, most of these studies were performed using one of many single-dose ionizing exposures at many stages. Because clinical irradiation therapy is virtually always delivered by multiple fraction techniques and to address questions about the effect of a dose of irradiation upon subsequent circadian dependence of radiotoxicity, SCHEVING et al. (1983) irradiated subgroups of mice standardized to 12 h

of light alternating with 12 h of darkness, at six different circadian stages with 2.25 Gy/day. Mortality was monitored for 30 days. More than 90% of the mice irradiated repeatedly with sublethal radiation fractions at one circadian stage (late-light/rest span) remained alive, whereas fewer than 30% irradiated at another circadian stage (mid-dark/ activity span) survived (Fig. 5.3). In most of the studies, death of the animals had been the endpoint. It should be noted, however, that circadian dependency of radiation injury at the cellular level has been reported for liver regeneration, blood leukocytes, intestinal crypt cell survival, and spleen colony-forming units (SCHEVING et al. 1988). Several reports have appeared in the literature relating the phenomenon of radiation-induced mitotic delay to circadian rhythms in cell division. According to RUBIN (1982), the mitotic delay induced by a single dose of radiation in mice varied significantly depending on when it was given along the 24-h time scale. All in all the evidence for the circadian dependence of radiosensitivity of normal host tissues in rodents is compelling and demands clinical investigation.

5.10 Summary

Infusional FUdR is one of the few chemotherapeutic alternatives with activity against metastatic renal cell cancer and gastrointestinal malignancies. Diarrhea and dehydration associated with long-term, constant rate infusion are dose limiting and may be severe and life threatening. Such toxicity can be reduced substantially by circadian patterning of the infusion shape if most of the daily dose is given late in the day. This therapy can be conveniently and automatically administered by a programmable, implantable Synchromed drug delivery system. Reduced toxicity allows dose escalations, which may result in greater antitumor activity. Treatment-related discomfort and complications are rare. Long-term ambulatory FUdR infusion offers cost-effective palliation and allows maintenance of a good quality of life.

Concomitant and time-coordinated radiation therapy and infusion of potentially radiosensitizing chemotherapeutic agents including – but not limited to – fluoropyrimidines may significantly improve response rates of malignancies that are now poorly controlled by either treatment modality. Such treatments can technically be facilitated by using programmable portable or implantable pumps, which allow optimal drug administration schedules regarding time of day and sequence and interval to other drugs or treatment modalities (e.g., radiation therapy, immunotherapy). This technologically advanced strategy creates new opportunity for improved multidisciplinary therapy.

References

Anderson N, Lokich J, Bern M, Wallach S, Moore C, Williams D (1989) A phase I clinical trial of combined fluoropyrimidines with leucovorin in a 14-day modulation. Cancer 63: 233–237

Byfield JE, Calabro-Jones P, Klisak I, Kulhanian F (1982) Pharmacologic requirements for obtaining sensitization of human tumor cells in vitro to combined 5-fluorouracil or ftorafur and x-rays. Int J Radiat Oncol Biol Phys 8: 1923–1933

Byfield JE, Frankel SS, Sharp TR, Hornbeck CL, Callipari FB (1985) Phase I and pharmacologic study of 72-hour infused 5-fluorouracil and hyperfractionated cyclical radiation. Int J Radiat Oncol Biol Phys 11: 791–800

Chabner BA (1982) Pyrimidine antagonists. In: Chabner BA (ed) Pharmacologic principles of cancer therapy. WB Saunders, Philadelphia, pp 183–212

Ensminger WD, Rosowsky A, Raso V et al. (1978) A clinical-pharmacological evaluation of hepatic arterial infusions of 5-fluoro-2'-deoxyuridine and 5-fluorouracil. Cancer Res 38: 3784–3792

Gonzales JL, Sothern RB, Thatcher G, Nguyen N, Hrushesky WJM (1989) Substantial difference in timing of murine circadian susceptibility to 5-fluorouracil and FUdR. Proc Am Assoc Cancer Res 30: 616

Hohn DC, Rayner AA, Economou JS, Ignoffo RJ, Lewis BJ, Staff RJ (1986) Toxicities and complications of implanted pump hepatic arterial and intravenous floxuridine infusion. Cancer 57: 465–470

Hrushesky WJM (1985) Circadian timing of cancer chemotherapy. Science 228: 73–75

Hrushesky WJM, Lanning R, Roemeling R von, Fraley E, Wesen C, Grage T (1989a) Circadian modified FUdR infusion controls progressive metastatic renal cell cancer. Proc Am Soc Clin Oncol 8: 134

Hrushesky WJM, Roemeling R von, Lanning RM Rabatin JT (1989b) Circadian shaped infusions of FUdR for progressive metastatic renal cell carcinoma. J Clin Oncol (in print)

Hryniuk WM, Figueredo A, Goodyear M (1987) Applications of dose intensity to problems in chemotherapy of breast and colorectal cancer. Semin Oncol 14 [Suppl 4]: 3–11

Kemeny N, Daly J, Reichman B, Geller N, Botet J, Oderman P (1987) Intrahepatic or systemic infusion of fluorodeoxyuridine in patients with liver metastases from colorectal carcinoma. Ann Intern Med 107: 459–465

Lanning RM, Rabatin J, Roemeling R von, Wesen C, Grage T, Hrushesky WJM (1989) Outpatient chemotherapy pump implantation is safe and cost effective. Proc Am Soc Clin Oncol 8: 146

Levi F, Boughattas NA, Blazsek I (1988) Comparative murine chronotoxicity of anticancer agents and related mechanisms. In: Reinberg A, Smolensky M, LaBrecque G (eds) Annual review of chronopharmacology, vol 4. Pergamon, Oxford, pp 283–332

Levi F, Soussan A, Adam R et al. (1989) Programmable-in-time pumps for chemotherapy of patients (PTS) with colorectal cancer with 5-day circadian modulated venous infusion of 5-fluorouracil (CVI-5FUra). Proc Am Soc Clin Oncol 8: 111

Lokich JJ, Sonneborn H, Paul S, Zipoli T (1983) Phase I study of continuous venous infusion of floxuridine (5-FUdR) chemotherapy. Cancer Treat Rep 67: 791–793

Lokich JJ, Ahlgren JD, Gullo JJ, Philips JA, Fryer JG (1989) A prospective randomized comparison of continuous infusion fluorouracil with a conventional bolus schedule in metastatic colorectal carcinoma: a Mid-Atlantic Oncology Program study. J Clin Oncol 7: 425–432

Nakajima Y, Miyamoto T, Tanabe M, Watanabi I, Terasima T (1979) Enhancement of mammalian cell killing by 5-fluorouracil in combination with x-rays. Cancer Res 39: 3763–3767

Nielsen OS, von der Maase H, Overgaard J (1988) Effect of combined 5-fluorouracil and radiation on murine hematopoetic tissue. Radiother Oncol 13: 145–152

Oberman RA (1983) Intra-arterial hepatic infusion chemotherapy in metastatic liver cancer. Semin Oncol 10: 206–214

Oken MM, Creech RH, Tormey DC, Horton J, Davis TE, McFadden ET, Carbone PP (1982) Toxicity and response criteria of the Eastern Cooperative Oncology Group. Am J Clin Oncol 5: 649–655

Patt YZ, Boddie A, Soski M, Claghorn L (1987) Arterial

therapy: percutaneous catheters or implantable infusion devices (Medtronics DADS, Infusaid Pump). In: Ensminger WD, Selam J-L (eds) Infusion systems in medicine. Futura, Mt. Kisco, NY, pp 189–199

Petrelli N, Stablein D, Bruckner H (1988) A prospective randomized phase III trial of 5-fluorouracil versus 5-FU plus high dose leucovorin versus 5-FU plus low dose leucovorin in patients with metastatic colorectal adenocarcinoma. A report of the Gastrointestinal Tumor Study Group. Proc Am Soc Clin Oncol 7: 94

Pinedo HM, Peters GFJ (1988) Fluorouracil: biochemistry and pharmacology. J Clin Oncol 6: 1653–1664

Reitemeier RJ, Moertel CG, Hahn RG (1965) Comparison of 5-fluorouracil and 2'-deoxy-5-fluorouridine in treatment of patients with advanced adenocarcinoma of the colon or rectum. Cancer Chemother Rep 44: 39–43

Roemeling R von, Hrushesky WJM (1988) Randomized toxicity and dose intensity (D.I.) comparison of constant rate vs. circadian modified continuous FUdR infusion. Proc Am Soc Clin Oncol 7: 67

Roemeling R von, Hrushesky WJM (1989) Circadian patterning of continuous FUdR infusion reduces toxicity and allows higher dose intensity. J Clin Oncol 7: 1710–1719

Roemeling R von, Hrushesky WJM (1990) Circadian FUdR infusion pattern determines its therapeutic index. J Natl Cancer Inst 82: 386–393

Roemeling R von, Mormont MC, Walker K et al. (1987a) Cancer control depends upon the circadian shape of continuous FUdR infusion. Proc Am Assoc Cancer Res 28: 326

Roemeling R von, Rabatin JT, Kennedy BJ, Hrushesky WJM (1987b) Circadian shaping of hepatic-arterial FUdR infusion (HAI) reduces or prevents severe liver toxicity. Chronobiologia 14: 227

Rubin NH (1982) Influence of the circadian rhythm in cell proliferation on radiation-induced mitotic delay in vivo. Radiat Res 89: 65–76

Scheving LE, Tsai TH, Scheving LA (1983) Chronobiology of the intestinal tract of the mouse. Am J Anat 168: 433–465

Scheving LE, Tsai TH, Sothern RB, Hrushesky WJM (1988) Circadian susceptibility-resistance cycles to radiation and their manipulation by methylene blue. Pharmacol Ther 39: 397–402

Steel GG (1988) The search for therapeutic gain in the combination of radiotherapy and chemotherapy. Radiother Oncol 11: 31–53

Steel GG (1989) Terminology of clinical combined radiotherapy-chemotherapy. Radiother Oncol 14: 315–316

Steel GG, Peckham MJ (1979) Exploitable mechanisms in combined radiotherapy-chemotherapy: the concept of additivity. Int J Rad Oncol Biol Phys 5: 85–91

Vietti T, Eggerding F, Valeriote F (1971) Combined effect of x-irradiation and 5-fluorouracil on transplanted leukemic cells. J Natl Cancer Inst 47: 865–870

Vogelzang NJ (1984) Continuous infusion chemotherapy: a critical review. J Clin Oncol 2: 1289–1304

Vogelzang N, Ruane M, DeMeester TR (1985) Phase I trial of an implanted battery-powered, programmable drug delivery system for continuous doxorubicin administration. J Clin Oncol 3: 407–414

von der Maase H (1987) Experimental studies on interactions of radiation and cancer chemotherapeutic drugs in normal tissues and a solid tumor. Radiother Oncol 7: 47–68

Weinberg MJ, Rauth AM (1987) 5-Fluorouracil infusions and fractionated doses of radiation: studies with a murine squamous cell carcinoma. Int J Radiat Oncol Biol Phys 13: 1691–1699

Wesen C, Olson G, Roemeling R, Grage T, Hrushesky WJM (1989) Circadian modified intra-arterial treatment of colo-rectal carcinoma metastatic to the liver allows higher dose intensity to be safely given. Proc Am Soc Clin Oncol 8: 105

6 Advances in the Technology of Continuous Infusion

Jose R. Marti

CONTENTS

6.1 Introduction

Since medicine demonstrated that chemotherapy could have an impact on the outcome of cancer, man has tried to improve on the techniques of delivery. Advances have been made, based on innovative concepts of applied anatomy and on an improved understanding of cell biology, but also based on pure technological progress at the mechanical level. In fact, continuous infusion of chemotherapy is just one of several techniques that reflect the level of multi-disciplinary approach available for the management of malignant disorders today. The basic requirements for establishing such a system consist of a large bore vein, a catheter with an entry site, and a mechanical device providing a constant flow. The technological advances, as well as their advantages over the traditional techniques, are reviewed below. The pitfalls and potential complications will also be briefly analyzed.

Jose R. Marti, MD, Associate Professor of Surgery-Suny, Chairman of Surgery, The Brooklyn Hospital, 121 Dekalb Ave., Brooklyn, NY 11201, USA

6.2 Advances Through Alternate Delivery System Routes

From an anatomical standpoint, the most frequent route for the administration of continuous infusion continues to be the superior vena cava (SVC). The approach to the SVC can be percutaneous, utilizing the internal jugular vein (IJ) or the subclavian vein (SC), or indirectly through the cephalic vein.

The SC approach has the advantage that it provides a quick, efficient, and direct route to the SVC. The technique for SC catheterization has been widely described and has changed little since being popularized many years ago by Dudrick and Copeland (1973) for the purpose of total parenteral hyperalimentation. The major disadvantage of this technique continues to be the possibility of an iatrogenic pneumothorax. The incidence of this complication in the U.S. approximates 1.4%, but it is directly related to the experience of the physician performing the procedure (Eisenhauer et al. 1982; Stillman 1986). Other complications include hematoma formation and subclavian arterial puncture, but they are usually relatively harmless. By paying careful attention to technical details, catastrophic events can be avoided (Marti 1986).

The IJ approach was designed to minimize the possibility of a pneumothorax. It must be acknowledged, however, that it is controversial whether the incidence is less or similar to that with a direct SC approach, and the fact remains that this technique does not eliminate that possibility altogether (Stillman 1986). This technique has also been widely described elsewhere (Daily et al. 1970). The disadvantage of the approach is that the route is less direct than the SC approach, and kinks in the catheter as well as a "positional flow" are potential undesirable consequences, defeating the whole purpose of a continuous infusion.

A third alternative is a cephalic vein cut-down. This technique is the safest of all three in reference

Table 6.1. Author's experience regarding the various approaches to the SVC

Approach	No.	Successful	Pneumo-thorax	Death
Subclavian vein	89	87	0	0
Internal jugular vein	7	6	0	0
Cephalic vein	5	3	–	0
Total	101	96	0	0

to serious complications, particularly the possibility of a pneumothorax. However, the disadvantages are numerous. It is a rather tedious technique, and more prolonged than a simple percutaneous approach. The route is much less direct, and the possibility of a positional flow is increased, again defeating the purpose of a continuous infusion. Lastly, not infrequently the cephalic vein will be absent, exceedingly small in caliber, or tortuous enough to obstruct any catheterization.

The author's experience is summarized in Table 6.1. These are the numbers accumulated from 1986 through 1989.

With the exception of five patients, all procedures were performed on an outpatient basis in an ambulatory surgery environment. Two patients had to be admitted due to suspicions of pneumothorax. However, upon admission pneumothorax was ruled out, and after careful observation both patients were discharged the next day.

In summary, the percutaneous SC approach, with careful attention to a meticulous technique, offers several advantages. It is fast, efficient, and the most direct route. It allows the patients to stay on as outpatients, and observing meticulous technical attention, complications are almost nonexistent.

6.2.1 External Catheters

As mentioned above, the SC approach was popularized approximately two decades ago by DUDRICK and COPELAND (1973). Their efforts were aimed toward parenteral hyperalimentation and the technique was designed for seriously ill patients in a hospital bed. The need for such a system in an outpatient population became obvious soon thereafter, and the Hickman and Broviac catheters were designed for that purpose (RIELLA and SCRIBNER 1976; HEIMBACK and IVEY 1976).

An ever-increasing number of reports began to appear in the literature reporting the experience with this technique. A meticulous account of the management and pitfalls for this procedure appear in a previous publication by the author (MARTI 1986). Since then, however, the market has seen a tremendous growth in the amount of central vein catheters for the infusion of chemotherapy (ROSENTHAL et al. 1983a,b; SIKIC 1986). The physician can now choose between a traditional single lumen catheter and double or even triple lumen versions. This will allow the continuous infusion of chemotherapy concomitantly with, for example, hyperalimentation of noncompatible drugs or even simultaneous transfusions of blood or blood products. A third lumen can be utilized for hemodynamic monitoring or blood-drawing purposes as well.

It must be understood, however, that while having more than one lumen on an external catheter might be desirable, the complication rate, particularly infection, is much higher. In fact, catheter sepsis on double lumen catheters approaches 30% in some reports (STILLMAN 1986; MARTI 1986). The incidence is higher if such catheters are utilized on outpatients. Other complications include a break in the external portion of the catheter on disconnection of the catheter, as previously reported (MARTI 1986). Such breaks, of course, carry the potential for an air embolism. The Groshong catheter is an innovative concept that has a valve

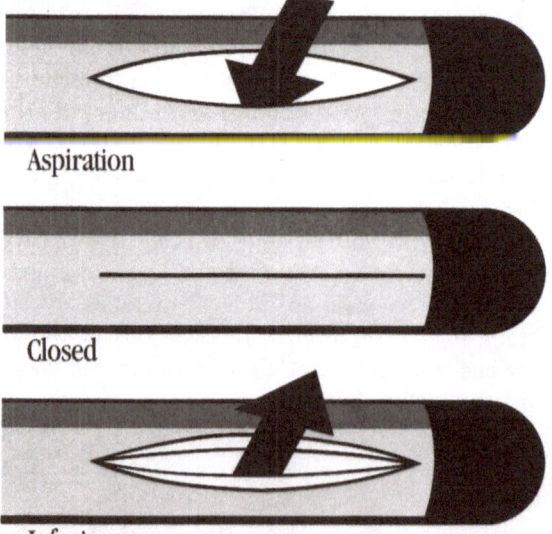

Fig. 6.1. Illustration of the way in which the valve system of the Groshong catheter functions

system on the tip of the catheter which remains open only during infusion, protecting the venous system from an embolus if a break occurs (Fig. 6.1).

6.2.2 Internal Ports

The most common complications of an external catheter consist of infection (either at the entry site or systemic) and air embolism due to catheter severance or disconnection, as previously reported (STILLMAN 1986; MARTI 1986). In addition, patients often find it awkward to have a catheter protruding from the middle of the chest wall, posing some restrictions in their daily routine. An internally placed port eliminates this aspect. Most ports consist of a small metallic reservoir covered by a sturdy synthetic diaphragm which is implanted in a subcutaneous pocket very similar to that of a pacemaker. The ports are much smaller and less bulky than a pacemaker, yet they are easily palpable. Noncoring needles are now standard equipment, and while they are essential to perform this technique, they usually come with the port.

The insertion technique is very similar to that for the external catheters. The IJ, the SC, and the cephalic vein all can be utilized for this purpose. After identification and catheterization of the appropriate vessel, the pocket is created subcutaneously, usually in the fourth or fifth intercostal space, medial to the midclavicular line. The port should be fixed to the fascia of the pectoralis major or to the connective tissue, depending on the obesity of the patient, and the incision is closed cosmetically in one or two layers, also depending on the amount of connective tissue.

Since it is a closed system, the incidence of

Table 6.2. Author's experience regarding the use of internal ports

Route	No.	Unable to pass catheter	Pneumo thorax	Delayed infection	Average duration
Internal jugular vein	87	1	0	2	20 wks
Subclavian vein	13	1	0	0	20 wks
Cephalic vein	5	1	N/A	0	15 wks

sepsis and/or thrombosis is not as great and the possibility of an air embolus is virtually eliminated. From a cosmetic point of view, a port is much more acceptable than a catheter. The author's experience is summarized in Table 6.2.

There are currently some products presenting the alternative of a double chamber port as well.

The most common complication is intramural thrombosis, the incidence of which is estimated to be 10%–20% (MARTI 1986). There is suggestive evidence that concomitant low dosage of coumadin can decrease intramural thrombosis without significant side-effects; however, at present no controlled studies have been reported in the literature (ROSENTHAL, personal communication).

6.2.3 Complications

The complications of these techniques have been briefly mentioned throughout the text and exhaustively described previously (MARTI 1986), but some of the most common potential complications can be summarized as follows:

1. Complications related to insertion
a) Inability to catheterize
b) Arterial puncture with hemothorax
c) Pneumothorax
d) Vessel transection

2. Chronic complications related to the catheter
a) Sepsis – entry site
          – [systemic
b) Embolism – [air
            – [intramural
c) Toxic complications (related to the product injection)

3. Complications related to the port
a) Sepsis
b) Mural thrombosis
c) Dislodgement of the port

6.3 Alternative Options for a Constant Flow System

The delivery of chemotherapy by constant infusion techniques is being performed with increasing frequency. This can carry significant advantages for various reasons (ROSENTHAL, personal communication). Logically, this technique is more likely to produce an impact on all phases of cellular reproduction than a bolus injection. The treatment is being delivered on an outpatient basis, contributing to the improvement in the quality of life for patients with cancer. Data suggest that the magnitude of undesirable side-effects is decreased when compared with those seen with repeated bolus injections. All this was made possible when small portable pumps became available. These pumps exist as internal implantable pumps or external portable pumps. Their use is relatively simple and basically safe, in contrast to their mechanism, which is highly sophisticated and ingenious. Their applications, as well as their advantages and pitfalls, are briefly reviewed below.

6.3.1 Internal Implantable Pumps

The Infusaid pump was the first of its kind to be developed, and it continues to be the model used more frequently (ENSMINGER et al. 1982). This pump consists of an implantable cylinder, made of titanium, with an external silicone rubber coating on the outside. It is slightly larger than an average pacemaker but is easily implanted subcutaneously through a pocket developed in the anterior abdo-

Fig. 6.2. The Infusaid pump (model 400: sagittal section) consists of a titanium cylinder in which the charging fluid is sealed between bellows and the shell. When the drug chamber is filled with medication and/or heparin and sterile water, the charging fluid is compressed into a liquid. As the patient's body temperature warms the charging fluid, it becomes a vapor. This vapor pressurizes the refill fluid, thereby releasing it from the drug reservoir

minal wall. Inside the cylinder, the drug chamber is filled through an inlet septum, not too different from that of an infusion port, which has been previously described. This drug chamber is expandable through a bellows mechanism. This is separated and sealed from a charging fluid chamber. This chamber is filled with a mixture of an inert fluid called Freon, that when compressed by filling the drug chamber with chemotherapy densifies into a liquid. As the patient's body temperature begins to warm this mixture, the Freon expands into a vapor that gradually forces the drug out of the reservoir through an outlet catheter (Figs. 6.2, 6.3).

This pump has been utilized almost exclusively for intrahepatic delivery, in contrast to the infusion ports utilized with an external portable pump, which are used for systemic therapy. The technique is still applied almost exclusively for the treatment of hepatic colorectal metastatic carcinoma (KEMENY et al. 1984; KEMENY and DALY 1986). The results of these studies are numerous and it would be beyond the scope of this chapter to review them. However, there are some potential dangers and pitfalls associated with the use of this pump which should be mentioned. The complications of the technique fall into two categories – pump failure and drug toxicity. Pump failure is uncommon and should not occur if both the patient and the medical team adhere to some very strict principles. The medical team consists of the surgeon implanting the pump, the medical oncologist supervising, and the nurse oncologist manipulating the injections.

The implantation of the pump is relatively easy,

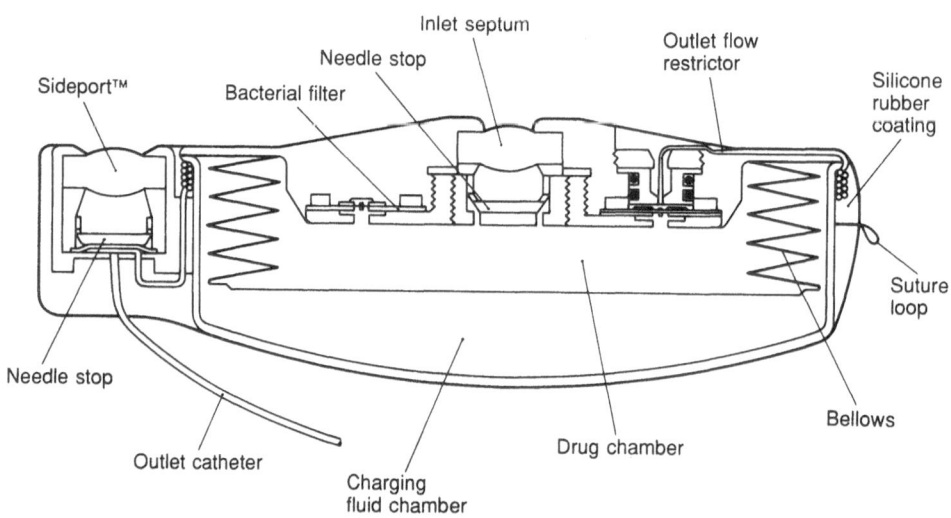

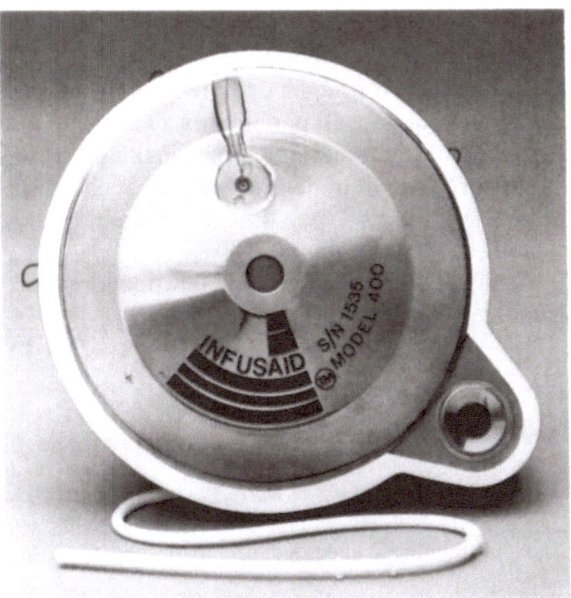

Fig. 6.3. Cross-section of the Infusaid pump

provided that the surgeon has adequate knowledge of the hepatic anatomy. A preoperative hepatic angiogram is *mandatory* since it is important to be aware of the patient's anatomy and the blood supply to the liver. There are Infusaid pumps with dual outlet catheters and side ports, and on occasion some patients might need two Infusaid pumps, depending on the extent of the disease and on the pattern of the blood supply to the liver. The surgeon must pay meticulous attention to the steps required to prime the pump. These steps are carefully explained by the manufacturer, and must be observed at the time of the procedure or at the time of the implantation to allow the physician to calculate the dose and the infusion flow rate. The patient must be made aware of the importance of keeping their refill appointments, since the pump must *never* be allowed to run empty. They must also be aware of temperature extremes (hot showers, sunbathing, saunas, etc.), high altitudes (travelling by plane), or any other activities that may cause a change in pump flow rate, such as strenuous exercise. If this occurs, they must notify their physician immediately. The medical oncologist and the nurse must understand some of the basic principles of the mechanism of the pump, such as *never* to aspirate directly from the pump through the inlet septum. This introduces blood into the pump mechanism, thus destroying it. However, it is important that the physician selects compliant pa-

tients who understand the commitment to this technique. Each patient's pump has an individual table of curves carefully calculated by the manufacturer for that patient. These are supplied to the surgeon by the company prior to the planned surgical procedure.

The complications related to drug toxicity consist primarily of an increased incidence of peptic ulcer disease, including diffuse gastritis and alterations in liver function (KEMENY and DALY 1986). Some authors have related this complication to a less than accurate technique in placing the tip of the catheter directly in the hepatic artery with careful interruption of the collateral blood supply returning to the gastric antrum (ENSMINGER et al. 1982).

Alterations in the liver function test are significant, and some patients might even develop biliary sclerosis. However, unlike with systemic chemotherapy, the incidence of gastrointestinal complications, such as diarrhea or colitis, is almost zero (KEMENY and DALY 1986). The procedure is expensive, meticulous, and demanding of proper care; however, it is safe and appears to produce a significant improvement in the quality of life of patients with hepatic colorectal metastatic carcinoma. There are, however, numerous data suggesting that despite an improvement in disease-free period, life expectancy remains unchanged (KEMENY and DALY 1986).

6.3.2 External Portable Pumps

A more frequently utilized continuous delivery system consists of an external portable pump which is attached to the patient's central venous catheter (i.e., Hickman, Broviac, Groshong, etc.). Rather than infusing the drug directly into an organ such as the liver, medication is delivered into the patient's venous circulatory system. A comparison between the alternatives (internal implantable vs external portable pumps) has been reported previously for metastatic hepatic disease (KEMENY and DALY 1986). However, external portable pumps are also frequently utilized for the control of other malignancies where continuous infusion is desired (SIKIC 1986).

The medication is delivered by the external portable pump via a peristaltic action over a preset length of time. Most of the complications of this particular technique are catheter related and have already been discussed earlier in this chapter.

Complications attributable to the pump itself are uncommon; they consist of either mechanical malfunction, which is extremely rare, or mistakes in the manipulation of the equipment. As such, patient teaching is essential, and must include care of the catheter, as well as care of the pump itself. Even though patient care and management of the pump are straightforward, in order to avert any potential problems, patients should be instructed with regard to the following:

1. How to turn the pump on and off.
2. The need to notify the physician if a constant humming is heard from the pump.
3. The need to notify the physician if the catheter is clotted or if there is any backflow in the tubing.
4. The fact that the presence of air leaks or bubbles is a cause for alarm. The patient should know how to check all connections. If the leakage continues, the patient should know how to disconnect the catheter, turn off the pump, and call for help immediately.
5. The fact that a persistent unexplained fever can be dangerous. The patient must know how to detect it.
6. How to protect the pump from getting wet or traumatized.
7. Any potential side-effects of the agents being delivered into the patient's system.

Most pumps have their own power pack. The average pump weighs just a few ounces and is smaller than a pack of cigarettes. The kits usually come with tubing and carrying devices, and their design is simple and easy to understand. Some pumps have a mechanism by which the patient can trigger a bolus injection. This is particularly useful for patients who are receiving analgesics through a continuous infusion (CHAPMAN and HILL 1989). Of course, this can also be a source of complications for obvious reasons.

6.4 Summary

In summary, continuous infusion chemotherapy is a viable alternative in the management of advanced malignant disease. It is frequently used concomitantly with radiation therapy. As such, and considering the different insertion techniques required for these methods, it reflects the multidisci-

plinary approach required for the treatment of patients with cancer today.

The technique offers a definite improvement in the quality of life of patients by decreasing the morbidity of the treatment and by making it possible to carry out treatment on an outpatient basis. Many authors also feel that it contributes to a prolonged life expectancy.

As the new century begins to dawn, undoubtedly more advances will be seen.

References

Chapman R, Hill HL (1989) Prolonged morphine self administration and additional liability. Cancer 63: 1636–1699

Daily PO, Griepp RB, Shumway NE (1970) Percutaneous internal jugular vein cannulation. Arch Surg 101: 534

Dudrick SJ, Copeland EM (1973) Parenteral hyperalimentation. In: Nyhus LM (ed) Surgery annual 1973. Appleton-Century-Crofts Medical, New York, p 69

Eisenhauer ED, Derveloy RJ, Hastings PR (1982) Prospective evaluation of central venous pressure (CVP) catheters in a large city-county hospital. Ann Surg 196: 560–564

Ensminger W, Niederhuber J, Gyves J, Thrall J, Cozzi E, Doan K (1982) Effective control of liver metastases from colon cancer with an implanted system for hepatic arterial chemotherapy. Proc ASCO 1: 94

Heimback DM, Ivey TD (1976) Technique for placement of a permanent home hyperalimentation catheter. Surg Gynecol Obstet 143: 634–636

Kemeny N, Daly J (1986) Preliminary results of a randomized study of intrahepatic infusion versus systemic infusion of FUDR for metastatic colorectal carcinoma. In: Rosenthal CJ, Rotman M (eds) Clinical applications of continuous infusion chemotherapy and concomitant radiation therapy. Plenum, New York, pp 73–78

Kemeny N, Daly J, Oderman P, Shike M, Chun H, Petroni G, Geller N (1984) Hepatic artery pump infusion: toxicity and results in patients with metastatic colorectal carcinoma. J Clin Oncol 2: 595–600

Marti JR (1986) Long term complications of the indwelling central line catheters. In: Rosenthal CJ, Rotman M (eds) Clinical applications of continuous infusion chemotherapy and concomitant radiation therapy. Plenum, New York, pp 239–242

Riella MC, Scribner BH (1976) Five years' experience with a right atrial catheter for prolonged parenteral nutrition at home. Surg Gynecol Obstet 143: 205–208

Rosenthal C, Bhutiani I, Choi K, Rotman M (1983a) Low dose Adriamycin by continuous intravenous infusion with and without concomitant radiation therapy. Proceedings of the 13th International Congress on Cancer; Abstr #3446: 603

Rosenthal CJ, Bhutiani I, Rotman M (1983b) Adriamycin by continuous infusion potentiates the effect of concurrent radiation therapy in soft tissue sarcomas and hepatomas. 13th International Congress of Chemotherapy 13: pp 1–10

Sikic BI (1986) Theoretical, clinical and pharmacokinetic aspects of cancer chemotherapy administered by continuous infusion. In: Rosenthal CJ, Rotman M (eds) Clinical applications of continuous infusion chemotherapy and concomitant radiation therapy. Plenum, New York, pp 3–12

Stillman R (1986) Potential complications of right atrial catheterization. In: Rosenthal CJ, Rotman M (eds) Clinical applications of continuous infusion chemotherapy and concomitant radiation therapy. Plenum, New York, pp 233–237

Section II
Radiosensitization and Radioprotection

7 Hypoxic Cell Sensitizers

C. Norman Coleman

CONTENTS

7.1 Introduction

The hypoxic cell radiosensitizers are included in the broad field of chemical modifiers of cancer treatment. The chemical modifiers of radiation include the radiation sensitizers and protectors, which are theoretically of no therapeutic value by themselves but are clinically active only when used in conjunction with irradiation. Combined modality therapy using radiation therapy with the standard cytotoxic chemotherapeutic agents is the major focus of this symposium. Such treatment may be designed to maximize the interaction between the radiation and chemotherapy rather than emphasizing one of the individual modalities. The radiation modifiers have also been developed as chemomodifiers, both chemosensitizers and normal tissue protectors. The overall field of chemical modifiers has been recently reviewed in detail (Coleman 1988, 1989; Coleman et al. 1988a, 1989a, b). This article will highlight some of the rationale for the clinical use of radiation and chemotherapy modifiers, with particular emphasis on the use of the hypoxic cell sensitizers as a continuous infusion.

C. Norman Coleman, MD, Professor and Chairman, Joint Center for Radiation Therapy, Harvard Medical School, 50 Binney Street, Boston, MA 02115, USA

7.2 Rationale for the Development of Hypoxic Cell Radiosensitizers

The energy of the x-ray used in radiation therapy is sufficient to eject electrons from the target tissues, hence the term ionizing irradiation. The critical lesion for cell death is felt to be double-strand breaks in DNA (Ward 1986). Ionizing radiation will produce many short-lived free radicals which are, conceptually, subject to two competitive processes: damage restoration and fixation (Coleman 1989; Coleman et al. 1989a, b). This model is called the competition model, which is useful for envisioning the potential role of radiation sensitizers and protectors. In this model, reducing agents such as thiols (-SH groups) can restore the radiation-induced radical by free radical scavenging or hydrogen donation, a process which can be called protection. When present, oxygen can interact with DNA radicals and form more permanent DNA-peroxy radicals. Therefore, oxygen is extremely important for cell killing. In the absence of oxygen, it is necessary to deliver two or three times the radiation dose to produce the same fraction of cell killing as occurs in room air (Hall 1988).

The ratio of radiation dose required to produce a certain fraction of cell killing under hypoxia compared with the dose required to kill the same fraction in air is the oxygen enhancement ratio (OER). At a clinically relevant dose per fraction of approximately 2 Gy, the OER is about 2 (Brown and Yu 1984; Skarsgard et al. 1986). Under hypoxia, the ratio of radiation dose required to kill a certain proportion of cells in the absence of sensitizer divided by the radiation dose to produce the same cell kill in the presence of sensitizer is called the sensitizer enhancement ratio (SER). When predicting the efficacy of sensitizers, it is important to remember that for the oxygen-mimetic sensitizers, the SER should be applied only to the hypoxic cells, which likely compose only 20% or so of the tumor. With the current sensitizers, about half the treatments can be sensitized. Therefore, an SER of 1.6 would not be applied to the total radiation dose, i.e., a dose of 60 Gy would not be made as effective as 96 Gy. An effective multiplier, given the above considerations, might be closer to 1.1–1.2, i.e., 60 Gy might be as effective against the tumor as 70 Gy. Since no oxygen-mimetic sensitizer is as efficient as oxygen (FINKLESTEIN and GLATSTEIN 1988), the OER should always be at least as great as the SER. However, should the sensitizer have effects beyond that of the "oxygen-mimetic" properties then, conceivably, the SER could exceed the OER. Lastly, normal tissues are probably well oxygenated; therefore, normal tissue sensitization would not be anticipated.

In general, most rodent tumors have hypoxic cells, usually in the range of 20% (MOULDER and ROCRWELL 1984). Given the relative radiosensitivity of the aerobic cells, it might be expected that the proportion of hypoxic cells would increase over the course of radiation, thereby leaving a tumor with 100% hypoxic cells. While the natural history of hypoxia during the course of treatment of human tumors is not known, in most murine tumors the proportion of hypoxic cells remains relatively constant during a course of irradiation.

This is due to a process operationally referred to as reoxygenation (HOWES 1969; HALL 1988). The precise mechanism for reoxygenation is not known but intermittence of blood flow within the tumor may be the important factor. Given the radiocurability of relatively large human tumors, it is likely that this process takes place in clinical radiotherapy. Thus, the sensitizers are designed to take over where reoxygenation leaves off.

Since reoxygenation takes place between fractions, radiotherapeutic regimens which use few, large fractions do not take best advantage of the potential sensitization by oxygen. Of note, due to technical or toxicity considerations, most of the early clinical investigations using hypoxic cell radiation sensitizers or hyperbaric oxygen used suboptimal radiotherapy fractionation regimens. Thus, the overall treatment administered in these trials did not fully exploit reoxygenation, which may account, in part, for their failure to show an improvement over standard radiation therapy.

Two mechanisms by which cells may become hypoxic or depleted of other critical nutrients are illustrated in Fig. 7.1 (COLEMAN 1989). In chronic hypoxia there is a limit on the diffusion distance of oxygen due to consumption of oxygen by the cells closest to the vessel (Fig. 7.1, left-hand side). In this setting it is assumed that the vessel is con-

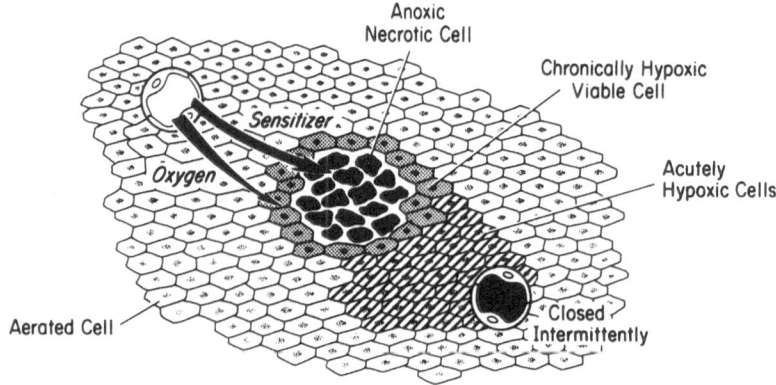

Approaches to Chronic Hypoxia

- Increase Oxygen Delivery
  Transfusion
  Hyperbaric Oxygen
  Perfluorochemical
  Altered Hgb Affinity for O_2
- Hypoxic Cell Sensitizers
  ± Thiol modification
- Bioreductive Agents
  Mitomycin C
  Nitroimidazoles
- ? Hyperthermia

Approaches to Acute Hypoxia

- Altered Oxygen Delivery
  Likely to have minimal impact
- Hypoxic Cell Sensitizers
  ± Thiol modification
- Bioreductive Agents
  Would need rapid action
  under hypoxia
- ? Hyperthermia
- ? Chemotherapy

Fig. 7.1. Chronic and intermittent hypoxia. Chronically hypoxic cells (*left-hand side*) are "diffusion limited." Intermittently hypoxic cells (*right-hand side*) are "perfusion limited" in that they are hypoxic only when the blood flow transiently stops in their nutrient vessel. The natural history of the two types of hypoxia during treatment and the relative clinical importance of each is unknown. Other nutrients may be subject to the same supply limitation. Possible methods of clinically approaching the different types of hypoxia are suggested (COLEMAN 1989)

tinuously perfused and that cells beyond the diffusion distance of oxygen, ~150 µm, are necrotic, while those surrounding this zone are hypoxic, yet clonogenic. The second type of hypoxia is intermittent hypoxia (CHAPLIN et al. 1986a, 1987) (Fig. 7.1, right-hand side). Intermittently hypoxic cells result from intermittent blood flow in the nutrient vessel. Cells irradiated when blood flow is present are sensitive, while those treated when flow temporarily ceases are relatively radioresistant. The validity of this model in clinical medicine remains to be established. Nevertheless, it is likely that both types of hypoxia are present. Better understanding of these processes should lead to an improvement in the therapeutic approach toward hypoxic cells.

Figure 7.1 includes possible approaches against the various hypoxic populations. Increasing oxygen delivery will affect predominantly chronically depleted cells. The hypoxic cell sensitizers should be effective against both types, as the drug will persist in the cells despite a cessation in blood flow. Bioreductive chemotherapeutic agents are being developed that are selectively toxic to hypoxic cells. These include mitomycin C, porfiromycin (SARTORELLI 1988), and novel compounds such as SR 4233 (ZEMAN et al. 1988) and RSU 1069 (CHAPLIN et al. 1986b). Hyperthermia appears to be especially toxic toward nutritionally deprived, hypoxic cells.

7.3 Development of SR 2508 (Etanidazole, Radinyl)

The class of hypoxic sensitizers which, to date, has been used exclusively in clinical trials are the 2-nitroimidazole compounds. For the oxygen-mimetic effect, the sensitizer must be present only at the time of irradiation. As with oxygen, the efficacy of a 2-nitroimidazole sensitizer increases with increasing drug concentration (BROWN 1984). Therefore, in the design of oxygen-mimetic radiation sensitizer trials consideration must be given to (a) the reoxygenation process, (b) the necessity to sensitize as many treatments as possible, and (c) the advantage to using as high a concentration of sensitizer as possible with each treatment (COLEMAN 1985; COLEMAN et al. 1989b). The ultimate schedule employed, as with all other drugs, is dictated by drug toxicity.

SENSITIZERS

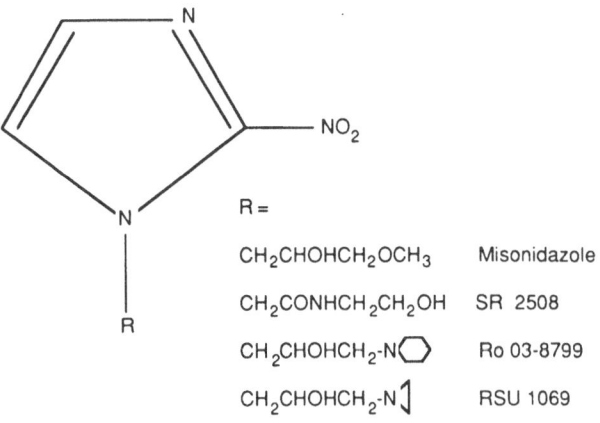

PROTECTORS

$NH_2CH_2CH_2CH_2NHCH_2SPO_3H_2$ WR-2721

Fig. 7.2. Structure of the 2-nitroimidazole sensitizers and the protector, WR-2721 (COLEMAN et al. 1989a)

The structures of the some of the current sensitizers of interest are shown in Fig. 7.2. Misonidazole was the first of the 2-nitroimidazoles to enter clinical trials (WASSERMAN et al. 1979). Its dose-limiting toxicity was a peripheral sensory neuropathy that occurred in approximately half the patients at a cumulative dose of $10-12 \, g/m^2$. The single dose of misonidazole used, $2 \, g/m^2$, was sufficient to produce an SER of 1.5 for the hypoxic cells (BROWN 1984). Given this toxicity, only five or six doses of misonidazole could be administered, leaving most of the radiation treatments in a curative regimen (usually 30–35 total treatments) to be administered without sensitizer. Therefore, in retrospect it is not surprising that most of the clinical trials did not show an advantage to the use of misonidazole (COLEMAN 1988; COLEMAN et al. 1988a). Recently, however, encouraging results have been reported from a Danish head and neck cancer trial demonstrating a statistically significant increase in local control and survival for men with pharyngeal squamous cell cancer (OVERGAARD et al. 1985).

A series of misonidazole analogs which were as effective as misonidazole in terms of radiation sensitization but which differed in pharmacokinetic properties were then developed (BROWN et al. 1981). As predicted, the less lipid soluble analog SR 2508 was less neurotoxic. The RTOG phase I study with SR 2508 demonstrated that peripheral neuropathy remains the dose-limiting toxicity. However, the cumulative dose with acceptable toxicity is $34 \, g/m^2$. Using a single dose of $2 \, g/m^2$, which will produce an SER of approximately 1.5–1.6 for hypoxic cells (BROWN 1984), will allow SR 2508 to be administered for approximately 17 treatments. Therefore, given the slight improvement in SER, the higher peak plasma and tumor level of intravenous SR 2508 compared with oral misonidazole, and the ability to deliver at least three times the total amount of drug, it is expected that SR 2508 would be about three to four times "better" than misonidazole. While still not ideal, SR 2508 is sufficiently better that a benefit might be seen in a clinical trial.

The toxicity of SR 2508 is predictable based on an assessment of drug exposure using the area under the plasma concentration versus time curve. By measuring each patient's pharmacokinetic profile, it is possible to estimate their individual risk of developing neuropathy and, therefore, to alter their drug treatment to avoid serious toxicity (COLEMAN et al. 1987). The morphological lesion of the peripheral neuropathy is an axonal degeneration (WASSERMAN et al. 1984). Recently, an in vitro model has been developed that should provide an insight into the mechanism of development of the sensitizer-induced neurotoxicity and which might provide a means of preventing it in the clinic (STEVENSON et al. 1989; COLEMAN et al. 1989b).

Currently, SR 2508 is being utilized with standard fractionated radiotherapy in phase II and III trials for patients with head and neck, prostate, esophageal and cancers. While efficacy data are not yet available, the rationale of the sensitizer trial design will be presented. The prostate cancer study for patients with large B2, C, and D1 lesions is using 66 Gy in 37 fractions, 17 of which are sensitized. The drug is given in a dose of $2 \, g/m^2$ three times a week. SR 2508 is excreted in high concentration in the bladder. Based on the high sensitizer concentration in bladder tumors (COLEMAN et al. 1984; AHWAD et al. 1988) and on responses observed in the phase I trials, both prostate and bladder trials will be conducted.

Pharmacokinetic parameters are measured on one of the first three doses. If the area under the curve (AUC) of plasma concentration is greater than 2.1 mM-h, the predicted cumulative exposure (total AUC) will exceed 36 mM-h (COLEMAN et al. 1987). At this level, the risk of neurotoxicity is about 50%; below it, the risk is < 10%. There-

fore, patients with a very high single-dose AUC, in excess of 4 mM-h, will have their single dose size halved so that a reasonable number of radiation treatments can be sensitized. In general, a patient who is destined to develop a neuropathy will develop early symptoms within 3 days of the last dose of drug. Therefore, as patients approach their predicted tolerance, 36 mM-h, the schedule is decreased to twice weekly. At the earliest indication of a persistent sensory change, albeit minor, drug is discontinued. Using these precautions, drug-induced neurotoxicity is now largely limited to very minor neuropathy which will resolve within 3–6 months. Persisting in drug treatment once unremitting symptoms have occurred can lead to a very debilitating neuropathy. The other toxicities encountered have been (a) a macular rash occurring in < 5% of patients, (b) an occasional complaint of joint discomfort that is not necessarily related to neurotoxicity, and (c) drug-induced neutropenia which has occurred in < 1% of patients to date.

Sensitizer head and neck cancer trials are being conducted in the United States, under the RTOG, and in Europe, under the support of VRG (Robert's Laboratories, Eatontown, New Jersey). Patients with T_3 and T_4 tumors are randomized to receive standard radiation ± SR 2508. The sensitizer is used as above. A phase I/II trial for esophageal cancer is being conducted at our institution. This is a multimodal study using cisplatin and 5-fluorouracil infusion during weeks 1 and 4 of radiation therapy. SR 2508 is administered during weeks 2, 3, and 5 (the latter is used only in nonsurgical patients who receive a higher total radiation dose). The concept of this protocol is to build on the Wayne State combined modality therapy approach wherein patients who achieved a complete response following presurgical radiation/chemotherapy had a somewhat superior outcome (HERSKOVIC et al. 1988). Since both SR 2508 and cisplatin are neurotoxic, the dose of SR 2508 is being escalated. Additionally, pharmacokinetics of both cisplatin (measured as non-protein-bound platinum) and SR 2508 are being monitored to see if a cumulative measure of both would be of predictive value in a manner analogous to that of SR 2508 alone. Operable patients will undergo surgery, which will allow a good assessment of efficacy. If the local control rate is high in the first cohort of patients, then more patients will be treated with a nonsurgical approach.

The bladder cancer trial is still under development and is designed as a bladder conservation study. It will use transurethral bladder resection, induction chemotherapy, and sensitized radiation. Following a dose of approximately 40 Gy, cystoscopy will be performed. Patients without evidence of disease will complete radiation therapy while those with persistent tumor will undergo cystectomy.

Other studies using sensitizer infusion, discussed below, are built on a somewhat different rationale than are the trials using bolus sensitizer. Clinical studies are planned using both bolus sensitizer with external beam and infusion sensitizer with brachytherapy.

Another sensitizer under clinical investigation for use with external beam irradiation is Ro-03-8799 (pimonidazole) (Fig. 7.2) (SAUNDERS et al. 1984; ROBERTS et al. 1986; MINCHINTON and STRATFORD 1986). Having a basic side chain, it accumulates in the acidic environment of tumors, producing a favorable tumor – plasma ratio of approximately 3:1 (SAUNDERS et al. 1984). Ro-03-8799 has a different dose-limiting toxicity than SR 2508. Rather than producing the cumulative peripheral neuropathy seen with SR 2508, it causes an acute central nervous system toxicity consisting of dizziness, nausea, and affective mental changes which last for 30–60 min after administration. A single dose of 750 mg/m^2 is tolerable and predicted to produce an SER of approximately 1.6 for hypoxic cells, similar to SR 2508.

Since it is desirable to administer as much sensitizer as possible and to give drug with each treatment, an effort has been made to administer both SR 2508 and Ro-03-8799 in combination. There is no pharmacokinetic interaction between the drugs. The total amount of SR 2508 that can administered is decreased slightly by the addition of Ro-03-8799 (MINCHINTON and STRATFORD 1986; NEWMAN et al. 1986, 1988).

Another approach to sensitization involves thiol depletion, with the focus having been on depletion of glutathione (GSH) (COLEMAN et al. 1988a). It is beyond the scope of this paper to discuss this approach in detail (COLEMAN et al. 1988a, 1989a). In essence, thiol depletion is designed to remove the endogenous radioprotection within a cell which will, in particular, increase the efficacy of the 2-nitroimidazole sensitizers (YU and BROWN 1984; MITCHELL et al. 1986). MEISTER (1983) has developed the compound buthione sulfoximine (L-BSO), which inhibits the de novo synthesis of GSH. A critical measurement in the assessment of the effect of BSO will be the GSH concentration within the target tissue.

Current radiosensitizer drug development is centering on non-nitro compounds and on dual function molecules. An example of the latter is RSU-1069, which contains an alkylating agent in the 2-nitroimidazole side chain (Fig. 7.2) (STRATFORD et al. 1986; AHMED et al. 1986). Such agents are still undergoing development with no clinical trials planned at present.

7.4 Reductive Metabolism of Sensitizers; Chemosensitization

In addition to their oxygen-mimetic properties, the 2-nitroimidazole sensitizers have other cellular properties related to their metabolism under hypoxic conditions. Prolonged exposure of hypoxic cells to the drugs can lead to (a) a reduction in the ability of the cells to repair radiation-induced DNA damage, as manifested by the reduction in the size of the shoulder of the survival curve, (b) direct cytotoxicity, (c) sensitization of the cells to alkylating agents and nitrosoureas, and (d) covalent binding to hypoxic cells, a property that is useful for labeling hypoxic cells (COLEMAN et al. 1988a, 1989a; STRATFORD et al. 1980; URTASUN et al. 1986). The precise mechanism(s) responsible for these effects is not known but involves the reductive metabolism of the nitro group, which is inhibited by oxygen (LADEROUTE et al. 1986; BIAGLOW 1981).

These additional properties are of potential therapeutic benefit. Both in vitro and in vivo data demonstrate that radiation sensitization may be enhanced beyond that seen from oxygen alone, that is, the SER may exceed the OER (TAYLOR and BROWN 1987; FU et al. 1980). Fig. 7.3 illustrates this phenomenon. Fu et al. studied radiosensitization of a mouse tumor using misonidazole plus low dose rate irradiation (1980). At the lower dose rate (0.0164 Gy/min) a longer time is required to administer a given radiation dose compared with the higher dose rate (0.042 Gy/min). This requires a more prolonged exposure to sensitizer. As seen in Fig. 7.3 (right), the enhancement observed is greater than that which is attributed to the oxygen-mimetic sensitization. Thus, due to multiple mechanisms, an SER can be obtained beyond the maximum predicted using the OER.

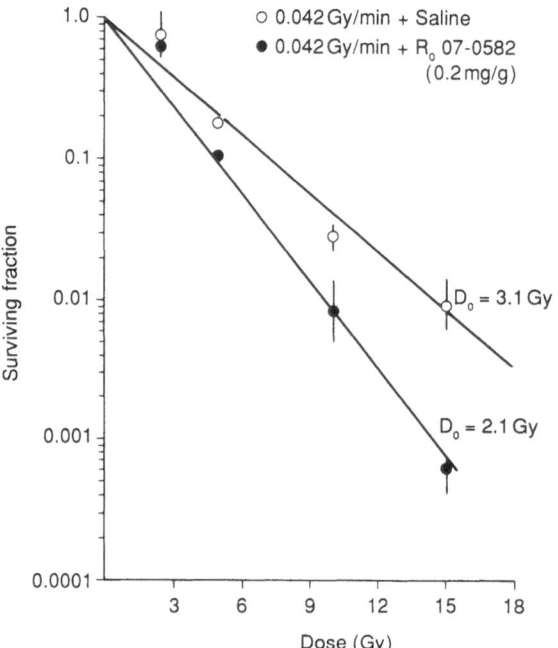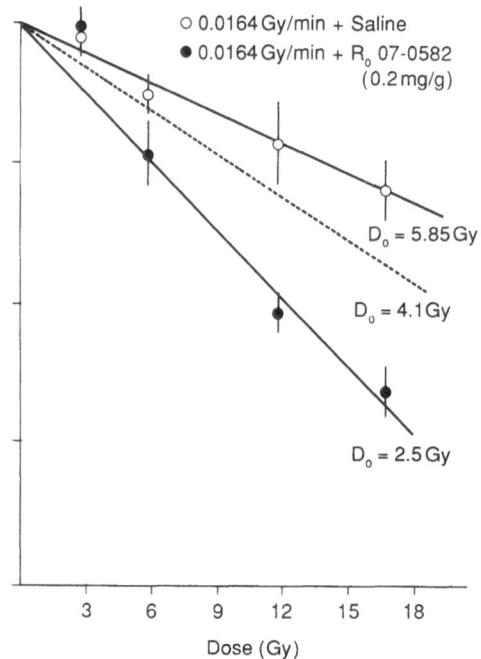

Fig. 7.3. Misonidazole with low dose rate irradiation. *Symbols* represent the mean of 4–16 EMT6/SF tumors; *bars* represent standard errors of the mean. Continuous irradiation was given with a ^{137}Cs irradiator. For the tumors given 0.042 Gy/min (*left-hand side*) the ER = 1.6. For the tumors given 0.0164 Gy/min (*right-hand side*) the ER attributed to the oxygen-mimetic effect is 1.4; however, the overall ER = 2.3. There is cell killing beyond that seen from the oxygen effect, possibly due to direct cytotoxicity, removal of the shoulder of the radiation survival curve, or inhibition of repair of radiation damage (Fu et al. 1980; Taylor and Brown 1987). Thus, the SER can exceed the OER. Brachytherapy sensitizer studies utilize a continuous infusion of sensitizer. With a clinically relevant dose rate of 0.6 Gy/h it will take 48–72 h to achieve the tumor dose desired, usually > 30 Gy. This may provide the opportunity to see the multiple sensitization effects of the 2-nitroimidazole drugs (Fu et al. 1980)

In order to exploit this potential therapeutically, developmental studies are in progress using SR 2508 as a 48-h continuous infusion with interstitial or intracavitary brachytherapy (Coleman et al. 1989c). In this trial, patients have received escalating doses of SR 2508 given by a 2 g/m² loading dose with the remainder of the sensitizer infused over 48 h. The current dose is 20 g/m², which has produced no toxicity.

Both phase I and II trials have been conducted investigating the property of chemosensitization, which is applicable to the alkylating agents and nitrosoureas (Coleman et al. 1988a; Mulcahy and Trump 1988). Most of the phase II trials did not

demonstrate a benefit compared with historical controls. Of interest, a randomized phase II trial using intravenous melphalan ± oral misonidazole for patients with non-small cell lung cancer demonstrated a statistically superior response rate in the sensitizer group (Coleman et al. 1988b).

Currently, SR 2508 is being studied in place of misonidazole, with phase I studies in progress. In designing these studies, it should be emphasized that it might not be necessary to give the sensitizer in its maximally tolerated singly dose. Rather, the duration of exposure may be as important as the peak plasma level. The efficacy of chemosensitization remains to be established. However, with the current interest in high dose alkylating agent treatment in situations such as autologous marrow transplantation, this approach may be of interest for conventional alkylating agent treatment and for use with supralethal chemotherapy doses.

Given the existence of hypoxia in tumors, strategies have been developed to exploit its presence. As noted above, a number of agents have been developed that are preferentially activated to toxic species within hypoxic cells (Coleman et al. 1988a, 1989a; Sartorelli 1988; Chaplin et al. 1986b; Zeman et al. 1988) Sartorelli and coworkers (1988) have shown that mitomycin C and porfiromycin are activated to alkylating intermediates in a low oxygen or reducing environment. Zeman et al. (1988) have developed a benzotriazine di-N-oxide compound, SR 4233, which in vitro is substantially more toxic to anoxic than to oxygenated human tumor cells. A less pronounced effect is observed in vivo (ZEMAN et al. 1988). Reductive activation is an attractive concept; however, its utility may be limited by the ability to deliver drug to hypoperfused cells and by the requirement for significant hypoxia and prolonged cell exposure to drug. The latter requirement may limit the efficacy of this approach for intermittently hypoxic cells, unless the damage from multiple short exposures to intermittent hypoxic cells is cumulative.

7.5 Summary

The field of chemical modifiers of cancer treatment is rather broad (COLEMAN et al. 1988a, 1989a, b), with 2-nitroimidazole hypoxic cell sensitization being only one aspect (Table 7.1). Hypoxic cell sensitizers that are superior to misonidazole have been developed but the clinical efficacy of this overall approach remains to be established. SR 2508 can be administered with irradiation as either a bolus or infusion. Due to reductive metabolism, the efficacy of the infusion might be such

that the SER will exceed the OER. Therefore, clinical trials addressing this approach are in progress. The relative importance of chronic versus intermittent hypoxia and the natural history of each during a course of treatment remain to be established. As further methods are developed to investigate the cellular and molecular biological aspects of hypoxia and nutritional deprivation, the clinical approaches will be appropriately modified. Chemosensitization by 2-nitroimidazole sensitizers is also being investigated. The progress made in this field has been steady. It is likely that the clinical trials with SR 2508 and Ro-03-8799 will yield important information in regard to cancer biology and therapeutic efficacy.

References

Ahmed I, Jenkins TC, Walling JM et al. (1986) Analogues of RSU-1069: radiosensitization and toxicity in vitro and in vivo. Int J Radiat Oncol Biol Phys 12: 1079–1081

Ahwad HK, El Badawy S, Zagloul M et al. (1988) Pharmacokinetics of Etanidazole (SR 2508) in bladder and cervical cancer: evidence of diffusion from urine. Proceedings from 6th Conference on chemical modifiers of cancer treatment, Paris (abstr 3–13)

Biaglow JE (1981) Cellular electron transfer and radical mechanisms for drug metabolism. Radiat Res 86: 212–242

Brown JM (1984) Clinical trials of radiosensitizers: What should we expect? Int J Radiat Oncol Biol Phys 10: 425–429

Brown JM, Yu Ny (1984) Radiosensitization of hypoxic cells in vivo by SR 2508 at low radiation doses. Int J Radiat Oncol Biol Phys 10: 1207–1212

Brown JM, Yu NY, Brown DM et al. (1981) SR-2508: a 2-nitroimidazole amide which should be superior to misonidazole as a radiosensitizer for clincal use. Int J Radiat Oncol Biol Phys 7: 695–701

Chaplin DJ, Durand RE, Olive PL (1986a) Acute hypoxia in tumors: implications for modifiers of radiation effects. Int J Radiat Oncol Biol Phys 12: 1279–1282

Chaplin DJ, Durand RE, Stratford IJ (1986b) The radiosensitizing and toxic effects of RSU-1069 on hypoxic cells in a murine tumor. Int J Radiat Oncol Biol Phys 12: 1091–1095

Chaplin DJ, Olive PL, Durand RE (1987) Intermittent blood flow in a murine tumor: radiobiological effects. Cancer Res 47: 597–601

Coleman CN (1985) Hypoxic cell radiosensitizers: expectations and progress in drug development. Int J Radiat Oncol Biol Phys 11: 323–329

Coleman CN (1988) Hypoxia in tumors: a paradigm for the approach to biochemical and physiologic heterogeneity. JNCI 80: 310–317

Coleman CN (1989) Chemical modification of radiation and chemotherapy. In: DeVita VT Jr, Hellman S, Rosenberg SA (eds) Cancer: principles and practice of oncology. JB Lippincott, Philadelphia pp 2436–2448, 1989

Table 7.1. Current clinical uses of chemical modifiers (COLEMAN et al. 1989a)

Clinical setting	Agent/maneuver
Radiation therapy	
Oxygen-mimetic sensitizers	SR 2508 (Etanidazole) Ro-03-8799
Increased oxygen delivery	Perfluorochemicals with hyperbaric oxygen Transfusion
Modulation of intracellular thiols	
– decrease glutathione (GSH)	BSO
– increase thiols: radio-protection	WR-2721
Altered radiosensitivity of DNA	IUdR, BUdR
Chemotherapy	
Chemosensitization	Misonidazole, SR 2508
Chemoprotection	WR-2721
Thiol depletion	BSO
Applicable to both	
Agents toxic to hypoxic cells	Mitomycin C and analogs Nitroimidazoles Nonnitro compounds, SR 4233
Hyperthermia	Various techniques

Coleman CN, Urtasun RC, Wasserman TH et al. (1984;
    Initial report of the phase I trial of the hypoxic cell
    radiosensitizer SR 2508. Int J Radiat Oncol Biol Phys 10:
    1749–1753
Coleman CN, Halsey J, Cox Rs et al. (1987) Prediction of
    the neurotoxicity of the hypoxic cell radiosensitizer SR
    2508 from the pharmacokinetic profile. Cancer Res 47:
    319–322
Coleman CN, Bump EA, Kramer RA (1988a) Chemical
    modifiers of cancer therapy. J Clin Oncol 6: 709–733
Coleman CN, Carlson RC, Halsey J et al. (1988b) En-
    hancement of the clinical activity of melphalan by the
    sensitizer misonidazole. Cancer Res 48: 3528–3532
Coleman CN, Glover DJ, Turissi AT (1990) Radiation and
    chemotherapy sensitizers and protectors. In: Chabner
    BA, Collins JM, Myers CE (eds) Cancer chemotherapy:
    principles and practice. W.B. Saunders, Philadelphia, pp
    424–448
Coleman CN, Looney WT, Hoskins H (1989) Radiation
    sensitizers. Semin Oncol 16: 169–175
Coleman CN, Noll L, Howes AE et al. (1989) Initial results
    of a phase I trial of continuous infusion SR 2508 (Etani-
    dazole). Int J Radiat Oncol Biol Phys 16: 1085–1087
Finklestein E, Glatstein E (1988) Seduced by oxygen
    (editorial). Int J Radiat Oncol Biol Phys 12: 1027–1032
Fu K, Hurst S, Begg AC, Brown JM (1980) The effects of
    misonidazole during continuous low dose rate irradia-
    tion. In: Brady L (ed) Radiation sensitizers, their use in
    the clinical management of cancer. pp 267–275 Masson
    Publishing Company, New York
Hall EJ (1988) Radiobiology for the radiologist. J.B. Lip-
    pincott, Philadelphia, 137–163
Herskovic A, Leichman L, Lattin P et al. (1988) Chemo/
    radiation with and without surgery in the thoracic
    esophagus: the Wayne State experience. Int J Radiat
    Oncol Biol Phys 15: 655–662
Howes AE (1969) An estimation of the changes in the
    proportions and absolute numbers of hypoxic-cells after
    irradiation of transplanted C3H mouse mammary
    tumors. Br J Radiol 42: 441–447
Laderoute KR, Eryavec E, McClelland RA et al. (1986)
    The production of strand breaks in DNA in the presence
    of the hydoxylamine of SR-2508 (1-[N-(2-hyd-
    roxylethyl)acetamido]-2-nitroimidazole) at neutral pH.
    Int J Radiat Oncol Biol Phys 12: 1215–1218
Meister, A (1983) Selective modification of glutathime
    metabolism. Science 220: 472–477
Minchinton AI, Stratford MRL (1986) A comparison of
    tumor and normal tissue levels of acidic, basic and neut-
    ral 2-nitroimidazole radiosensitizers in mice. Int J Radiat
    Oncol Biol Phys 12: 1117–1120
Mitchell JB, Phillips TL, DeGraff W ct al. (1986) The
    relationship of SR-2508 sensitizer enhancement ratio to
    cellular glutathione levels in human tumor cell lines. Int J
    Radiat Oncol Biol Phys 12: 1143–1146
Moulder JE, Rockwell S (1984) Hypoxic fractions of solid
    tumors: experimental techniques, methods of analysis,
    and a survey of existing data. Int J Radiat Oncol Biol
    Phys 10: 695–712
Mulcahy RT, Trump DL (1988) Clinical chemosensitiza-
    tion by misonidazole and related compounds: a critical
    evaluation (editorial). J Clin Oncol 6: 569–573
Newman H, Bleehan NM, Workman P (1986) A phase I
    study of the combination of two hypoxic cell radiosensi-

tizers, Ro 03-8799 and SR 2508: toxicity and pharmaco-
    kinetics. Int J Radiat Oncol Biol Phys 12: 1113–1116
Newman H, Workman P, Bleehan NM (1988) The multi-
    dose clinical tolerance and pharmacokinetics of the com-
    bined radiosensitizers, Ro 03-8799 (Pimonidazole) and
    SR 2508 (Etanidazole). Int J Radiat Oncol Biol Phys 15:
    1073–1083
Overgaard J, Sand Hansen H, Anderson AP et al. (1985)
    Misonidazole as an adjuvant to radiotherapy in the treat-
    ment of invasive carcinoma of the larynx and the
    pharynx. 2nd interim analysis of the Danish Head and
    Neck Cancer Study (personal communication and Pro-
    ceedings of the Conference on Chemical Modifiers of
    Cancer Treatment, Clearwater, FL 1-23 (abstr)
Roberts JT, Bleehan NM, Walton JI et al. (1986) A clinical
    phase I toxicity study of Ro 03-8799; plasma, urine,
    tumour and normal brain pharmacokinetics. Br J Radiol
    59: 107–116
Sartorelli AC (1988) Therapeutic attact of hypoxic cells of
    solid tumors: presidential address. Cancer Res 48: 775–
    778
Saunders MI, Anderson PJ, Bennett MH et al. (1984) The
    clinical testing of Ro 03-8799 – pharmockinetics, toxicol-
    ogy, tissue and tumor concentrations. Int J Radiat Oncol
    Biol Phys 10: 1759–1763
Skarsgard LD, Harrison I, Durand RE et al. (1986)
    Radiosensitization of hypoxic cells at low doses. Int J
    Radiat Oncol Biol Phys 12: 1075–1078
Stevenson MA, Calderwood SK, Coleman CN (1989)
    Effects of nitroimidazoles on neuronal cells in vivo. Int J
    Radiat Oncol Biol Phys 16: 1225–1230, 1989
Stratford IJ, Adams GE, Horsman MR et al. (1980) The
    interaction of misonidazole with radiation, chemother-
    apeutic agents, or heat. Cancer Clin Trials 3: 231–236
Stratford IJ, O'Neill P, Sheldon PW et al. (1986) RSU
    1069, a nitroimidazole containing an aziridine group.
    Biochem Pharmacol 35: 105–109
Taylor YC, Brown JM (1987) Radiosensitization in multif-
    raction schedules: II. Greater sensitization by 2-
    nitroimidazoles than by oxygen. Radiat Res 112: 134–
    145
Urtasun RC, Chapman JD, Raleigh JA et al. (1986) Bind-
    ing of ^{3}H-misonidazole to solid human tumors as a
    measure of tumor hypoxia. Int J Radiat Oncol Biol Phys
    12: 1263–1267
Ward JF (1986) Mechanisms of DNA repair and their
    potential modification for radiotherapy. Int J Radiat
    Oncol Biol Phys 12: 1027–1032
Wasserman TH, Phillips TL, Johnson RJ et al. (1979)
    Initial United States clinical and pharmacologic evalua-
    tion of misonidazole (RO-07-0582), and hypoxic cell
    radiosensitizer. Int J Radiat Oncol Biol Phys 5: 775–786
Wasserman TH, Nelson JS, WonGerichton K (1984)
    Neuropathy of nitroimidazole radiosensitizers: clinical
    and pathological description. Int J Radiat Oncol Biol
    Phys 10: 1725–1730
Yu NY, Brown JM (1984) Depletion of glutathione in vivo
    as a method of improving the therapeutic ratio of misoni-
    dazole and SR 2508. Int J Radiat Oncol Biol Phys 10:
    1265–1269
Zeman EM, Hirst VK, Lemmon MJ et al. (1988) Enhance-
    ment of radiation-induced tumor cell killing by the hypo-
    xic cell toxic SR 4233. Radiother Oncol 12: 209–218

8 Glutathione, a Determinant of Response to Cancer Treatment

DWIGHT KAUFMAN, JAMES B. MITCHELL, and ANGELO RUSSO

The ability to cure a limited number of cancer types with drugs has existed for only the past 25 years. Although success has been limited primarily to lymphomas and leukemias and more recently, testicular cancer, analyses of common factors in successful treatment and of the reasons for failure in both the responsive tumor types and the much broader spectrum of malignancies in which chemotherapy usually plays at best a palliative role have allowed the establishment of a number of principles that may allow the rational design of curative treatment for most cancer. These principles, consequents of the mutual interactions of treatments with tumors and of the effects of the treatments on normal tissues, may be applied not only to the established therapeutic modalities of surgery, chemotherapy, and radiation, but also to the newer immunotherapies and biological response modifiers:

1. Foremost, treatment is most likely to be successful when applied early – metastasis and tumor bulk, and consequently both biochemical and anatomic resistance, increase with time.
2. Localized disease should be treated with local modalities when possible.
3. At least one highly active agent must be included in a successful systemic regimen.
4. Treatment should be as frequent as can be tolerated and with agents having disparate intracellular targets, means of transcellular transport, mechanisms of activation and detoxification, and toxicities to normal tissues.
5. Potential tumor sanctuary sites should be treated ("prophylactically") with added intensity and with alternative modalities.
6. Since both the dose–response and the dose–toxicity curves for many essential anticancer agents are steep, potentially life-threatening normal tissue toxicity is accepted and justified when the the quest for cure is realistic.

These principles have been exploited in the treatment of virtually all tumor types. Primary extirpative debulking surgery prior to intensive chemotherapy or radiation therapy, the use of "adjuvant" therapy, increasing the number of effective drugs, increasing their doses, and decreasing the intervals between cycles, the use of so-called non-cross-resistant drug combinations, local organ infusion, and prophylaxis of potential pharmacological sanctuaries have all been extensively investigated in attempts to improve responses and cure rates. Still, success is elusive; innate and acquired tumor cell resistance to existing agents appears to be the most common reason for failure. Development of new and better agents with different points of attack is one approach to overcoming this barrier to therapeutic progress, the expectations of which, unfortunately, have been largely unrealized over the past 15 years. Immunotherapy is a nascent glow on the near horizon. For now, discovery of the reasons for tumor cell resistance and development of means for overcoming resistance remain the predominant goal of much laboratory and clinical research and will be the focus of this chapter.

Resistance to the cytotoxic effects of chemotherapeutic drugs or radiation may be due to anatomical or local physiological effects, to pharmacological barriers, to growth kinetics resistance, or to biochemical resistance. Inadequate tumor vascularity may not only preclude the accumulation of sufficient concentrations of active drug in the vicinity of the tumor cell, but can also result in hypoxia and alterations of local pH, which can alter the cells' responses to drugs or ionizing radia-

DWIGHT KAUFMAN, MD, PhD, JAMES B. MITCHELL, PhD, Head, Radiation Biology Section.
ANGELO RUSSO, MD, PhD, Head, Experimental Phototherapy Section, Radiation Oncology Branch, National Cancer Institute, National Institutes of Health, Bldg. 10, Room B3-B69, Bethesda, MD 20892, USA

tion. Both radiation and most cytotoxic drugs are cidal primarily to cycling cells, some having action only in specific stages of the cell cycle; thus, non-cycling cells or cells that never reach the most susceptible portion of the cycle during exposure to potentially cidal levels of the therapeutic agent may be said to be kinetically resistant. Stable acquired biochemical resistance is a genetic event, now thought by most to be random; thus, the probability of acquisition of resistance via a specific biochemical mechanism to one or to a similar class of agents increases with increasing cell number, hence, with increasing time since tumorigenesis, and is independent of previous exposure to the toxic agent. Resistance may be through alterations in drug transport, either increased egress or decreased ingress, decreased drug activation or increased detoxification of the active species or of a toxic metabolite, increases in amounts of specific enzyme targets, alteration of drug/active site binding affinity, or by increased repair of potentially lethal damage. An understanding of these mechanisms is a fundamental prerequisite to treatment designed to overcome resistance.

A common xenobiotic detoxifying pathway is the glutathione-dependent scheme. Glutathione (GSH) is a sulfhydryl-containing tripeptide (γ-glutamylcysteinylglycine) which comprises the major proportion of intracellular nonprotein sulfhydryl function (0.5–10 mM) (MEISTER 1983; MEISTER and ANDERSON 1983b). The γ-glutamyl group provides relative biological stability by limiting peptide hydrolysis, whereas the sulfhydryl group provides one of nature's most efficient nucleophiles, which, especially in its thiolate anion form, can function independent of enzyme catalysis by reacting directly with electrophilic alkylating agents. It is also a powerful reducing agent capable of reacting with toxic oxygen species or organic free radicals and peroxides produced by antineoplastic agents or by radiation. GSH and the assorted GSH-dependent detoxifying enzymes – glutathione-S-transferase, selenium-dependent and selenium-independent glutathione peroxidases, glutathione reductase, and glutaredoxin – are all potentially involved in drug metabolism and radiation protection and repair. The effect of alteration in GSH metabolism on the handling of chemotherapy agents by normal and malignant cells will be dictated in part by the chemical reactions of GSH and the means by which other detoxifying systems adapt to alterations in GSH concentration and in part by the chemotherapy compound itself. GSH

and its related enzymes may function to modify chemotherapeutic response by (a) noncatalyzed nucleophilic reactions with carbon-centered electrophils such as alkylating agents, (b) enzyme-catalyzed nucleophilic reaction through glutathione-S-transferase, (c) detoxification of hydrogen peroxide and organohydroperoxides through glutathione peroxidase and glutathione-S-transferase, (d) activation of certain drugs to reduced toxic species, (e) maintenance of cellular structural integrity and function during and after toxic assault by reduction of oxidized moieties, and (f) participation in DNA repair by reduction of oxidized nucleotides.

Although it is established that GSH or its related GSH-dependent enzymes can be elevated in the face of resistance, usually one- to two-fold increases, a fundamental question remains whether GSH may be actually responsible for induced radiation or drug resistance. The already high intracellular concentrations of GSH, at least tenfold higher than the K_m for all of its related detoxifying enzymes, makes suspect the unqualified assertion that minimal increases in intracellular GSH could provide markedly enhanced detoxification through enzymatic pathways of any particular drug or radiation intermediate, especially considering the small number of toxic moieties that the cell is likely to encounter. On the other hand, if the majority of intracellular GSH is strictly compartmentalized, then protective GSH concentrations may not necessarily be available at biologically crucial or specific cellular sites; if this be the case, then resistance due to moderately increased GSH levels is plausible. What is the evidence that GSH mediates resistance against antineoplastic drugs and radiation? Does an increase in activity of the GSH detoxification pathways occur? Do alterations of GSH within malignant cells result in cellular resistance? How does one go about proving the importance of GSH in radiation and drug resistance? Since changes in intracellular concentration of GSH could have an effect on many other intracellular biochemical systems, it may be difficult or impossible to attribute directly an encompassing end-point phenomenon, such as death, membrane derangement, or altered biosynthetic function to a simple change in GSH concentration.

To study the effects of changing intracellular GSH concentrations on drug or radiation response, nonspecific sulfhydryl-oxidizing agents such as diamide (KOSOWER et al. 1972; HARRIS and

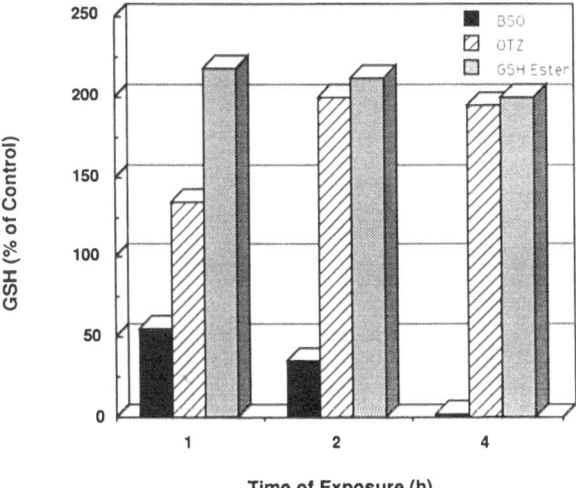

Fig. 8.1. Modulation of cellular GSH levels in Chinese hamster V79 cells by treatment with 10 mM BSO, 10 mM OTZ, or 5 mM GSH monoethyl ester. Control V79 GSH levels were 25 nmol/mg protein. These agents over the time course employed were not cytotoxic and did not affect normal growth rate or cell cycle distribution

BIAGLOW 1972; KOSOWER and KOSOWER 1978) or general sulfhydryl-binding agents such as diethyl maleate (CHASSEAUD et al. 1976) can be used. Unfortunately, other than their being of historical interest, these reagents, because of their general effects on all sulfhydryl-containing compounds, are less than ideal for studying GSH-dependent detoxification dependency. Thus, the capability of specifically inhibiting GSH synthesis with resultant depletion of glutathione would be much more informative: buthionine sulfoximine (BSO) provides such a function (GRIFFITH and MEISTER 1979). BSO acts to inhibit the synthesis of γ-glutamylcysteine, the precursor of GSH. The depletion of intracellular GSH/GSSG (oxidized glutathione) by BSO is demonstrated in Fig. 8.1. High concentrations (10 mM) of BSO were used to effect rapid GSH depletion and thereby avoid the more profound effects of chronic GSH depletion on diverse intracellular processes. Obversely, the effects of increasing intracellular GSH can be studied by employing the sulfhydryl-masked, latent cysteine moiety, 2-oxothiazolidine-4-carboxylate (OTZ) (WILLIAMSON et al. 1982). OTZ functions as a compulsory, enzymatically mediated substrate source which results in elevations of GSH up to 200% of control without exposing the cell to high levels of cysteine-containing sulfhydryl (Fig. 8.1). A second means of rapidly increasing intracellular GSH without dependence on an enzymatic process

is to expose cells to GSH monoesters (PURI and MEISTER 1983; ANDERSON and MEISTER 1989). These esters, unlike GSH, can readily cross the cell membrane and be hydrolyzed to GSH. Depending on the ester used, high levels of GSH can be positioned intracellularly in a short time (Fig. 8.1). In Fig. 8.2 the effects of manipulating GSH concentration on the responsiveness of V79 cells to several agents is demonstrated. It has been shown that a breast cancer cell line MCF-7[ADR] that has become multidrug resistant displays a marked increase in glutathione-S-transferase (~40–80 fold higher than the wild type MCF-7) and a moderate ten-to fourteenfold increase in glutathione peroxidase activity (this line also expresses the MDR phenotype) (BATIST et al. 1986; SINHA et al. 1987; ALEGRIA et al. 1989). Adriamycin cytoxicity has been postulated to result from, among other things, a reduced Adriamycin semiquinone radical intermediate that subsequently reacts with oxygen to initiate a cascade of active oxygen species. Therefore, GSH functioning either by itself or in conjunction with glutathione-S-transferase or glutathione peroxidase might be expected to participate in "mopping-up" the Adriamycin-produced hydrogen peroxide and hydroxyl radicals. As is seen in Fig. 8.2, alterations in the intracellular levels of glutathione do change the *de novo* response of cells to Adriamycin.

The major detoxifying scheme for melphalan is said to be hydrolysis by hydrolase enzymes of the chloro groups from the 2-chloroethylamino side chain. Although this reaction may occur, the effect of alteration of the intracellular GSH concentration on the cellular response to melphalan, as is seen in Fig. 8.2, suggests that enzymatic or nonenzymatic nucleophilic GSH conjugation is a major detoxifying mechanism, and perhaps, with hydrolysis, one of several possible alternative or back-up pathways for detoxifying the nitrogen mustard class of chemotherapeutic agents.

The importance of defining the mechanisms of detoxifying or activating a given chemotherapeutic agent is seen in the case of bleomycin. It has been stated that bleomycin is dependent on activation by GSH in order to produce toxic species (ANTHOLINE et al. 1981; RUSSO et al. 1984). If that were the case, then bleomycin cytotoxicity might be anticipated to be directly related to the GSH content; i.e., within limits, bleomycin's toxicity might increase with increased levels of GSH. However, as is demonstrated in Fig. 8.2, bleomycin's cytoto-

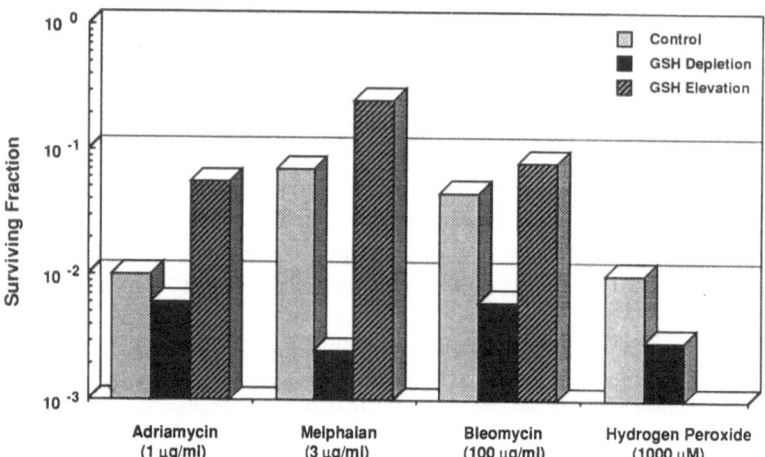

Fig. 8.2. The effects of GSH modulation on the survival of Chinese hamster V79 cells exposed for 1 h to Adriamycin (1 µg/ml), melphalan (3 µg/ml), bleomycin (100 µg/ml), and hydrogen peroxide (1000 µM). GSH depletion employed BSO pretreatment for 4 h (see Fig. 8.1) which yielded GSH levels <5% of control prior to drug exposure. GSH elevation was accomplished by pretreatment with OTZ for 2 h, which resulted in GSH levels ≈200% of control values (see Fig. 8.1). Cell survival was assessed by the clonogenic assay

xicity is increased by depletion of the GSH with BSO, whereas OTZ provides significant protection. These results suggest that under the conditions employed, activation of bleomycin proceeds uninhibited and that the predominant observed effects result from GSH's scavenging of toxic oxygen metabolites resulting from active bleomycin reacting with oxygen.

In all cases shown, GSH depletion results in increased cytotoxicity by the chemotherapeutic agents used. In contrast, as is demonstrated, an increase in GSH results in a survival benefit. The last agent, hydrogen peroxide, was chosen as a model agent to mimic the effects of radiation. GSH depletion increases hydrogen peroxide cytotoxicity (RUSSO et al. 1984). This is particularly interesting in light of the effect of modulating GSH on the radiation response. As we have previously shown, modulating GSH levels from 5% to 200% does not have a significant impact on radiation survival (MITCHELL et al. 1983; RUSSO and MITCHELL 1984; RUSSO et al. 1985a). Such a finding regarding hypoxic cells was most intriguing, particularly when one considers the well-known resistance to radiation conferred on hypoxic cells within tumors (RUSSO et al. 1985b), generally a threefold greater survival of hypoxic cells when compared with aerobic cells. Although there is no proof that hypoxia is an issue in human tumors, in experimental rodent models hypoxic areas have been demonstrated. There have been several approaches to circumvent the hypoxia-induced radiation resistance of tumors; among these has been the development of nitroimidazole hypoxic cell radiosensitizers (FOWLER et al. 1976; ADAMS and STRATFORD 1986). These compounds have been shown to be effective *in vitro*, but trials in humans have been unimpressive. One of the primary reasons for the failure of the nitroimidazole radiosensitizers is their inherent toxicity and the resultant inability to achieve effective intracellular concentrations. In addition to the pharmacological problems associated with the use of nitroimidazole compounds, another possible mechanism that would thwart the effectiveness of nitroimidazole radiation sensitization has been identified: *in vitro*

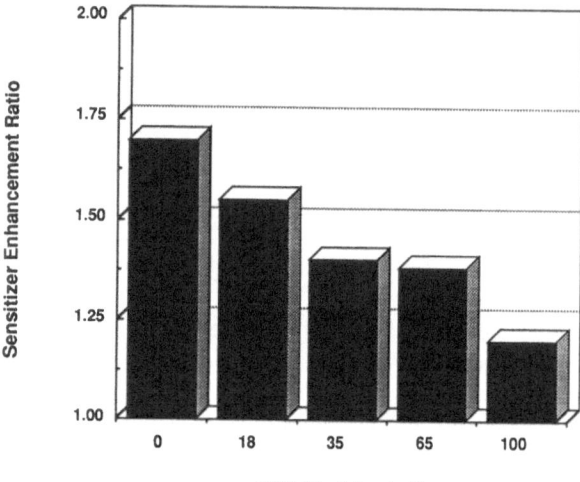

Fig. 8.3. Radiosensitization off hypoxic human lung adenocarcinoma A549 cells by the nitroimidazole SR 2508 as a function of intracellular GSH levels. The sensitizer enhancement ratio (SER) was determined by taking the ratio of radiation doses to yield 1% survival for hypoxic irradiation alone versus hypoxic irradiation with 1 mM SR 2508. An SER of 1.0 means that no hypoxic radiosensitization has occurred, while an SER of 3.0 means that hypoxic cells are fully sensitized. Full dose radiation survival curves (for hypoxia alone and with sensitizer) were determined for cells with different levels of GSH as a result of variable treatment times prior to irradiation with 10 mM BSO. SR 2508 treatment alone yields an SER of 1.18; however, depleting GSH results in a significant increase in the SER (MITCHELL et al. 1986)

growing human tumor cells have high levels of GSH and the higher the GSH level the more resistant cells are to many nitroimidazole radiation sensitizers (MITCHELL et al. 1986; PHILLIPS et al. 1989; DEGRAFF et al. 1989).

As is demonstrated in Fig. 8.3, BSO-initiated depletion of GSH results in restoration of nitroimidazole radiation sensitization. If GSH is shown to be high in critical hypoxic tumor cells and if BSO can deplete GSH from these cells, there might be a use for BSO in the clinical setting. The key questions other than GSH depletion in the tumor are: Will there be any selectivity? and How long and with what consequences can GSH depletion be sustained in humans? Preclinical trials indicate that BSO can be used in doses that will produce GSH depletion in normal tissue without causing undue host toxicity (CARMICHAEL et al. 1986; OZOLS et al. 1987). For the normal treatment of animals with BSO to achieve decreased levels of GSH, BSO must be given over longer periods of time than the few hours given in an *in vitro* setting. This will probably be particularly true for the use of multiple fractionation ionizing radiation given over several weeks. Moreover, the normal detoxifying pathways for nitroimidazole radiation sensitizers may be altered by GSH depletion; therefore, accentuated routine or unexpected toxicities may become manifest.

References

Adams GE, Stratford IJ (1986) Hypoxia-mediated nitro-heterocyclic drugs in the radio- and chemotherapy of cancer. Biochem Pharmacol 35: 71–76

Alegria AE, Samuni A, Mitchell JB (1989) Free radicals induced by Adriamycin-sensitive and Adriamycin-resistant cells: a spin-trapping study. Biochemistry 28: 8653–8658

Anderson ME, Meister A (1989) Glutathione monoesters. Anal Biochem 183: 16–20

Antholine WE, Petering DH, Saryuan LA, Brown CE (1981) Interaction among iron (II), bleomycin, lewis bases, and DNA, Proc Natl Acad Sci USA 78: 7515–7520

Batist G, Tulpule A, Sinha BK (1986) Overexpression of a novel anionic glutathione transferase in multidrug-resistant human breast cancer cells. J Biol Chem 261: 15544–15549

Carmichael J, Friedman N, Tochner Z (1986) Inhibition of the protective effect of cyclophosphamide by pretreatment with buthionine sulfoximine. Int J Radiat Oncol Biol Phys 12: 1191–1193

Chasseaud LF (1976) Properties of the glutathione S-alkenetransferase system catalyzing the conjugation of glutathione with diethyl maleate. In: Arias IM, Jakoby WB (eds) Glutathione: metabolism and function. Raven New York, pp 281–284

DeGraff WG, Russo A, Gamson J, Mitchell JB (1989) Evaluation of nitroimidazole hypoxic cell radiosensitizers in a human tumor cell line high in intracellular glutathione. Int J Radiat Oncol Biol Phys 16: 1021–1024

Fowler JF, Adams GE, Denekamp J (1976) Radiosensitizers of hypoxic cells in solid tumors. Cancer Treat Rev 3: 227–256

Griffith OW, Meister A (1979) Potent and specific inhibition of glutathione synthesis by buthionine sulfoximine (S-n-butyl homocysteine sulfoximine). J Biol Chem 254: 7558–7560

Harris JW, Biaglow JE (1972) Non-specific reactions of the glutathione oxidant "diamide" with mammalian cells. Biochem Biophys Res Commun 46: 1743–1749

Kosower EM, Correa W, Kinon BJ, Kosower NS (1972) Glutathione. VII. Differentiation among substrates by the thiol-oxidizing agent, diamide. Biochim Biophys Acta 264: 39–44

Kosower NS, Kosower EM (1978) The glutathione status of cells. Int Rev Cytol 54: 109–159

Meister A (1983) Selective modification of glutathione metabolism. Science 220: 442–447

Meister A, Anderson MA (1983) Glutathione. Annu Rev Biochem 52: 711–760

Mitchell JB, Russo A, Biaglow JE, McPherson S (1983) Cellular glutathione depletion by diethyl maleate or buthionine sulfoximine: no effect of glutathione depletion on the oxygen enhancement ratio. Radiat Res 96: 422–428

Mitchell JB, Phillips TL, DeGraff WG, Carmichael J, Rajpal RK, Russo A (1986) The relationship of SR-2508 sensitizer enhancement ratio to cellular glutathione levels in human tumor cell lines. Int J Radiat Oncol Biol Phys 12: 1143–1146

Ozols RF, Louie KG Plowman J (1987) Enhanced melphalan cytotoxicity in human ovarian cancer *in vitro* and in tumor-bearing nude mice by buthionine sulfoximine depletion of glutathione. Biochem Pharmacol 36: 147–153

Phillips TL, Mitchell JB, DeGraff WG (1986) Variation in sensitizing efficiency for SR-2508 in human cells dependent on glutathione content. Int J Radiat Oncol Biol Phys 12: 1627–1635

Puri RN, Meister A (1983) Transport of glutathione as gamma-glutamylcysteinylglycyl ester into liver and kidney. Proc Natl Acad Sci USA 80: 5258–5260

Russo A, Mitchell JB (1984) Radiation response of Chinese hamster cells after elevation of intracellular glutathione levels. Int J Radiat Oncol Biol Phys 10: 1243–1247

Russo A, Mitchell JB, McPherson S, Friedman N (1984) Alteration of bleomycin cytotoxicity by glutathione depletion or elevation. Int J Radiat Oncol Biol Phys 10: 1675–1678

Russo A, Mitchell JB, Finkelstein E (1985a) The effects of cellular glutathione elevation on the oxygen enhancement ratio. Radiat Res 103: 232–239

Russo A, Mitchell JB, Kinsella T (1985b) Determinants of radiosensitivity. Semin Oncol 12: 332–349

Sinha BK, Katki AG, Batist G (1987) Differential formation of hydroxyl radicals by Adriamycin in sensitive and resistant MCF-7 human breast tumor cells: implications for the mechanism of action. Biochemistry 26: 3776–3781

Williamson JM, Boettcher B, Meister A (1982) Intracellular delivery system that protects against toxicity by promoting glutathione synthesis. Proc Natl Acad Sci USA 79: 6246–6249

9 Radiosensitization of Nonhypoxic Cells by Halogenated Pyrimidines

Timothy J. Kinsella

Halogenated pyrimidine analogs such as iododeoxyuridine (IdUrd) have been recognized as potential clinical radiosensitizers for over two decades (Djordjevic and Szybalski 1960; Erikson and Szybalski 1963; Kaplan and Tomlin 1960; Kinsella et al. 1984a). More recently, in vitro studies suggest these analogs may sensitize certain chemotherapy agents such as bleomycin and cisplatinum (Russo et al. 1986; Ackland et al. 1988), although the mechanism(s) of chemosensitization, like those of radiosensitization, are not clearly understood. However, incorporation into DNA is felt to be necessary for both types of sensitization (Ackland et al. 1988; Kinsella et al. 1987). IdUrd has been shown to be as effective a clinical radiosensitizer as bromodeoxyuridine (BrdUrd), with less systemic skin toxicity (Kinsella et al. 1985; Kinsella et al. 1984b). This skin toxicity is felt to result from photosensitization with fluorescent light and sunlight (Mitchell et al. 1984). Several clinical trials of IdUrd as a radiosensitizer show encouraging results and will be summarized later. Clinical testing of IdUrd as a chemosensitizer with bleomycin is underway as a phase I study sponsored by NCl (R. Schilsky, personal communication, 1990).

Iododeoxyuridinc is an analog of the nucleoside thymidine (dThd) and competes with dThd for incorporation into DNA (Goz 1978; Sirotnak and Barruesco 1987). dThd replacement is believed to result from stereochemical similarities between the Van der Waals's radius of the iodine atom (2.15 Å) and the methyl group (2.0 Å) at the 5-position of the uridine molecule (Fig. 9.1).

Iododeoxyuridine, like dThd, must undergo sequential phosphorylations prior to incorporation into DNA. In Fig. 9.2, a schema for the endogenous (de novo) and exogenous (salvage) pathways for dThd is illustrated. The key enzyme in the salvage pathway is dThd kinase (TK), which is the first and rate-limiting step in the phosphorylation of both dThd and IdUrd. The key enzyme in the de novo pathway of dThd is thymidylate synthase (TS). Catabolic reactions of importance in the intracellular pools of dThd and IdUrd, as well as their monophosphate forms, are cytoplasmic 5'-nucleotidase and nucleoside phosphorylase.

The salvage pathway of thymidine triphosphate (dThd) is regulated by end-product [(dTTP), IdUTP] feedback inhibition of TK (Breitman 1983), which would limit the activation of drugs such as IdUrd and fluorodeoxyuridine (FdUrd) (Cohen and Ullman 1984) (Fig. 9.2). 5'-Aminodeoxythymidine (5'-AT) (Fig. 9.1) represents a new class of compounds capable of reducing this feedback regulatory mechanism by a direct interaction with the enzyme, TK (Fischer and Baxter 1982). The interaction between TK and 5'-AT is critically dependent on the presence of dTTP. In the absence of dTTP, 5'-AT competitively inhibits enzyme activity (Cheng and Prusoff 1974), whereas in the presence of dTTP, 5'-AT antagonizes the dTTP-induced inhibition of TK (Fischer and Baxter 1982) (Fig. 9.2). 5'-AT is an interesting drug for exploitation of potential clinical radiosensitization and chemosensitization with IdUrd since it is not a substrate of the mammalian TK (Chen et al. 1980) and is very nontoxic in small animals (Pavan-Langstom et al. 1987). Additionally, 5'-AT has been shown to enhance the uptake of IdUrd in a human bladder carcinoma cell line (647V) but not in normal human urothelial cells propagated in vitro (Fischer et al. 1986a), suggesting a potential for differential sensitization in humans (Fischer et al. 1986b). Recent published data suggest that this differential response of the 647V tumor cells compared with normal urothelial cells of IdUrd incorporation by cotreatment with 5'-AT results from differences in regulation of TK activity which may be pH dependent (Vazquez-Padua et al. 1989). No studies on

Timothy J. Kinsella, MD, Professor and Chairman, Department of Human Oncology, University of Wisconsin School of Medicine, Clinical Cancer Center, K4/312–600 Highland Avenue, Madison, WI 53792, USA

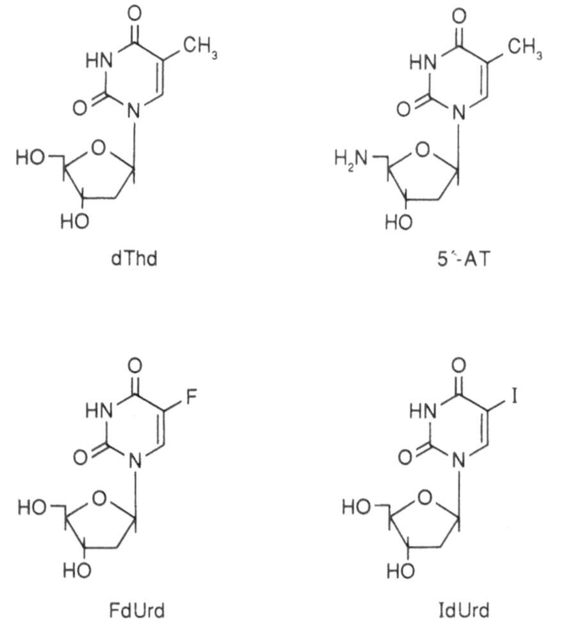

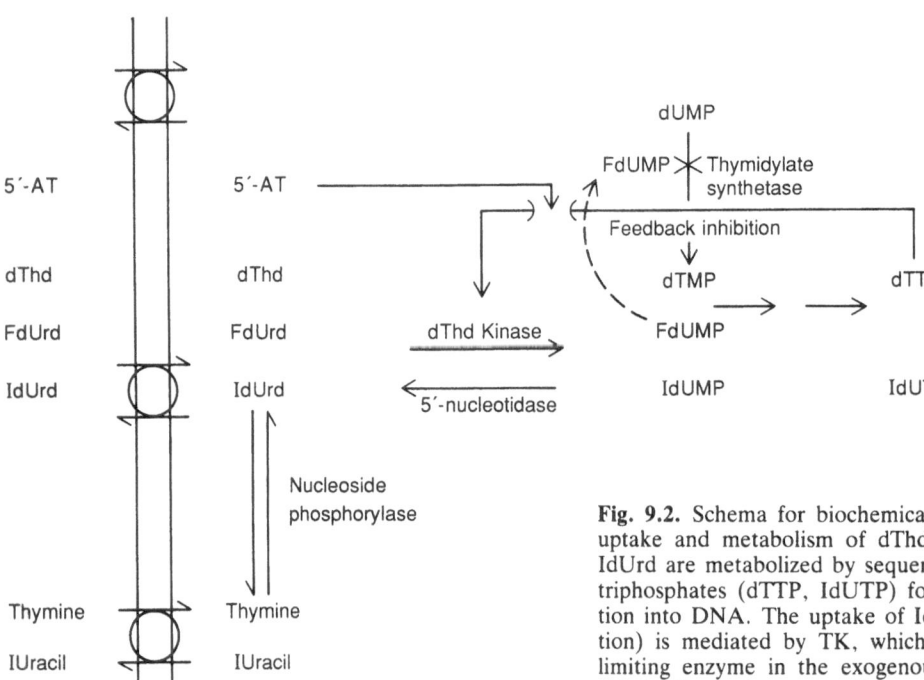

Fig. 9.1. Structure of dThd and related analogs relevant to this project. The various analogs differ only in one substitution from dThd. FdUrd and IdUrd have a halogen substitution for the methyl group at position 5, while 5'-AT has an amino group instead of the hydroxyl at the 5 position

in vitro or in vivo chemosensitization or radiosensitization with 5'-AT have been reported in the literature to date.

The de novo pathway of dThd synthesis is also illustrated, in part, in Fig. 9.2. Since IdUrd competes directly with dThd for DNA incorporation, modulation of the de novo pathway (i.e., decreased dThd synthesis) may also be important for increasing IdUrd incorporation and sensitization. The key enzyme in the de novo pathway is TS. There are several drugs, including FdUrd, 5-fluorouracil (FUra), methotrexate (MTX) and leucovorin, that inhibit TS either directly (FdUrd, FUra) or indirectly (MTX and leucovorin via dihydrofolate reductase) (O'DWYER et al. 1987). Both FdUrd and FUra inhibit TS following metabolism to fluorodeoxyuridine monophosphate (FdUMP) (SPEARS et al. 1982). FdUrd is also a substrate of TK (Fig. 9.2). Interestingly, the pattern of uptake of FdUrd differs from that of other nucleosides (dThd, IdUrd) because its active metabolite (FdUMP) inhibits TS, resulting in the depletion of dTTP pools. This depletion of dTTP by FdUrd is an attractive characteristic to study in

Fig. 9.2. Schema for biochemical pathways affecting the uptake and metabolism of dThd and IdUrd. dThd and IdUrd are metabolized by sequential phosphorylations to triphosphates (dTTP, IdUTP) for subsequent incorporation into DNA. The uptake of IdUrd (i.e., phosphorylation) is mediated by TK, which is the initial and rate-limiting enzyme in the exogenous (salvage) pathway of dThd. The endogenous (de novo) pathway of dThd is mediated by TS

vitro/in vivo mechanisms of potentiation of IdUrd sensitization for two reasons: first, it can be used to evaluate the importance of regulation TK by dTTP in the action of 5'-AT; and second, pretreatment of cells with FdUrd can deplete dTTP pools to allow preferential conversion of IdUrd to IdUMP when IdUrd treatment follows FdUrd. Obviously, the timing of treatment with FdUrd and IdUrd will need careful study in vitro and in vivo. A recent clinical study of concomitant continuous infusions of FdUrd and IdUrd suggests that one can enhance IdUrd incorporation into tumor cell DNA (colorectal liver metastases) by up to twofold compared with normal human liver using FdUrd (SPETH et al. 1988a, 1989; CHANG et al. 1989).

Several recent in vitro investigations by the author and others have focused on mechanisms of IdUrd radiosensitization with potential clinical application. Incubation of exponentially growing V79 cells with IdUrd at $10^{-7}-10^{-5}$ M (clinically relevant plasma steady state range) for two population doublings showed a progressive increase in the % thymidine replacement and in radiosensitization (MITCHELL et al. 1984). The extent of radiosensitization ($\approx 2 \times$ over control cells) appeared directly correlated with an increase in single strand (SSBs) and double strand breaks (DSBs) using filter elution techniques. No differences in the kinetics of SSB and DSB repair (MITCHELL et al. 1984) were found during 3 h of postirradiation repair. Interestingly, a higher than predicted ratio of SSBs to DSBs (BRADLEY and KOHN 1979) was found, suggesting that some excess SSBs produced in IdUrd-substituted DNA were DSBs. The increased production of DSBs in IdUrd-treated cells immediately following x-irradiation and the persistence of more DSBs after 3 h of repair compared with irradiated controls are consistent with the hypothesis that cellular lethality is directly related to unrepaired DSB. One possible mechanism for the increased DSB is the attack of a complementary DNA strand by radical intermediates (possibly uracilyl radicals) (WARD 1975; ZIMBRICK et al. 1969) produced in the IdUrd-containing strand by reaction of a radiation-induced hydrated electron with IdUrd.

PHILLIPS et al. (1989) have used the same in vitro cell system (exponentially growing V79 cells with a population doubling time of 7–8 h) to correlate exposure time, drug concentration, and cellular incorporation of IdUrd with radiation response. At concentrations of $\geq 1 \mu M$, the sensitizer enhancement ratio (SER) peaked after 48–72 h of exposure, but it required 72–96 h at lower concentrations ($0.1-1.0 \mu M$). An important, but not surprising, finding by this same group was that there can be considerable variation in the concentration and exposure time ($C \times T$) for maximum radiosensitization between different cell lines. Using a human lung adenocarcinoma line (A549), they found the highest SER with a 10-μM exposure for only one cell cycle time. This finding underscores the need to investigate carefully how IdUrd is metabolized compared with dThd in different human tumor and normal cell lines. Such studies may have clear clinical implications, as recently reported (SPETH et al. 1988a, b, 1989).

Another potential limitation to the clinical application of IdUrd as a radiosensitizer (and possibly as a chemosensitizer) is whether any sensitization can result of IdUrd is incorporated into only one DNA strand. No previous in vitro study had compared x-radiosensitization with unifilar versus bifilar DNA substitution in the clinically relevant range ($1-10 \mu M$). In a recent study presented by the author at the 1988 AACR meeting, significant radiosensitization was found using exponentially growing V79 cells following 10 μM IdUrd for one (8% thymidine replacement) and two (16% thymidine replacement) population doublings. By differential labelingg of IdUrd in DNA strands, an enhancement in x-ray induced SSBs occurred in unsubstituted DNA in the strand base pairing with the IdUrd strand and to a lesser extent in unsubstituted duplex DNA in the same cell (data summarized in Fig. 9.3). These data demonstrate that the radiolysis of IdUrd-DNA produces mobile reactive intermediates which cause intermolecular damage, i.e., DNA SSBs in unsubstituted DNA and resultant DSBs as postulated in our previous study (MITCHELL et al. 1984). These intermediates (? uracilyl radical) must be small and mobile to travel substantial distances and cause damage in adjacent unsubstituted DNA duplexes. Since IdUrd incorporation into one strand can enhance radiation damage in adjacent unsubstituted DNA strands, it has greater potential as a clinical radiosensitizer. These issues have definite clinical implications since the reported doubling times of poorly radioresponsive solid tumors such as glioblastoma multiforme are 1 or more weeks (HOSHINO et al. 1985) and unifilar substitution is a definite clinical reality.

	SSB[1]			DSB[2]	%dThd Replacement	D₀ (Gy)	ñ
	IdUrd[3]	Unsub. complement[4]	Unsub. duplex[5]				
2 cycles of IdUrd	2.1	-	-	2.0	16	1.20	4.0
1 cycle of IdUrd	2.4 (A)	1.9 (B)	-	1.5	8	1.35	5.8
1 cycle of IdUrd, 1 cycle no IdUrd			1.4 (C)				
No IdUrd			1	1.0	0	1.70	8.5

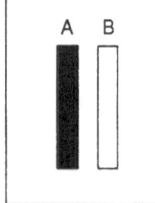

1 cycle IdUrd

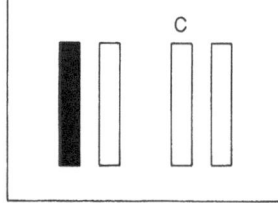

1 cycle IdUrd, 1 cycle no IdUrd

Fig. 9.3. Summary of enhancement of radiation-induced strand breaks in V79 cells substituted with IdUrd. *1*, DNA single strand breaks; *2*, DNA double strand breaks; *3*, IdUrd-labeled DNA strand; *4*, unsubstituted complementary strand DNA; *5*, unsubstituted duplex DNA. *Shaded portions* of figure indicate DNA single strands containing IdUrd

The author has conducted several pharmacological and phase I/II studies assessing IdUrd alone as a clinical radiosensitizer (KINSELLA et al. 1985, 1987, 1988; HOSHINO et al. 1985; KLECKER et al. 1985; BELANGER et al. 1986; JACKSON et al. 1987; TOCHNER et al. 1989; CHANG et al.1989). The overall results of these studies will be summarized briefly to serve as a background to support the potential clinical significance of this treatment approach. First, IdUrd, when given as a continuous intravenous infusion, shows linear pharmacokinetics over the dose range used (250–1200 mg/m²/day), with a maximum tolerated dose (MTD) of 1000 mg/m²/day × 14 days (KINSELLA et al. 1985; KLECKER et al. 1985). Steady state arterial plasma ("tumor bed") levels are 4–6 µM at the MTD (throughout the entire 14-day infusion). This is a drug concentration associated with significant radiosensitization (enhancement ratios › 1.5) both in vitro (MITCHELL et al. 1984) and in vivo in patients (using bone marrow CFU-C taken before and after the infusion) (KINSELLA et al. 1984a; MITCHELL et al. 1983). Systemic toxicity primarily to the bone marrow limited the period of continuous infusion to approximately 2 weeks, but bone marrow recovery was prompt, allowing for a second 2-week infusion in most patients.

Second, two different techniques were developed to measure incorporation of IdUrd into cellular DNA in normal (skin, peripheral granulocytes) and tumor cells (when available) in these clinical studies. In vitro staining of human tissue biopsy sections (skin, tumor) with an anti-IdUrd monoclonal antibody and immunohistochemistry demonstrated significantly greater tumor (high grade sarcoma) cell incorporation (up to 50% cells were counterstained positive) compared with normal skin (≈10% cells were positive by visual inspection) (KINSELLA et al. 1985). The second technique involves more quantitative analysis of IdUrd incorporation into DNA using high-performance liquid chromatography (HPLC) (BELANGER et al. 1987). In one study, up to 17% of thymidine bases in DNA of peripheral granulocytes (doubling time of 7–10 days) were substituted with IdUrd following a 14-day continuous infusion using 1000 mg/m²/day (BELANGER et al. 1986). More recently, in a clinical study of continuous infusions of IdUrd for patients with liver metastases, we combined these techniques for assaying IdUrd incorporation by using flow cytometry to sort monoclonal antibody positive tumor cells (employing a fluorescent conjugate) and the HPLC technique to measure thymidine substitution (SPETH et al.1988a). Using duplicate pellets of single cell suspensions off biopsies of colorectal tumor metastases and normal liver parenchyma after a 3-day intravenous infusion of IdUrd at 1000 mg/m²/day, a median of 32% of tumor cells incorporated IdUrd using flow cytometry while the thymidine substitution in tumor DNA averaged 3% by HPLC (SPETH et al. 1988a). These data suggest a potential doubling time of approximately 10 days for these tumor metastases. For comparison, normal liver parenchyma showed a 5% median incorporation by monoclonal staining with ‹ 1% thymidine substitution. Additionally, TS activity in tumors was 20-fold greater than in normal liver while TK activity was twofold greater in tumors. Thus, IdUrd in this trial exhibited selective incorporation into hepatic metastases compared with normal liver parenchyma (hepatocytes).

Finally, and most importantly, the clinical outcome in patients on these IdUrd studies suggests that clinical radiosensitization was achieved (KINSELLA et al. 1987, 1988; JACKSON et al. 1987; TOCHNER et al. 1989; CHANG et al. 1989). These studies were designed to focus on human tumors that are poorly radioresponsive (clinically "radioresistant") and are surrounded by normal tissues with low mitotic activity. Tumors selected for study included glioblastoma multiforme (labeling index of 12%–15%) (HOSHINO et al. 1985), high grade (grade 3) bone and soft tissue sarcomas (pathologically graded by extent of mitotic activity), and colorectal liver metastases (tumor doubling time of ≈10 days as above). Clinical radiosensitization was suggested by an improvement in local tumor control and survival (compared with historical controls of patients treated with radiation alone) without any associated increase in acute and late radiation effects on normal tissue (brain, bone and soft tissue, liver). However, the design of phase I/II studies does not involve a direct comparison of similar patients treated with standard therapy. Such phase III studies of IdUrd in high grade gliomas and sarcomas are being performed by the Radiation Therapy Oncology Group and the National Cancer Institute.

The basic strategy in these recent clinical studies was postulated by Dr. Henry Kaplan nearly three decades ago (SZYBALSKI 1974) and attempted to exploit differences in the proliferation rate of tumor compared with surrounding normal tissue. In the near future, it may be possible to better "select" patients for IdUrd sensitization based on high labeling indices of tumor versus normal tissue using the monoclonal antibody technique (SPETH et al. 1988a; GRATZNER 1982; MORSTYN et al. 1983, 1984; WILSON et al. 1985). It may also be possible to reduce systemic toxicity to IdUrd by inhibiting DNA synthesis in normal self-renewal tissues (such as bone marrow) using pretreatment with hydroxyurea ["reversed-role chemotherapy" as proposed by BAGSHAWE (BAGSHAWE 1986; BAGSHAWE et al. 1987)]

Exploiting biochemical differences in IdUrd metabolism in tumor versus normal tissue will be a major focus of clinical research in the next few years. The clinical potential of biochemical modulation using inhibitors of TK and TS will be studied in vitro and in vivo. Preliminary analysis of our clinical study combining infusions of both IdUrd and FdUrd (to block thymidylate synthase) in patients with colorectal liver metastases demonstrates that biochemical modulation is feasible in humans.

References

Ackland SP, Schilsky RL, Bedcett, Weichselbaum RR (1988) Synergistic cytotoxicity and DNA strand break formation by bromodeoxyuridine and bleomycin in human tumor cells. Cancer Res 48: 4244–4289

Bagshawe KD (1986) Reversed-role chemotherapy for resistant cancer. Lancet 2: 778–781

Bagshawe KD, Boden J, Boxer GM, et al. (1987) A cytotoxic DNA precursor is taken up selectively by human cancer xenografts. Br J Cancer 55: 299–30

Belanger K, Klecker RW Jr., Rowland J, Kinsella TJ, Collins JM (1986) Incorporation of iododeoxyuridine (IdUrd) into cellular DNA in patients receiving continuous intravenous infusion. Cancer Res 46: 6509–6512

Belanger K, Colline JM, Klecker RW Jr. (1987) Technique for detection of DNA nucleobases by reversed-phase high-performance liquid chromatography optimized for quantitative determination of thymidine substitution by iododeoxyuridine. J Chromatogr 47: 57–63

Bradley MO, Kohn KW (1979) x-ray induced DNA double strand break production and repair in mammalian cells as measured by neutral filter elution. Nucleic Acids Res 7: 793–804

Breitman TR (1983) The feedback inhibition of thymidine kinase. Biochem Biophys Acta 67: 153–158

Chang AE, Collins JM, Speth PA, et al. (1989) A phase I study of intra-arterial iododeoxyuridine in patients with colorectal liver metastases. J Clin Oncol 7: 662–668

Chen MS, Shiau FT, Prusoff WH (1980) 5'-Amino-5'-deoxythymidine: Synthesis, specific phosphorylation by herpes virus thymidine kinase, and stability to pH of the enzymically formed diphosphate derivative. Antimicrob Agents Chemother 18: 433–436

Cheng YC, Prusoff WH (1974) Mouse ascites sarcoma 180 deoxythymidine kinase. General properties and inhibition studies. Biochemistry 13: 1179–1185

Cohen A, Ullman B (1984) Role of intracellular dTTP levels in fluorodeoxyuridine toxicity. Biochem Pharmacol 33: 3298–3301

Djordjevic B, Szybalski W (1960) Genetics of human cell lines III. Incorporation of 5'-bromo- and 5-iododeoxyuridine into the deoxyribonucleic acid of human cells and its effect on radiation sensitivity. J Exp Med 112: 509–531

Erikson RL, Szybalski W (1963) Molecular radiobiology of human cell lines V. Comparative radiosensitizing properties of 5-halodeoxycytidines and 5-bromouracil. Cancer Res 23: 122–130

Fischer PH, Baxter D (1982) Enzyme regulatory-site directed drugs: modulation of thymidine triphosphate inhibition of thymidine kinase by 5'-amino-5'-deoxythymidine. Mol Pharmacol 22: 231–234

Fischer PH, Vazquez-Padua MA, Reznikoff CA, Ratschan WJ (1986a) Preferential stimulation of iododeoxyuridine phosphorylation by 5'-aminothymidine in human bladder cancer cells in vitro. Cancer Res 46: 4522–4526

Fischer PH, Vazquez-Padua MA, Reznikoff, CA (1986b) Perturbation of thymidine kinase regulation: A novel chemotherapeutic approach. Adv Enzyme Regul 25: 21–34

Fischer PH, Fang T-T, Lin T-S, Hampton A, Bruggink J (1988) Structure activity analysis of antagonism of the feedback inhibition of thymidine kinase. Biochem Pharmacol 37: 1293–1298

Goz B (1978) The effects of incorporation of 5-halogenated deoxyuridines into the DNA of eukaryotic cells. Pharmacol Rev 29: 249–272

Gratzner HG (1982) Monoclonal antibody to 5-bromo and 5-iododeoxyuridine; a new reagent for detection of DNA replication. Science 218: 474–475

Hoshino T, Nagashima T, Murovic J, Levin EM, Levin VA, Rupp SM (1985) Cell kinetic studies of in situ human brain tumours with bromodeoxyuridine. Cytometry 6: 627–632

Jackson D, Kinsella TJ, Rowland J, et al (1987) Halogenated pyrimidines as radiosensitizers in the treatment of glioblastoma multiforme. Am J Clin Oncol 10: 437–443

Kaplan HS, Tomlin PA (1960) Enhancement of x-ray sensitivity of E. coli by 5-bromouracil. Radiat Res 12: 447–448

Kinsella TJ, Glatstein E (1987) Clinical experience with intravenous radiosensitizers in unresectable sarcomas. Cancer 59: 908–915

Kinsella TJ, Mitchell JB, Russo A, Morstyn G, Glatstein E (1984a) The use of halogenated thymidine analogs as clinical radiosensitizers: rationale, current status, and future prospects: nonhypoxic cell sensitizers. Int J Radiat Oncol Biol Phys 10: 1399–1406

Kinsella TJ, Mitchell JB, Russo A, et al. (1984b) Continuous intravenous infusion of bromodeoxyuridine (BUdR) as a clinical radiosensitizer. J Clin Oncol 2: 1144–1150

Kinsella TJ, Russo A Mitchell JB, Collins JM, Rowland J, Wright D, Glatstein E (1985) Phase I study of intravenous iododeoxyuridine as a clinical radiosensitizer. Int J Radiat Oncol Biol Phys 11: 1941–1946

Kinsella TJ, Collins JM, Rowland J, et al. (1988) Pharmacology and Phase I/II study of continuous intravenous infusions of iododeoxyuridine (IdUrd) and hyperfractionated radiotherapy in patients with glioblastoma multiforme. J Clin Oncol 6: 871–879

Kinsella TJ, Dobson PP, Mitchell JB, Fornace AJ Jr (1987) Enhancement of x-ray induced DNA damage by pretreatment with halogenated pyrimidine analogs. Int J Radiat Oncol Biol Phys 13: 733–739

Klecker RW Jr, Jenkins JF, Kinsella TJ, Fine RL, Strong JM, Collins JM (1985) Clinical pharmacology of 5-iodo-2'-deoxyuridine and 5-iodouracil, and endogenous pyrimidine modulation. Clin Pharmacol Therapeutics 38: 45–51

Mitchell JB, Kinsella TJ, Russo A, et al. (1983) Radiosensitization of hematopoietic precursor cells (CFU-C) in glioblastoma patients receiving intermittent intravenous infusions of bromodeoxyuridine (BUdR). Int J Radiat Oncol Biol Phys 9: 457–463

Mitchell JB, Morstyn G, Russo A, Kinsella TJ, Fornace AJ Jr, McPherson S, Glatstein E (1984) Differing sensitivity to fluorescent light in Chinese hamster cells containing equally incorporated quantities of BUdR versus IUdR. Int J Radiat Oncol Biol Phys 10: 1447–1452

Morstyn G, Hsu SM, Kinsella TJ, Gratzner H, Russo A, Mitchell JB (1983) Bromodeoxyuridine in tumors and chromosomes detected with a monoclonal antibody. J Clin Invest 72: 1844–1850

Morstyn G, Kinsella TJ, Hsu S-M, Russo A, Gratzner H, Mitchell JB (1984) Identification of bromodeoxyuridine

in malignant and normal cells following therapy: relationship to complications. Int J Radiat Oncol Biol Phys 10: 1441–1445

O'Dwyer PJ, King SA, Hoth DF, Leyland-Jones B (1987) Role of thymidine in biochemical modulation: a review. Cancer Res 47: 3911–3919

Pavan-Langstom D, Park NH, Lass J et al. (1987) 5'-Amino-5'-deoxythymidine: Topical therapeutic efficacy in ocular herpes and systemic teratogenic and toxicity studies (41386). Proc Soc Exp Biol Med 170: 1–7

Phillips TL, Bodell WJ, Uhl V, Ross GY, Rasmussen J, Mitchell JB (1989) Correlation of exposure time, concentration and incorporation of IdUrd in V79 cells with radiation response. Int J Radiat Oncol Biol Phys 16: 1251–1255

Russo A, DeGraff W, Kinsella TJ, Gamson J, Glatstein E, Mitchell JB (1986) Potentiation of chemotherapy cytotoxicity following iododeoxyuridine incorporation of Chinese hamster cells. Int J Radiat Oncol Biol Phys 12: 1371–1374

Sirotnak FM, Barrueco JR (1987) Membrane transport and the antineoplastic action of nucleoside analogues. Cancer Metastasis Rev 6: 459–480

Spears CP, Shahinian AH, Moran RG, Heidelberger C, Corbett TH (1982) In vivo kinetics of thymidylate synthetase inhibition in 5-fluorouracil-sensitive and -resistant murine colon adenocarcinomas. Cancer Res 42: 450–456

Speth PA, Kinsella TJ, Chang AE, Klecker RW, Belanger K, Collins JM (1988a) Selective incorporation of iododeoxyuridine into DNA of hepatic metastases versus normal human liver. Clin Pharm Therapeutics 44: 369–375

Speth PA, Kinsella TJ, Belanger K, Klecker RW, Smith R, Rowland JB, Collins JM (1988b) Fluorodeoxyuridine modulation of the incorporation of iododeoxyuridine into DNA of granulocytes: a phase I and clinical pharmacological study. Cancer Res 48: 2933–2937

Speth PA, Kinsella TJ, Chang AE, et al. (1989) Iododeoxyuridine (IdUrd) incorporation into DNA of human hematopoietic cells, normal liver and hepatic metastases in man as a radiosensitizer and as a marker for cell kinetic studies. Int J Radiat Oncol Biol Phys 16: 1247–1250

Szybalski W (1974) x-ray sensitization by halopyrimidines. Cancer Chemother Rep 58: 539–557

Tochner Z, Kinsella TJ, Rowland J, Glatstein E (1989) Treatment of unresectable sarcomas of adults with hyperfractionated irradiation and iododeoxyuridine. Br J Radiol 19: 107–111

Vazquez-Padua MA, Fischer PH, Christian BJ, Reznikoff CA (1989) Basis for the differential modulation of IdUrd uptake by 5'-AdThd among various cell types. Cancer Res 49: 2415–2421

Ward JF (1975) Molecular mechanisms of radiation-induced damage to nuleic acid. Adv Radiat Biol 5: 181–239

Wilson GD, McNally NJ, Dunphy E, Kiarcher H, Pfragner R (1985) The labelling index of human and mouse tumours assessed by bromodeoxyuridine staining in vitro and in vivo and flow cytometry. Cytometry 6: 641–647

Zimbrick JD, Ward JF, Myers LS Jr (1969) Studies on the chemical basis of cellular radiosensitization by 5-bromouracil substitution in DNA. II. Pulse and steady-state radiolysis of bromouracil-substituted and unsubstituted DNA. Int J Radiat Biol 16: 525–534

10 Perfluorocarbon Emulsion and Oxygen with Concomitant Radiation Therapy in Primary High Grade Brain Tumors

Richard G. Evans, Bruce F. Kimler, Robert A. Morantz, Tribhawan S. Vats, Vici Liston, and Norma L. Lowe

CONTENTS

10.1 Introduction

High grade gliomas represent 40%–50% of primary intracranial tumors, and the prognosis for these patients remains poor, with a median survival time of <1 year (Karlsson and Brady 1987). The Brain Tumor Study Group's clinical trial, BTSG 69–01, was the first randomized trial to show that postoperative radiation therapy significantly increased median survival time in patients with high grade gliomas when compared with neurosurgical treatment alone (Walker et al. 1978). Although the quality of life in these patients treated with high dose radiation therapy is accept-

Richard G. Evans, PhD, MD, Professor and Chairman, Department of Radiation Oncology, University of Kansas Medical Center, 39th and Rainbow Blvd., Kansas City, KS 66103, USA

Bruce F. Kimler, PhD, Professor and Director, Radiation Biology Laboratory, Department of Radiation Oncology, University of Kansas Medical Center, Kansas City, KS 66103, USA

Robert A. Morantz, MD, Brain Tumor Institute, 2316 E. Meyer Boulevard, Kansas City, MO 64132, USA

Tribhawan S. Vats, MD, Professor and Chief, Section of Pediatric Oncology, Department of Pediatrics, University of Kansas Medical Center, Kansas City, KS 66103, USA

Vici Liston, RN, Department of Radiation Oncology, University of Kansas Medical Center, Kansas City, KS 66103, USA

Norma L. Lowe, PhD, Alpha Therapeutics Corporation, 5555 Valley Boulevard, Los Angeles, CA 90032, USA

able, the vast majority of patients succumb to their tumors within 1 year from the termination of treatment. Since the observation over 30 years ago that poorly oxygenated cells are approximately two to three times more resistant to radiation, many attempts have been made to overcome this relative radioresistance of the radiobiologically hypoxic cells thought to exist in many human tumors. A recent study examining the patterns of failure following radiation treatment for high grade brain tumors revealed that 78% of unifocal tumors recurred within 2 cm of the enhancing edge of the tumor, as demonstrated by the CT scan (Wallner et al. 1989). This study highlights the failure of high doses of radiation to sterilize pockets of presumably radiobiologically hypoxic cells. It has been hypothesized that either the tumor has outgrown its blood supply or the external pressure of the tumor has caused capillaries to become collapsed. The failure, therefore, of radiotherapy in the treatment of high grade gliomas has been attributed, at least in part, to the presence of radiobiologically hypoxic areas (Nelson et al. 1986). The first evidence that human brain tumors contained regions of hypoxia was provided by direct electrode measurements in 16 patients with malignant glioma (Kayama 1988). A whole host of approaches have been attempted to overcome this relative hypoxia, including the use of hyperbaric oxygen breathing, hypoxic cell radiosensitizers such as misonidazole, and high linear energy transfer radiation such as neutrons with their minimal dependence on the oxygen effect, but all of these approaches have proved futile due to, respectively, further restriction of the capillaries, toxicity of the drug, or unacceptable damage to the normal brain tissues.

Fluosol-DA 20% (Fluosol) is a perfluorocarbon (PFC) emulsion manufactured by the Green Cross Corporation (Osaka, Japan), currently under investigation by Alpha Therapeutic Corporation (Los Angeles, CA). Fluosol is a PFC oxygen transport emulsion consisting of perfluorodecalin and perfluorotri-*n*-propylamine in a 7:3 ratio. The average particle size of Fluosol is 0.175 μm. The PFC emulsion particles absorb, transport, and release oxygen and carbon dioxide in relation to each gas's partial pressure in the surrounding region. Oxygen and carbon dioxide are directly soluble in Fluosol with rapid uptake and release. Studies in various animals showed the half-life of a single intravenous injection of Fluosol to be in the range of 13–29 h but it may be as low as 8 h in humans. The PFC in Fluosol is essentially all expired from the body as a gas, with small amounts excreted in bile and in feces. However, >98% of the dose of Fluosol is excreted via the lungs as unmetabolized PFC. PFC emulsions, in view of their small particle size and ability to carry large amounts of oxygen in a high PO_2 environment and rapidly release this oxygen when the environmental PO_2 is low, have been explored in numerous animal tumors (TEICHER and ROSE 1984; SONG et al. 1985). Fluosol has been extensively tested in normal human volunteers and investigated in clinical trials with anemic patients and patients who refused blood transfusions on religious grounds. The first study carried out in patients with cancer was most encouraging and showed few acute and late side-effects when Fluosol was used with oxygen as an adjuvant to radiation in the treatment of advanced squamous cell tumors of the head and neck (LUSTIG et al. 1989).

A phase I/II study of Fluosol was initiated in March 1987 in patients with primary high grade brain tumors. The main objective of the study was to evaluate the safety and efficacy of Fluosol with short-term high inspired oxygen tension as an adjuvant to radiation therapy. Fluosol is not a cytotoxic agent but is hypothesized to act in an adjunctive manner by preferentially sensitizing hypoxic cells to radiation with no effect on well-oxygenated normal tissues. We report here the first 18 patients treated on this Fluosol dose-escalating study, who now have a median follow-up time from the date of surgery of 56 weeks.

10.2 Methods and Materials

The study design was a nonrandomized, Fluosol dose-ranging (cumulative) study. Radiation was delivered to the whole brain at 1.8 Gy/daily treatment for 5 weeks to a total dose of 45 Gy. The radiation portals were then reduced in size to encompass the known volume of tumor, as determined by the presurgical contrast-enhancing ring on computed tomography, plus a 3-cm margin. An additional ten treatments of 2 Gy each were given to the smaller volume to bring the total tumor dose to 65 Gy in 7 weeks. To date, 18 patients have been entered onto the study. The first four patients received 8 ml/kg Fluosol on the Monday of weeks 1, 2, 3, 6, and 7 of radiation treatment; three patients received the same concentration of Fluosol at the beginning of weeks 1, 2, 3, 5, 6, and 7; and the last 11 patients received Fluosol prior to each of the 7 weeks of treatment. Immediately following Fluosol administration on a Monday, patients breathed 100% oxygen through a non-rebreathing mask for at least 45 min prior to and throughout their radiation treatment. On each subsequent day of the week on which they received Fluosol, the patients breathed 100% oxygen for at least 45 min prior to and during radiation treatment. The patients underwent a detailed neurological examination and Karnofsky evaluation weekly during treatment and subsequent follow-up times at 1 and 3 months and at 3-month intervals thereafter. At each follow-up interval, a CT scan with and one without contrast were obtained, together with a full neurological examination and Karnofsky assessment. An MRI was obtained prior to treatment and at 6 months following completion of radiation therapy. Tumor status was recorded as either stable disease or progressive disease. Hematological and blood chemistry analyses were also performed prior to Fluosol treatment, each Friday during treatment, and at the 2-week, 3-month, and 6-month follow-up visits.

The median age of the patients was 45 years (16–72); 13 patients were male; 15 carried the diagnosis of glioblastoma multiforme (three had anaplastic astrocytoma). Seven patients had gross total removal of tumor, seven partial resection, and four biopsy only. The initial Karnofsky performance status was 80 in six patients, 90 in seven patients, and 100 in five patients. The median follow-up time from the date of surgery was 56 weeks (39–100 weeks).

10.3 Results

Two-thirds of the patients had an initial allergic reaction to the Fluosol, consisting of back pain, shortness of breath, and flushing, but all responded to 50–100 mg Benadryl, which they received at all subsequent infusions. During radiation therapy, all patients developed scalp erythema and complete alopecia by the end of 3 weeks, but with the application of Alphaderm (started at the end of the 3rd week) no patient required a treatment rest. The serum levels of SGOT, SGPT, and alkaline phosphatase were examined throughout the Fluosol treatment and, by week 5, half of the patients had increased values of all three enzymes in the range of 20%–50%. These increases persisted through the end of treatment, but most values returned to essentially normal by 1 month following completion of radiation therapy. An MRI obtained on all patients at 6 months following completion of all treatment failed to show any paraventricular changes or leukoencephalopathy, and in only one patient was white matter edema appreciated. The scalp erythema that was most marked at the end of therapy resolved in all patients by the 1-month follow-up visit. Although all patients were noted to have complete alopecia at the end of their course of treatment, hair growth had returned in the whole brain field by 6 months in the majority of patients, although patches of alopecia persisted in several patients within the high dose boost field.

At the time of this report (March 1989), ten patients are alive with stable disease, as judged by CT or MRI and physical examination. Seven patients survived >1 year from diagnosis; two of them subsequently died, at 86 and 88 weeks. We have been impressed by the quality of life following the treatment of these patients with Fluosol and oxygen with concomitant radiation therapy and have detected no long-term side-effects in the seven patients who survived >1 year from diagnosis. Although the number of patients is too small to carry out a statistical analysis, it appears that the patients surviving tend to be those who are 45 years of age and younger, having an initial Karnofsky score of 90 or 100. Interestingly, all three patients with grade III tumors have succumbed to their disease, at 46, 49, and 88 weeks. The median survival in the group of 18 patients has not been reached but will be in excess of 46 weeks.

10.4 Discussion

We feel we have accomplished the main objective of this study, which was to evaluate the safety of Fluosol with short-term high inspired oxygen tension as an adjuvant to radiation therapy in the treatment of high grade tumors of the brain. Fluosol given once a week to a total dose of 56 ml/kg over 7 weeks in conjunction with "standard" radiation therapy has been well tolerated, with only minimal acute side-effects. The initial allergic reaction to Fluosol noted in two-thirds of the patients, consisting of shortness of breath, flushing, and back pain, was easily managed with 50–100 mg Benadryl, which they received at all subsequent infusions, and did not cause any patients to be removed from the study. The transient elevations of serum levels of SGOT, SGPT, and alkaline phosphatase demonstrated by week 5 in half of the patients were marked only in those with heavy alcohol abuse prior to initiation of treatment and, even in this small group, values had returned essentially to normal by 1 month following completion of radiation therapy. No significant increases in creatinine were noted, and no significant hematological toxicity was seen in any patients.

Having seen no significant acute or long-term toxicity from a total dose of 56 ml/kg given in seven equal fractions over 7 weeks, we have escalated the total dose of Fluosol to 70 ml/kg in the second phase of the study, through a twice-weekly regimen in weeks 2 and 7. Early results presented here are encouraging, with an apparent plateau appearing at approximately 50 weeks, and appear to be marginally superior to the results in a historical group of patients treated at the same institution with equivalent doses and fields of radiation (Miller et al. 1990). Whether this combination of Fluosol and oxygen with concomitant radiation will eventually prove superior to conventional radiation therapy remains to be seen.

References

Karlsson UL, Brady LW (1987) Primary intracranial neoplasms. In: Perez CA, Brady LW (eds) Principles and practice of radiation oncology. JB Lippincott, Philadelphia, pp 408–436

Kayama T (1988) A study of intratumoral oxygen pressure in brain tumors. In: Suzuki J (ed) Treatment of glioma. Springer, Tokyo Berlin Heidelberg New York, pp 125–133

Lustig R, McIntosh-Lowe N, Rose C, Haas J, Krasnow S, Spaulding M, Prosnitz L (1989) Phase I/II study of Fluosol®-DA and 100% oxygen as an adjuvant to radiation in the treatment of advanced squamous cell tumors of the head and neck. Int J Radiat Oncol Biol Phys 16: 1587–1593

Miller PJ, Hassanein RS, Giri PGS, Kimler BF, O'Boynick PL, Evans RG (1990) Univariate and multivariate analysis of the response of highgrade gliomas to radiation therapy. Int J Radiat Oncol Biol Phys 19: 275–280

Nelson DF, Urtasun RC, Saunders WM, Gutin PH, Sheline GE (1986) Recent and current investigations of radiation therapy of malignant gliomas. Semin Oncol 13: 46–55

Salazar O, Rubin P, McDonald J, Feldstein M (1976) Patterns of failure in intracranial astrocytomas after irradiation: analysis of dose and field factors. Radiology 126: 279–292

Song CW, Zhang WL, Pence DM, Lee I, Levitt SH (1985) Increased radiosensitivity of tumors by perfluorochemicals and carbogen. Int J Radiat Oncol Biol Phys 11: 1833–1836

Teicher BA, Rose CM (1984) Oxygen-carrying perfluorochemical emulsion as an adjuvant to radiation therapy in mice. Cancer Res 44: 4285–4288

Walker MD, Alexander E, Hunt WE, MacCarty CS, Mahaley MS, Mealey J, Norrell HA, Owens G, Ransohoff J, Wilson CB, Gehan EA, Strike TA (1978) Evaluation on BCNU and/or radiotherapy in the treatment of anaplastic gliomas. A cooperative clinical trial. J Neurosurg 49: 333–343

Wallner KE, Galicich JH, Krol G, Arbit E, Malkin MG (1989) Patterns of failure following treatment for glioblastoma multiforme and anaplastic astrocytoma. Int J Radiat Oncol Biol Phys 16: 1405–1409

11 Chemo- and Radioprotection: Clinical Trials Combining WR-2721 with Cisplatin and Cyclophosphamide

Donna Glover[1], Clare Weiler, and Stephen Grabelsky

CONTENTS

11.1 Introduction

WR-2721 [S-2-(3-aminopropylamino) ethylphosphorothioic acid] was one of the most effective and least toxic of over a thousand sulfhydryl radioprotectors tested. Yuhas and Storer first reported that WR-2721 could increase the radiation resistance of murine skin and bone marrow by factors of 2.5 and 2.7, respectively, without increasing the radiation resistance of the animals' solid mammary tumors. (Yuhas 1980a) Preclinical data on WR-2721 have been expanded to include five additional species, 11 additional normal tissues, and 16 additional transplanted or spontaneous tumors. Differential protection in favor of normal tissues has resulted in little or no protection in the majority of experimental tumors. The basic proposal that WR-2721 can improve the effectiveness of solid tumor radiotherapy remains intact, except that it does not protect the central nervous system (Coleman et al. 1989; Yuhas 1980a).

In the animal model, WR-2721 selectively protects normal tissues against the cytotoxicites of cisplatin, cyclophosphamide, nitrogen mustard, and L-phenylalanine mustard. Renal tolerance to cisplatin is improved by factors of 1.3–1.7 (Chabner 1989). Bone marrow tolerance to cyclophosphamide and nitrogen mustard is improved by factors of 1.5–2 and 2–4, respectively (Coleman et al. 1989; Yuhas 1980a; Wasserman et al. 1981). Thus, combining WR-2721 with alkylating agents at higher doses leads to greater fractional tumor cell kill with the advantage of decreased toxicity.

11.2 General Mechanisms of Action and Cellular Pharmacology of WR-2721

The mechanisms by which WR-2721 protects against radiation and alkylating agent toxicity are not clear. Two frequently proposed hypotheses are (a) scavenging of free radicals and (b) competition with oxygen by hydrogen donation to the free radicals. The cytotoxicity of cisplatin complexes can be reduced by thiol compounds, which inactivate the platinum binding site. Thiols may react with either the chloride or aquo platinum species to prevent DNA cross-linking (Chabner 1989).

Sulfhydryl radioprotectors can inhibit indirect damage from radiation, repair direct and indirect radiation effects, and enhance recovery. At the molecular level, these compounds may scavenge free radicals, donate hydrogen ions, bind to critical biological targets, and form mixed disulfides. At the biochemical level, they may protect by producing hypoxia, by releasing nonprotein sulfhydryls, or by producing biochemical shock or hypothermia (Giambbarresi and Jacobs 1987).

The phosphate group which covers the sulfhydryl portion of WR-2721 reduces its toxicity and facilitates differential absorption in normal tissues. The dephosphorylated metabolite, WR-1065, is

---

[1] Dr. Glover is a recipient of an American Cancer Society Faculty Research Award

Donna Glover, MD, Chief of Hematology and Oncology, Clare Weiler, RN, Stephen Grabelsky, Section of Hematology/Oncology, Presbyterian Medical Center, 39th and Market Streets, Philadelphia, PA 19104, USA

thought to be the active protective agent. Intact WR-2721 is unable to protect various cultured cell lines, whereas WR-1065 protects cultured cells (COLEMAN et al. 1989).

Alkaline phosphatase is the primary enzyme responsible for the distribution and metabolism of WR-2721. This plasma membrane enzyme is the catalyst responsible for hydrolysis of WR-2721 to WR-1065 and subsequent uptake of WR-1065 by cells in vivo. High concentrations of alkaline phosphatase are found in the plasma membrane of endothelial cells in small blood vessels and the brush border of the kidney proximal tubules (COLEMAN et al. 1989). Modulation of alkaline phosphatase activity may potentiate normal tissue protection. Shortly after WR-2721 is administered, the highly reactive free sulfhydryl compound, WR-1065, appears as the major non-protein-bound metabolite. WR-1065 is probably rapidly converted into other metabolites, including cysteamine, sulfinite and sulfonate oxidation products, mixed disulfides with low molecular weight substances (such as cysteine and glutathione), and proteins containing reactive sulfhydryl groups (SHAW et al., in press).

In the animal model, intraperitoneal WR-2721 provides significant radioprotection to most normal tissues, except for the brain and spinal cord (COLEMAN et al. 1989; WASSERMAN et al. 1981). Normal tissues are protected against radiation toxicity to a varying degree. The radiation dose modification factors range from 1.2 for lung to 2.7 for bone marrow. The difference in normal tissue protection may be due to differences in (a) the quantity and distribution of WR-1065, (b) tissue oxygenation, or (c) the tissue distribution and catalytic activity of alkaline phosphatase (COLEMAN et al. 1989; SHAW et al., in press).

WR-2721's differential protection in normal versus malignant cells may be related to several factors. WR-2721 is actively transported into normal tissues by facilitated diffusion, while solid tumors absorb the drug slowly by passive diffusion (YUHAS 1980b). Selective protection may also be due to (a) reduced drug absorption in the tumor due to deficient vasculature, (b) decreased protection of hypoxic tumor cells, and (c) the tumor's less efficient metabolic function. Drug hydrophilicity is a major factor underlying WR-2721's ability to be selectively absorbed into normal tissues. Less hydrophilic sulfhydryl compounds (e.g., cysteine and dephosphorylated disulfide and thiol derivatives of WR-2721) more readily crossed tumor cell membranes (YUHAS 1980b).

11.3 Clinical Trials of WR-2721

Based on preclinical studies, phase I-II studies of WR-2721 were conducted. Separate phase I studies were performed in which over 250 patients with advanced malignancies received WR-2721 prior to cyclophosphamide, nitrogen mustard, cisplatin, or radiotherapy.

11.3.1 WR-2721 and Cisplatin

The preliminary data from the phase I trials of WR-2721 and cisplatin with mannitol diuresis suggest that WR-2721 may provide some protection against cisplatin's nephrotoxicity, neurotoxicity, and ototoxicity. When AL-SARRAF (cited by COLEMAN et al. 1989) used hydration and mannitol diuresis with cisplatin $100 \, mg/m^2$, 32% of their 34 patients experienced renal dysfunction, and one patient died with renal failure. The clinical trial of WR-2721 and cisplatin with mannitol diuresis was initiated to determine whether cisplatin doses above $100 \, mg/m^2$ could be safely administered. In this trial, patients received WR-2721 $740 \, mg/m^2$ over 15 min. Cisplatin was given over 30 min, beginning 15 min after the WR-2721 infusion was complete. All patients had hematological profiles, electrolytes, and renal function studies twice a week. Audiograms, detailed neurological examinations, and creatinine clearances were measured prior to each course of therapy. Patients were retreated every 3–4 weeks (COLEMAN et al. 1989).

Transient nephrotoxicity was observed in 11% of courses. In all cases, the patients' renal function returned to normal values. The incidence of transient nephrotoxicity with WR-2721 and cisplatin doses of $120 \, mg/m^2$, $135 \, mg/m^2$, and $150 \, mg/m^2$ were 7%, 11%, and 29%, respectively.

Hematological toxicity was mild and infrequent. Granulocyte counts less than $1000/mm^3$ and white blood cell nadirs less than $2000/mm^3$ were seen in 9% and 10% of courses, respectively. Only 6% of courses had platelet nadirs less than $50\,000/mm^3$. No patient had an infectious complication or required platelet transfusions (COLEMAN et al. 1989).

Grade 1–2 peripheral neuropathies occurred in 14% of patients after a median cumulative cisplatin dose of $825 \, mg/m^2$ (COLEMAN et al. 1989). Results from a prospective study suggest that WR-

2721 may offer some protection against cisplatin's peripheral neuropathy. All patients receiving cisplatin had detailed neurological examinations performed prior to cisplatin therapy and serially after each course. Patients who received WR-2721 pretreatment had a significantly lower incidence of peripheral nerve dysfunction compared with patients treated with cisplatin alone or in combination with other antineoplastic agents. Forty-seven percent of patients treated with Adriamycin 50 mg/m^2, cyclophosphamide 500 mg/m^2, and cisplatin 50 mg/m^2 developed neuropathy following a cumulative cisplatin dose of 358 mg/m^2. When patients received five daily doses of cisplatin 40 mg/m^2 with hypertonic saline and cyclophosphamide, 100% of patients experienced significant peripheral nerve damage after a median cumulative cisplatin dose of 327 mg/m^2. However, with WR-2721 pretreatment, only 14% of patients treated with 120–150 mg/m^2 doses of cisplatin developed mild-to-moderate neuropathies after a mean cumulative cisplatin dose of 825 mg/m^2 (COLEMAN et al. 1989).

WR-2721 does not appear to protect against the antitumor efficacy of cisplatin. In the phase I trials of WR-2721 and cisplatin with mannitol diuresis, objective, partial or complete responses were observed in 47 of 105 (45%) patients with measurable disease. Objective responses occurred in 25 of 53 (47%) patients with metastatic melanoma, 12 of 22 (55%) patients with locally recurrent or metastatic head and neck cancer, and 7 of 13 (54%) patients with metastatic breast cancer refractory to conventional therapy. Four patients with melanoma and two with head and neck cancer had complete responses (COLEMAN et al. 1989).

11.3.2 WR-2721 and Cyclophosphamide

Preliminary data from our phase I trial of WR-2721 and cyclophosphamide suggest that WR-2721 protects against cyclophosphamide-induced granulocytopenia (COLEMAN et al. 1989). Since variable drug doses and infusion rates were used in these early studies, a controlled trial using constant drug doses was initiated to establish more precisely WR-2721's level of protection. Initially, 21 patients received cyclophosphamide 1500 mg/m^2 alone and were retreated 4 weeks later after hematological recovery was complete with WR-2721 740 mg/m^2 before the same dose of cyclophosphamide. With WR-2721 pretreatment, 19 of 21 (90%) patients had improved white blood counts and granulocyte

counts. The mean granulocyte nadir increased from 541/mm^3 with cyclophosphamide to 1247/mm^3 with WR-2721 and cyclophosphamide ($p < 0.005$). Following cyclophosphamide alone, neutropenic fevers developed in three patients. No patient experienced a febrile episode following WR-2721 and the same dose of cyclophosphamide. Platelet nadirs below 100 000/mm^3 were only noted in two patients treated with cyclophosphamide alone. No patient experienced thrombocytopenia when they were retreated with the same cyclophosphamide dose with WR-2721 pretreatment. These data suggest that WR-2721 provides significant protection against cyclophosphamide-induced hematologic toxicity (GLOVER et al. 1986).

11.4 Clinical Pharmacology

Several pharmacokinetic assay systems have been developed to measure WR-2721 and its metabolites. A dual mercury gold amalgam electrochemical detection system has been developed employing high pressure liquid chromatography for the detection and measurement of WR-2721, WR-1065, and the symmetrical disulfide, WR-33278 in urine, blood, and tissues (COLEMAN et al. 1989; SHAW et al., in press).

Pharmacokinetic studies have been performed following WR-2721 given as a 150 mg/m^2 i.v. bolus to patients with advanced malignancies. Less than 10% of WR-2721 is in the plasma compartment 6 min following a bolus injection. The short distribution half-life of 0.88 min, the rapid plasma clearance of 2.17 liters/min, and the fact that the drug is rapidly cleared from the plasma compartment indicate that WR-2721 is rapidly absorbed in man. The low steady state volume of distribution (6.44 liters) indicates that the unmetabolized drug is largely confined to the extravascular space (COLEMAN et al. 1989; SHAW et al., in press). The urinary excretion values for WR-2721, WR-1065, and WR-33278 in the 1-h pharmacologic study period were 1.05%, 1.38%, and 4.1%, respectively (COLEMAN et al. 1989; SHAW et al., in press).

Pharmacokinetics of WR-2721 given at a dose of 740 mg/m^2 over 15 min were investigated in ten patients. Most of the pharmacokinetic parameters were similar to those following a bolus injection. Over 90% of WR-2721 was cleared from the plasma within 6 min following the completion of the 15-min infusion. Since a 740 mg/m^2 dose of WR-

2721 is almost five times that used in the bolus study, these data supply further evidence for the rapidity and predominance of the distribution phase for WR- 2721 (SHAW et al., in press).

11.5 Toxicity

WR-2721 is generally well tolerated with transient side-effects including nausea, vomiting, sneezing, a warm or flushed feeling, mild somnolence, hypocalcemia, and rarely, allergic reactions. The only potentially dose-limiting side-effect of WR-2721 pretreatment is hypotension. Although WR-2721 produces transient hypocalcemia due to inhibition of parathyroid hormone secretion and direct inhibition of bone resorption, only three patients experienced symptoms of hypocalcemia (COLEMAN et al. 1989).

The most serious toxicity is hypotension, defined as a decrease in systolic blood pressure of more than 20 mm Hg lasting over 5 min. Only 5% of patients required drug interruption because of a decrease in blood pressure. Hypotension occurs more often when WR-2721 is given at slower infusion rates. The incidence of hypotension appears to increase among patients with cancers of the head and neck, esophagus, or lung; prior neck irradiation; carotid artery disease; or hypercalcemia (COLEMAN et al. 1989). The single WR-2721 dose for phase II studies with chemotherapy is 910 mg/m^2 for low risk patients and 740 mg/m^2 for patients with high risk for hypotension. A daily 340 mg/m^2 WR-2721 dose given four times a week for 5 weeks prior to radiation therapy is recommended for phase II radiation studies (COLEMAN et al. 1989).

References

Chabner BA (1989) Pharmacologic principles of cancer treatment. WB Saunders, New York

Coleman CN, Glover D, Turrisi AT (1989) Radiation and chemotherapy sensitizers and protectors. In: Chabner BA (ed) Pharmacologic principles of cancer treatment. WB Saunders, New York, (in press)

Giambbarresi L, Jacobs AJ (1987) Radioprotectants: In: Conklin JJ, Walker RI (eds) Military radiology. Academic, New York, pp 265–301

Glover D, Glick J, Weiler C, Kligerman MM (1986) WR-2721 protects against the hematologic toxicity of cyclophosphamide: a controlled phase II trial. J Clin Oncol 4: 584–588

Shaw LM, Turrisi AT, Glover DJ, Bonner HJ, Glick JH, Kligerman MM (in press) Pharmacokinetics and radioprotectors. Pharmacol Ther

Yuhas JM (1980a) On the potential application of radioprotective drugs in radiotherapy. In: Sokol GH (ed) Radiation–drug interaction in cancer management. Wiley, New York, pp 113–135

Yuhas JM (1980b) Active versus passive absorption kinetics as the basis for selective protection of normal tissues by S-2-(3-aminopropylamino) ethyl phosphorothioic acid. Cancer Res 40: 1519–1524

Wasserman TH, Phillips TL, Ross G, Kane LJ (1981) Protection against cytotoxic chemotherapeutic effects on bone marrow colony forming units by the radioprotector, WR-2721. Cancer Clin Trials 4: 4–6

12 Biological Modifiers' Potential for Radioprotection

GARY B. THURMAN and ROBERT K. OLDHAM

CONTENTS

12.1 Introduction

Accidental or intentional (therapeutic) exposure of humans to large doses of ionizing radiation or chemotherapeutic drugs often causes major detrimental effects on essential bodily functions. The hematopoietic and immune systems are most susceptible to lethal radiation damage. The gastrointestinal system is also sensitive to radiation damage but the lethal dose of irradiation is usually much higher than in the case of the hematopoietic or immune system. If the dose received is not sufficient to produce irreversible lethal damage to other organs, but is sufficient to cause lethal hematopoietic and immune system damage, the exposed individual can be rescued from death by reconstitution with a bone marrow graft. However, allogeneic grafts often lead to severe graft-versus-host disease and closely matched or autologous bone marrow is often not available. Alternative methods of restoration of the hematopoietic and immune systems without using cellular grafts would be desirable. Currently, the best candidates to generate such desirable effects on bone marrow regeneration are biological response modifiers

GRAY B. THURMAN, PhD, Dept. Biochemistry, Vanderbilt University School of Medicine, Nashville, TN 37232-0146, USA

ROBERT K. OLDHAM, MD, Director, Biological Therapy Institute, Hospital Drive, Franklin, IN 37064, USA

(BRMs) such as cytokines. These factors are involved in controlling the production and activation of hematopoietic and immune cell populations. This review is intended to summarize the current knowledge regarding the abilities of these factors either to potentiate the effects of radiation damage or to help ameliorate and resolve the effects of radiation damage that would otherwise be lethal.

There are two major aspects to be considered in regard to radiation damage. Either the radiation exposure is part of a planned and well-controlled therapeutic procedure designed to treat a disease, or it is accidental as the result of an occupational hazard or a nuclear accident. Use of BRMs to ameliorate the effects of accidental exposure to radiation requires that the factors must be effective when given subsequent to the radiation exposure. Those factors which must be given prior to the irradiation will only be useful for modifying the effects of therapeutic irradiation. This obvious point must be kept in mind during the discussion of the potential use of cytokines to alter effects of ionizing irradiation.

A survey of the literature has revealed that our knowledge in this field is still in its infancy. Many questions regarding the effects of cytokines on the production of radiation or drug damage, the recovery from that damage, and the mechanisms of action of these cytokines remain to be answered. However, the recent observations and significant effects are encouraging and indicate that cytokines may play an important role in modifying damage caused by radiation or drugs, allowing more aggressive radiotherapy and chemotherapy to be considered. Radioprotective and therapeutic effects of a number of purified recombinant cytokines predict that these agents will play an important role in therapies currently being designed for future treatment.

However, concomitant utilization of cytokines and radiation therapy could have detrimental effects if the cytokines' mode of action causes the affected cells to be more radiosensitive. Several recent reports indicate that in certain diseases combined use of certain cytokines with radiotherapy is contraindicated.

12.2 Radiomodulating Effects of Cytokines

Cytokines are natural biochemical factors which are produced by cells of the reticuloendothelial system and secreted into extracellular fluids, and which serve as intercellular messengers. These factors can induce a number of biological responses in cells of a variety of types, provided these cells have appropriate cell surface receptors. The changes induced may range from simple surface changes and induction of the production and secretion of another cytokine, to the differentiation of cell types into functionally mature cells leading to extensive biological changes. The fact that cytokines can induce cellular changes would indicate that they might also induce some change

Table 12.1. Summary of the effects of cytokines on radiation sensitivity and recovery from radiation damage

	References
IL-1	
Has a major radioprotective effect both in vivo and in vitro	NETA et al. 1986a; GALLICCHIO et al. 1989
Has a major radioprotective effect both pre- and postirradiation	NETA and Oppenheim 1988
Gives dose reduction factors of 1.17–1.25	NETA 1988
May act by increasing expression of CSF receptors and stimulating CSF production	MOORE and WARREN 1987; VOGEL et al. 1987
IL-2	
No radioprotective effect in vivo or in vitro	NETA et al. 1987a; GALLICCHIO et al. 1989
IL-3	
Accelerates hematopoiesis in sublethally irradiated mice	SIEFF 1987
No radioprotective effect in vitro	GALLICCHIO et al. 1989
IL-6	
Increases radiation sensitivity when given before irradiation	NETA et al. 1988a
Synergizes with IL-1 to give a radio-protective effect when given before irradiation	NETA et al. 1988a
IFN-α	
Appears to be a radiosensitizing agent when given prior to irradiation	DRITSCHILO et al. 1982; REAL et al. 1985; MATTSON et al. 1985
May increase radiosensitivity of some types of tumor	MOSSMAN et al. 1982
IFN-β	
Sensitizes human bronchogenic carcinoma cells to radiation cytotoxicity	GOULD et al. 1984
IFN-γ	
No radioprotective effect when given prior to irradiation	NETA et al. 1986b
Substantially increases survival of irradiated mice if given after irradiation	NETA and OPPENHEIM 1988
TNF	
Has major in vivo radioprotective effect both pre- and postirradiation	NETA et al. 1988b
Gives a dose reduction factor of 1.13	NETA 1988
Requires 50-fold higher dose than IL-1 and gives lesser effect	NETA and OPPENHEIM 1988
Synergizes with IL-1 to give greater effect than either alone	NETA et al. 1988b
GM-CSF	
No effect of single dose given before or after irradiation	NETA et al. 1986b
Radioprotective when given in multiple doses after irradiation	CASTELLI et al. 1988
Synergizes with suboptimal doses of IL-1 when given prior to irradiation	NETA et al. 1988b
Other CSFs	
Little testing has been done. G-CSF appears to have effects similar to GM-CSF	NETA and OPPENHEIM 1988

in sensitivity to radiation. Multiple recent reports suggest that this is the case (Table 12.1).

12.2.1 Induction of Radiosensitization by Cytokines

REAL et al. (1985) reported two cases of severe radiation mucositis due to radiation therapy to the oral mucosa of two homosexual males with Kaposi's sarcoma and acquired immune deficiency (AIDS). These patients were undergoing treatment with human recombinant leukocyte A interferon (IFN) given systematically at a daily dose of 36 million units intramuscularly. The mucositis appeared within 5 days of the initiation of radiotherapy and at radiation doses of 9 and 10.5 Gy. Radiomucositis usually does not appear until after 14 days of treatment with an accumulative dose of 35–40 Gy (RUBIN and CASARETT 1968). The rapid appearance of mucositis at much lower radiation doses was felt to be directly related to the concomitant IFN treatment. The impaired immunity of the AIDS patients may have contributed to the increased radiation sensitivity, but other AIDS patients treated with pharyngeal irradiation, who were not being treated with IFN, did not show this degree of radiation sensitivity or the rapidity of onset evident in these cases.

MATTSON et al. (1985) reported unexpected severe radiation pneumonitis in three of five patients with small cell lung cancer treated with human leukocyte IFN-α and radiation therapy. Their results suggested that the (IFN) treatment delayed the growth of small cell lung cancer but also radiosensitized normal lung tissue, leading to excessive lung radiation damage. GOULD et al. (1984) showed that human IFN-β sensitized human A549 bronchogenic carcinoma cells to radiation damage and DRITSCHILO et al. (1982) reported that Swiss mouse 3T3 cells, exposed to murine IFN in culture, were more sensitive to radiation damage.

VALTER (1977) demonstrated similar increased sensitivity to radiation caused by incubation of murine L cells with IFN. These observations contrast with the report that mice treated with murine IFN 24 h after lethal irradiation showed a significant increase in survival time (ORTALDO and MCCOY 1980), indicating a radioprotective effect when IFN treatment is given after the radiation damage has been incurred.

12.2.2 Induction of Radioresistance by Cytokines

12.2.2.1 Interleukin-1

Substantial work has been done investigating the radioprotective effects of interleukin-1 (IL-1) since the initial report by NETA et al. (1986a) that a single treatment of mice with IL-1, 20 h prior to irradiation, produced a marked increase in survival in lethally irradiated mice. The initial results seemed to indicate that this protective effect was dependent on the IL-1 being given 20 h prior to the radiation treatment. However, subsequent work by NETA and OPPENHEIM (1988) using a single bolus injection 1–3 h after irradiation and by CASTELLI et al. (1988) using multiple injections of IL-1 beginning 2 h after irradiation indicated that IL-1 can produce a restorative effect from radiation-induced injury, even when administered after the radiation.

The ability of IL-1 to produce beneficial effects when administered after radiation exposure greatly increases the potential for clinical utilization of IL-1 and makes it a candidate for use in therapy of people exposed to substantial doses of radiation through nuclear accidents (provided that the dose was insufficient to produce lethal gastrointestinal injury).

To date, IL-1 is the most impressive cytokine in showing restorative effects following radiation injury. The currently known optimal use of IL-1 in irradiated mice gives a dose reduction factor of approximately 1.2, indicating that IL-1 loses its effectiveness when the lethal radiation dose is exceeded by 20%. This also indicates that IL-1 utilization in patients receiving whole body radiation therapy could allow the radiation therapy dosage to be increased by 20% and still allow recovery. In cancer therapy, that 20% increase could substantially augment therapeutic benefit, but only if the IL-1 treatment does not also reduce radiosensitivity of the tumor cells. The fact that IL-1 does have tumorostatic properties (NAKAMURA et al. 1986) indicates that decreased mitotic activity in tumor cells induced by IL-1 would cause them to be more radiosensitive.

Another point to consider is that IL-1 administration to mice following irradiation prevents regeneration of thymus gland cellularity (MORRISSEY et al. 1988), even though it hastens recovery of the myeloid compartment (MORRISSEY et al. 1987). This, coupled with the report that in vivo IL-1 administration is immunosuppressive and inhibits cell-mediated reactions such as contact sensitivity (ROBERTSON et al. 1987), indicates that IL-1 treatment may cause the rescued survivors of lethal irradiation to remain, at least initially, immunosuppressed. This possibility has not been reported in the literature and, to our knowledge, remains to be tested. If it exists, such IL-1-induced immunosuppression following recovery from substantial doses of irradiation might be rectified by treatment with other lymphokines and thymic hormones.

12.2.2.2 Interleukin-2

Interleukin-2 (IL-2) has consistently been unable to increase survival of lethally irradiated mice (NETA et al. 1987a). Substantial testing of IL-2 for inducing increased radiation sensitivity has not been reported. Since IL-2 is mitogenic for thymocytes, lymphokine-activated killer cells, natural killer cells, and activated T cells, it is not unreasonable to speculate that IL-2 treatment in vivo may increase radiosensitivity.

12.2.2.3 Interleukin-3

Interleukin-3 (IL-3) has been reported to have a radioprotective effect in sublethally irradiated mice by accelerating hematopoiesis (SIEFF 1987) but has no modulating effect on the radiosensitivity of murine bone marrow cells in vitro (GALLICCHIO et al. 1989).

12.2.2.4 Other Interleukins

To our knowledge, IL-6 is the only other interleukin to be reported to modify cellular sensitivity to radiation. The production of IL-6 has been found to be induced by IL-1 (BILLIAU 1987). However, NETA et al. (1988a) have shown that the radioprotective effect of IL-1 is not effected through production of IL-6. When IL-6 was given 20 h before lethal irradiation, no increase in survival was evident. If IL-6 was given 20 h prior to a sublethal dose of radiation, increased mortality was observed, indicating that IL-6 increased radiosensitivity. However, when IL-6 was given concomitantly with IL-1, 20 h before irradiation, it synergized with the radioprotective effect of the IL-1, through an unknown mechanism, and caused

survival of a larger percentage of the irradiated mice.

12.2.2.5 Colony-Stimulating Factors (CSFs)

Single doses of either GM-CSF or G-CSF do not cause a radioprotective effect when given alone (NETA et al. 1986b). This is surprising, since these factors appear to be involved in the IL-1-induced recovery from radiation-caused hematopoietic injury. Treatment of mice with IL-1 induces high titers of CSF in the circulation (VOGEL et al. 1987) and both GM-CSF and G-CSF can combine with IL-1 (given at a suboptimal level) to enhance synergistically the survival of irradiated mice (NETA et al. 1988b). Also, the observed cycling of bone marrow cells after in vivo IL-1 treatment, particularly those cells of the myeloid series (NETA et al. 1987b), suggests the involvement of CSFs in IL-1's action. This growth-stimulating effect of the CSFs would suggest they actually induce greater sensitivity to subsequent radiation.

Although a single dose of any of the CSFs may not be radioprotective, 15 daily doses of GM-CSF given beginning 2 h after lethal irradiation of C57BL/6 mice induced a 40% survival at 38 days ($P = 0.001$, CASTELLI et al. 1988). This response was higher and more statistically significant than the responses seen with three different doses of IL-1 administered on the same schedule.

12.2.2.6 Tumor Necrosis Factor

The close similarity of the biological activities of tumor necrosis factor (TNF) to those of IL-1 is also evident in its radioprotective effects (NETA et al. 1988b). However, it appears that 10-50 times more TNF is required to produce a maximal radioprotective effect. It is also evident that the response seen may be dependent on the strain of mice used. In the work just referenced, three strains of mice were used: C57BL/6, B6D2F1, and C3H/HeN. TNF gave an equivalent radioprotective effect in all three types of mice, with maximal protection ranging from 41% to 55% survival at doses from 5.0 to 7.5 μg/mouse. With C57BL/6 and B6D2F1 mice, IL-1 treatment gave more protection (70%-85% survival) at lower doses (100-150 ng/mouse range) than TNF. Results in C3H/HeN mice, however, showed that IL-1 was less protective (28% survival), even at higher doses

(300–500 ng/mouse), than it was in the other two strains. In this case, with the doses given, IL-1 would be considered inferior to TNF (which gave 50% survival at a dose of 5 µg/mouse) in the C3H/HeN strain of mice. It was not determined whether higher doses of IL-1 in C3H/HeN mice gave more radioprotection but it was shown that suboptimal doses of IL-1 and TNF synergized together to give near the maximal radioprotection effect that could be reached with optimal doses of IL-1 alone in the other mouse strains. The combination of IL-1 and TNF in C3H/HeN mice gave two to three times more protection than either cytokine alone (88% survival at 200 ng/mouse IL-1 + 7.5 µg/mouse TNF).

12.2.2.7 Interferons

Interferons (IFNs) appear to be able to cause both radiation-sensitizing and radiation-protective effects (Mossman et al. 1982). Their radiomodulatory effects seem to be dependent on the timing of their administration relative to radiation. When given prior to irradiation, the IFNs seem to be radiosensitizers (see Sect. 12.2.1). However, there is some indication that when IFN is given subsequent to the irradiation, a restorative effect is observed (Ortaldo and McCoy 1980). This especially appears to be true with IFN-γ, where 1.25 µg/mouse in C3H/HeN mice gave 75% survival (Neta and Oppenheim 1988) given an LD95/30 dose of radiation. This contrasts with their previous report (Neta et al. 1986b) in which IFN-γ was not radioprotective when used either 3 h or 20 h before lethal irradiation (Neta et al. 1986c).

12.3 Mechanisms of Action

Little is known about the mechanisms of action for cytokines in either radiosensitization or radioprotection. A substantial amount of work needs to be done in vitro to help distinguish which observed effects are direct actions of cytokines on specific cells and which effects may be mediated through a variety of cells and intermediate factors. Three broad types of mechanisms are apparent:

1. Mechanisms that directly help promote repair of intracellular radiation damage
2. Mechanisms that stimulate cellular prolifera-

tion to replace essential cellular bone marrow components for hematopoiesis
3. Mechanisms that promote regeneration of immunological reactivity to environmental microorganisms

It appears obvious that direct answers to mechanistic questions will not be obtained by in vivo experimentation. Recent work by Gallicchio et al. (1989) has shown that IL-1 has an in vitro radioprotective effect on murine bone marrow progenitors (CFU-GM and CFU-Meg). These experiments showed that 10 units/ml IL-1, added to bone marrow cells along with GM-CSF, showed a radioprotective effect up to a radiation dose of 3 Gy. At 5 Gy, the effect was lost and GM-CSF alone had no protective effect at any dose. IL-2 and IL-3 did not show a similar synergistic radioprotective effect with GM-CSF. IL-1 alone, without added GM-CSF, did not stimulate colony formation by the bone marrow cells.

These results suggest that IL-1's radioprotective effect is not mediated completely through GM-CSF and that IL-1 may have a direct effect on hematopoietic progenitors. Moore and Warren (1987) speculated that one of IL-1's mechanisms of action is the stimulation of the expression of more CSF receptors on hematopoietic progenitor cells. This would increase their ability to respond to the CSFs. The fact that IL-1 alone had no effect indicates that the GM-CSF production in vivo induced by IL-1 (Vogel et al. 1987) probably occurs outside of the bone marrow and is delivered to the hematopoietic precursor cells in the bone marrow via the circulation.

Initial observations of IL-1's radioprotective effect (Neta et al. 1986a) appeared to indicate that IL-1 had to be given 20 h before irradiation for the radio-protective effect to be exercised. This led to speculation that the mechanisms of action may involve cellular migration, induction of bone marrow progenitors to cycle into a more radioresistant phase, generation of radioresistant hypoxic conditions caused by increases in fibrinogen in the circulation, increased oxygen metabolism resulting in radioresistance due to depleted intracellular oxygen levels, or induction of acute phase proteins that exert radioprotective effects. The observations by two groups that IL-1 and GM-CSF can produce restorative effects on lethally irradiated mice, even when administered after irradiation (Castelli et al. 1988; Neta and Oppenheim 1988), and the report by Gallicchio et al. (1989) that

IL-1 has a radioprotective effect in vitro, make these putative mechanisms seem less likely to play a major role in the radioprotective effects induced by IL-1.

The fact that IL-1 has now been shown to have restorative effects after irradiation would seem to favor the hypothesis that IL-1 acts via a mechanism that stimulates the growth of progenitor cells rather than by inducing mechanisms that interfere with or protect from direct radiation damage.

12.4 Summary

The recent development of the ability to produce recombinant cytokines has aided greatly in determining which BRMs are involved in inducing recovery from radiation damage. BRMs such as lipopolysaccharides (LPSs) (SMITH et al. 1957), muramyl dipeptide (MDP) (BEHLING 1983), and glucans (PATCHEN and MACVITTIE 1986) have been known to have radioprotective effects and are now felt to operate mainly through the induction of beneficial cytokines that actually cause the radioprotective effect. Using purified cytokines, clinicians should soon be able to induce radioprotective effects with much less toxicity than would be experienced with BRMs such as LPSs. Although purified cytokines such as IL-1 and IFNs cause side-effects themselves, they often are not as broad and difficult to deal with as are those caused by nonphysiological BRMs such as LPSs, MDP, or glucans.

Preliminary reports indicate that the same cytokines that are effective in producing hematopoietic restoration following irradiation may also be helpful in inducing hematopoietic recovery from cytotoxic drugs such as cyclophosphamide (CASTELLI et al. 1988; BENJAMIN et al. 1989) and 5-fluorouracil (MOORE and WARREN 1987). These reports indicate that cytokines such as IL-1 may serve a useful role in cancer chemotherapy by allowing larger doses of cytotoxic drugs to be used in treatment.

Although these studies are still preliminary, and mostly have been done in mice, the observation that certain cytokines help improve recovery from radiation damage or from cytotoxic drug treatment should lead to human trials that will test their potential for beneficial use in man. A phase I trial for interferon-α in combination with radiation therapy has already been reported (TORRISI et al. 1986) and other studies are underway. These stu-

dies should help provide the necessary information that will allow us to realize further the potential for utilization of cytokines in conjunction with radiation in the treatment of disease.

Acknowledgments. The skilled assistance of JEAN COATS, JANE FIGG, and BRIAN GANNON was essential in the preparation of this manuscript. Dr. R. NETA graciously provided some of the background material used in reviewing the literature.

References

Behling UH (1983) The radioprotective effect of bacterial endotoxin. In: Nowotry A (ed) Beneficial effects of endotoxins. Plenum, New York, p 127

Benjamin WR, Tare NS, Hayes TJ, Becker JM, Anderson TD (1989) Regulation of hemopoiesis in myelosuppressed mice by human recombinant IL-1. J Immunol 142: 792–799

Billiau A (1987) Interferon 2 as a promoter of growth and differentiation of B cells. Immunol Today 8: 84–87

Castelli MP, Black PL, Schneider M, Pennington R, Abe F, Talmadge JE (1988) Protective, restorative, and therapeutic properties of recombinant human IL-1 in rodent models. J Immunol 140: 3830–3837

Dritschilo A, Mossman K, Gray M, Sreevalsan T (1982) Potentiation of radiation injury by interferon. Am J Clin Oncol 5: 79–82

Gallicchio VS, Hulette BC, Messino MJ, Gass C, Biesche MW, Doukas MA (1989) The effect of various interleukins (IL-1, IL-2, and IL-3) on the in vitro radioprotection of bone marrow progenitors (CFU-GM and CFU-MEG). J Biol Resp Modif 8: 479–487 1989

Gould MN, Kakria RC, Olson S, Borden EC (1984) Radiosensitization of human bronchogenic carcinoma cells by interferon. J Interferon Res 4: 123–128

Mattson K, Holsti LR, Niiranen A, Kivisaari L, Iivanainen M, Sovijarvi A, Cantell K (1985) Human leukocyte interferon as part of a combined treatment for previously untreated small cell lung cancer. J Biol Resp Modif 4: 8–17

Moore MAS, Warren DJ (1987) Synergy of interleukin 1 and granulocyte colony-stimulating factor: in vivo stimulation of stem cell recovery and hematopoietic regeneration following 5-fluorouracil treatment of mice. Proc Natl Acad Sci USA 84: 7134–38

Morrissey PJ, Charrier K, Bressler L, Alpert A (1987) The influence of IL-1 treatment on the reconstitution of the hematopoietic and immune systems following sublethal radiation. J Immunol 140: 4204

Morrissey PJ, Charrier K, Alpert A, Bressler L (1988) In vivo administration of IL-1 induces thymic hypoplasia and increased levels of serum corticosterone. J Immunol 141: 1456–1463

Mossman KL, Hill LT, Dritschilo A (1982) Utility of interferons in clinical radiotherapy. J Natl Med Assoc 74: 1083–1087

Nakamura S, Nakata K, Kashimoto S, Yoshida H, Yamada M (1986) Antitumor effect of recombinant human interleukin 1 alpha against murine syngeneic tumors. Jpn J Cancer Res 77: 767–773

Neta R (1988) Cytokines in radioprotection and therapy of radiation injury. Biotherapy 1: 41–45

Neta R, Oppenheim JJ (1988) Cytokines in therapy of radiation injury. Blood 72: 1093–1095

Neta R, Douches S, Oppenheim JJ (1986a) Interleukin 1 is a radioprotector. J Immunol 136: 2483–2485

Neta R, Vogel SN, Oppenheim JJ, Douches SD (1986b) Cytokines in radioprotection. Comparison of the radioprotective effects of IL-1 to IL-2, GM-CSF, and IFN-gamma. Lymphokine Res 5: s105–s110

Neta R, Oppenheim JJ, Douches SD, Giclas PC, Imbra RJ, Karin M (1986c) Radioprotection with interleukin-1: comparison with other cytokines. In: Cinader B, Miller RG (eds) Progress in immunology VI. Academic, New York, p 900

Neta R, Douches SD, Oppenheim JJ (1987a) Radioprotection by interleukin-1. In: Goldstein G, Bach JF, Wigzal H (eds) Immune regulations by characterized polypeptides. Alan R. Liss, New York, p 429

Neta R, Sztein MB, Oppenheim JJ, Gillis S, Douches SD (1987b) The in vivo effects of interleukin 1. I. Bone marrow cells are induced to cycle after administration of interleukin 1. J Immunol 139: 1861–1866

Neta R, Vogel SN, Sipe JD, Wong GG, Nordan RP (1988a) Comparison of in vivo effects of human recombinant IL 1 and human recombinant IL 6 in mice. Lymphokine Res 7: 403–412

Neta R, Oppenheim JJ, Douches SD (1988b) Interdependence of the radioprotective effects of human recombinant interleukin 1, tumor necrosis factor, granulocyte colony-stimulating factor, and murine recombinant granulocyte-macrophage colony-stimulating factor. J Immunol 140: 108–111

Ortaldo JR, McCoy JL (1980) Protective effects of interferon in mice previously exposed to lethal irradiation. Radiat Res 81: 262–266

Patchen ML, Macvittie TJ (1986) Comparative effects of soluble and particulate glucans on survival in irradiated mice. J Biol Resp Modif 5: 45–60

Real FX, Krown SE, Nisce LZ, Oettgen HF (1985) Unexpected toxicity from radiation therapy in two patients with Kaposi's sarcoma receiving interferon. J Biol Resp Modif 4: 141–146

Robertson BA, Gahring LC, Newton R, Daynes RA (1987) In vivo administration of interleukin 1 to normal mice depresses their capacity to elicit contact hypersensitivity responses: prostaglandins are involved in the modification of immune function. J Invest Dermatol 88: 380–388

Rubin P, Casarett GW (1968) Clinical radiation pathology. WB Saunders, Philadelphia, p 120

Sieff CA (1987) Hematopoietic growth factors. J Clin Invest 79: 1549–1560

Smith WW, Alderman IM, Gillespie RI (1957) Increased survival in irradiated animals treated with bacterial endotoxins. Am J Physiol 191: 124–130

Torrisi J, Berg C, Harter K et al. (1986) Phase I combined modality clinical trial of alpha-2-interferon and radiotherapy. J Radiat Oncol Biol Phys 12: 1453–1456

Valter S (1977) The study of the effect of interferon on the radiosensitivity of cells. Radiobiologiia 17: 105–108

Vogel SN, Douches SD, Kaufman EN, Neta R (1987) Induction of colony stimulating factor in vivo by recombinant interleukin 1 and recombinant tumor necrosis factor. J Immunol 138: 2143–2148

Section III
5-Fluorouracil Radiopotentiation and Its Modulation by Other Agents

13 Theoretical Basis and Clinical Applications of 5-Fluorouracil as a Radiosensitizer – an Overview

John E. Byfield

CONTENTS

13.1 Introduction

During the past decade, several institutions have combined an infusion of the antimetabolite 5-fluorouracil (5-FU) and radiation in the treatment of various human cancers. The results of these studies are thus far uniformly promising. However, no randomized investigations have been completed as yet. The stimulus to these pilot studies came from two disparate sources. The first was the empirical observation by Nigro et al. (1974) that an infusion of 5-FU (combined with porfiromycin or mitomycin C), coupled in part with radiation, led to rapid preoperative regression of squamous anal cancer. These results led to an application of this type of preoperative program against other cancers (Leichman et al. 1984; Carey et al. 1986; Steiger et al. 1981). The second stimulus was the author's identification of the scheduling requisites for the application of infused 5-FU as a true radiosensitizer of human tumors (Byfield et al.

John E. Byfield, MD, PhD, Medical Director, Radiation Therapy Associates Medical Group, 3550 Q Street, Suite 106, Bakersfield, CA 93301, USA

1977). Our preclinical observations then led to a variety of clinical applications described below in which infused 5-FU was used as a radiosensitizer in the nonsurgical therapy for epithelial cancers (Byfield 1989). The current data suggest that the use of slowly infused 5-FU in conjunction with radiation may offer substantial improvement in the control of diverse epithelial cancers (Byfield 1989). A clear understanding of the fundamental radiobiological and pharmacological principles employing infused 5-FU radiosensitization (RS) is necessary if one is to utilize it optimally in clinical practice.

13.2 Radiobiological Basis of 5-Fluorouracil Radiosensitization

5-Fluorouracil has been known to be a radiosensitizer for about two decades. The RS properties of 5-FU were first demonstrated in tissue culture by Bagshaw (1961) soon after its discovery (Heidelberger 1975). Mouse leukemia cells were subsequently shown to be strikingly radiosensitized in vivo (Vietti et al. 1971). These original, preclinical studies stimulated a wealth of early clinical trials using various combinations of 5-FU and external beam radiation. Some of these early studies suggested clinical benefit (Lo et al. 1976; Moertel et al. 1969), others did not. All employed bolus 5-FU, usually in some variant of the original Wisconsin regimen, in which daily bolus 5-FU to toxicity (usually myelosuppression) was given, followed by lower-dose maintenance bolus 5-FU. Interest in bolus 5-FU combined with radiation declined steadily in the 1970s because of difficulties in managing its marrow toxicity and doubt as to the magnitude of its clinical benefit.

However, it was subsequently shown in the author's laboratory (Byfield et al. 1977) that bolus 5-FU cannot radiosensitize because of the pharmacological requirements of the RS phenomenon. Basically, the radiosensitized state is a cellular condition that develops gradually in the 24 h or more of *continuous* 5-FU exposure *after* each radiation exposure (BYFIELD et al. 1982). Moreover, it occurs only if the cell is exposed to an adequate concentration of 5-FU (BYFIELD et al. 1982). Exposure of the cells to 5-FU prior to radiation has no sensitizing effect, although additive toxicity (and tumor response) may occur. At the cellular level, it appears possible that the radiation exposure actually may be sensitizing the cells to 5-FU (BYFIELD et al. 1982). All of these observations showed that radiosensitization could be achieved only by infusing 5-FU slowly throughout the period of irradiation, plus at least 24 h.

We also demonstrated that RS by 5-FU is not an arcane cellular event. It requires a substantial cytotoxic effect of the drug itself to become significant (BYFIELD et al. 1982). In tissue culture (Fig. 13.1), this means RS is found only when there is sufficient drug [on a concentration $(C) \times$ time (T) basis] to produce a kill of about 30% of the cells by drug alone, i.e., without any added x-rays

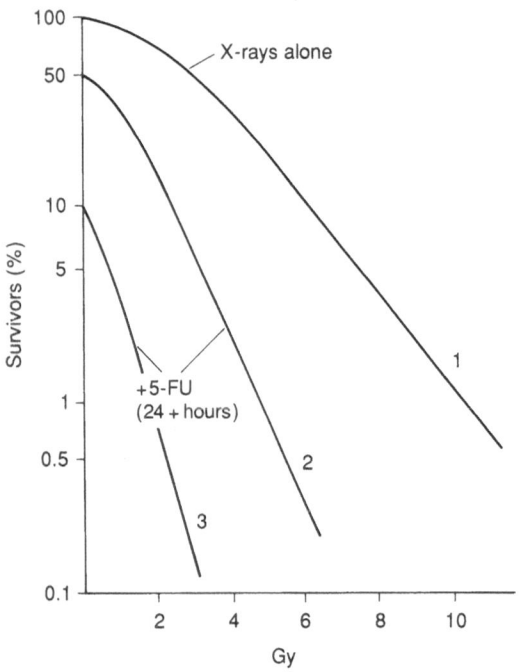

Fig. 13.1. Radiosensitization by 5-FU. *Curve 1* is a radiation survival curve of human tumor cells without added 5-FU. *Curves 2* and *3* show the effects of progressively greater concentrations of 5-FU present for 24 h after the radiation exposure. *Curve 2*, 50% cytotoxicity by 5-FU (zero Gy dose). *Curve 3*, 90% cytotoxicity by 5-FU (zero Gy dose)

(BYFIELD et al. 1982; CALABRO-JONES et al. 1982). In terms of clinical applications, RS can probably always be anticipated if enough infused 5-FU can be given to achieve a partial response (50% tumor volume reduction). 5-FU therefore can be expected to radiosensitize any tumor which shows primary sensitivity to the drug. Contrarily, 5-FU cannot sensitize tumors which are 5-FU resistant. Clinically, this makes 5-FU RS therapy most useful in the epithelial tissues that are sensitive to both 5-FU and radiation (PRICE 1987). During therapy, the administration of the 5-FU infusion to at least a low level of clinical toxicity is theoretically desirable since this is the only means by which the clinician can gauge 5-FU "dosimetry" in any individual patient (BYFIELD 1989).

The exact reasons why bolus-equivalent 5-FU does not radiosensitize are not known. This failure well may stem from the mode of action of the drug in some cells. Infused 5-FU may poison some types of tissues (and their derivative cancers) through its accumulation in cellular RNA rather than inhibiting thymidylate synthetase (ARDALAN et al. 1980; BELLAMY and HILL 1984; CALABRO-JONES et al. 1982; HEIDELBERGER 1975). This interpretation is consistent with both the temporal sequence for RS (drug after x-ray) and the relatively slow development of RS in irradiated cells. However, it lacks experimental proof. On the other hand, cellular RNA containing 5-FU may well provide a pool of 5-FU metabolites prolonging thymidylate synthetase inhibition to create a lethal state. The weight of biochemical evidence supports the latter hypothesis. Whatever its origin, it is clear from toxicity studies that human tissue sensitivity to 5-FU has a great dependence on the schedule of 5-FU administration (ANSFIELD et al. 1977; MOERTEL et al. 1968; SIEFERT et al. 1975). The most obvious demonstration of this phenomenon was made by SIEFERT et al., who first clearly demonstrated the schedule-dependent reversal of toxicity dominance described below.

13.3 Clinical Scheduling Requisites of 5-Fluorouracil Radiosensitization

Once it was understood that RS requires a significant postradiation period of time to develop, it became apparent that only slowly infused 5-FU could radiosensitze (BYFIELD et al. 1977). This stems from the short half-life of 5-FU in the bloodstream. When 5-FU is administered as a bolus injection, its half-life in the blood is only about 10 min, most of the drug being degraded rapidly by the liver (ALMERSJÖ et al. 1980; MYERS 1981; PINEDO and PETERS 1988). In order to create the conditions required for RS (a reasonably constant exposure to extracellular 5-FU for about 24 h after *each* exposure), it is necessary to renew the extracellular supply of drug constantly. Currently, this can only be done adequately by a slow, continuous infusion. Accordingly, the clinical toxicity of slowly infused 5-FU becomes quite relevant.

As noted, the importance of scheduling in the normal tissue sensitivity ot 5-FU was first pointed out by SEIFERT et al. (1975). They showed that the limiting toxicity of 5-FU reversed itself when the schedule of administration was changed from bolus injection to a 5-day infusion. During bolus 5-FU therapy, bone marrow toxicity is almost always limiting and is sometimes lethal (MOERTEL et al. 1972). However, when a 5-FU infusion is given for 4–5 days to toxicity, stomatitis becomes dose limiting and marrow suppression is usually very mild (SEIFERT et al. 1975). This inversion effect on the dose-limiting tissue is relative rather than absolute. Thus, the incidence and severity of each toxic reaction increases as the dose rate increases for 5-day 5-FU infusions. This is illustrated

in Fig. 13.2, where the incidence of toxicity for 120-h infusions is plotted versus the daily 5-FU dose. It can be seen that the reaction generated in all three tissues evidencing toxicity (i.e., mucosa, skin, and marrow) increases with 5-FU infusion dose. However, both the skin and the marrow have significantly higher thresholds than the oral mucosa. This small difference in threshold is, nevertheless, sufficient to convert a potentially lethal schedule (bolus 5-FU) to a program that is clinically tolerable and safe (a continuous 5-FU infusion to toxicity). This aspect is quite important for the combination of the drug with radiation, especially for pelvic cancers.

These observations illustrate the three central requisites for applying 5-FU as a radiosensitizer in humans:

1. 5-FU RS is a postradiation phenomenon and requires that 5-FU be available to the cells for 24 h after *each* radiation exposure. This requires a slow, constant infusion.
2. The more drug that is present (i.e., the higher the concentration for any given period), the greater the likelihood of tumor response to the drug and therefore the greater chance that RS will develop.
3. There is also the reasonable possibility that many tumors, particularly those derived from squamous and squamous-like epithelial tissues, are more likely to respond to slowly infused 5-FU than to bolus 5-FU (BYFIELD 1989; LOKICH et al. 1981).

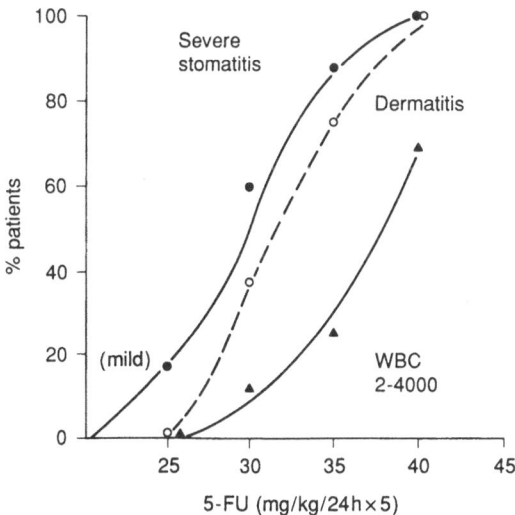

Fig. 13.2. Dose–toxicity relationship of infused 5-FU. The incidence of mucosal (stomatitis), skin (dermatitis), and marrow (WBC) toxicity seen with increasing daily doses of continuously infused 5-FU (5-day infusions). (SEIFERT et al. 1975)

These three prerequisites are interdependent but all must be recognized in the development of ideal clinical regimens. At this stage of research, there is no reason to believe that the optimal $C \times T$ factor using infused 5-FU against all human tumor types will have a constant value. Since the turnover times of both normal tissues and cancers can very significantly, the optimal $C \times T$ factors for inducing 5-FU RS in different tumor sites probably also vary. LOKICH et al. (1981) have shown that protracted 5-FU infusions (greater than 5 days in duration) are feasible and can be combined readily with radiation (RICH et al. 1985). The important point is that only 5-FU infusions can radiosensitize and that any schedule supplying sufficient drug in a prolonged fashion (>24 h after each x-ray exposure) should be at least partially effective.

13.4 Pharmacology of Infused 5-Fluorouracil

When humans are infused with 5-FU, one encounters an unusual phenomenon. The clearance of the drug is nonlinear (COLLINS et al. 1980; FLOYD et al. 1982). This means that the serum 5-FU levels obtained are not a simple function of the amount of drug administered. At low infusion rates (anything significantly below 15 mg/kg/day), little to no drug is found in the plasma (FLOYD et al. 1982). Rather, the drug "disappears." We have proposed that this is due to its total removal from the bloodstream (by incorporation in growing cells) at a single pass during low dose infusions. In this model, the drug is actually accumulating within cycling cells rather than being degraded by the liver or other organs (ALMERSJO et al. 1980). This seems likely since the maximum clearance is essentially the cardiac output at daily doses under 10 mg/kg (BYFIELD et al. 1985a).

As the infusion rate increases above 10–15 mg/kg/day, 5-FU begins to appear in the blood on a linear dose-concentration basis (BYFIELD 1989; BYFIELD et al. 18985a, c). Since it is quite clear that the toxicity of 5-FU relates to both the extracellular 5-FU level and the duration of tumor cell exposure to the drug (CALABRO-JONES et al. 1982), it is apparent that both the dose rate of an infusion *and* its duration are critical in the development of 5-FU RS. Table 13.1 shows the predicted effect on 5-FU cytoxicity of the common time–dose reductions encountered in various clinical studies. The reductions in cell kill are predicted by the author's preclinical and pharmacological studies (BYFIELD et al. 1985c; CALABRO-JONES et al. 1982). This appears to be borne out in clinical practice. Both the author (BYFIELD et al. 1984) and TAYLOR et al. (1989) found reduced response rates in patients receiving less 5-FU. In Table 13.2, one may find the respective response rate for 4-day (JACOBS et al. 1988) versus 5-day (TAPAZOGLOU et al. 1986) infusions of 5-FU. If these comparative data are correct, it would certainly seem unwise to reduce

Table 13.2. Five-day versus 4-day infused 5-FU: effect on response rate in advanced head and neck cancer

Authors	Infusion duration	Response rate
JACOBS et al. (1988)	4 days (96 h)	18%
TAPAZOGLOU et al. (1986)	5 days (120 h)	100%

the duration of an infusion to 4 days, as is commonly done.

13.5 Status of Current Clinical Studies

To date, the combination of infused 5-FU and radiation has been applied in several cancers, including esophagus, head and neck, lung, rectal, bladder, and squamous anal carcinoma. A related drug, 5-fluorouridine deoxyriboside (5-FUdR), has been used with radiation in metastatic colon cancer to the liver but will not be discussed further here because 5-FUdR does not radiosensitize. Although our first clinical observations were made in the mid 1970s (the scheduling requirement for 5-FU RS was first described by our group in 1976), there is still a paucity of data and no published phase III (randomized) studies. In the studies that are available, a second and even third chemotherapeutic agent almost invariably has been employed, rendering it difficult to interpret whether or not the 5-FU and the radiation component have been "optimized." Nevertheless, in almost all cases, the results are encouraging enough to warrant further trials. The existing studies now will be evaluated in the context of what this writer believes to be the established prerequisites to the *correct* use of 5-FU as a radiosensitizer.

13.5.1 Head and Neck Cancer

The data available for this group of cancers are limited but of interest since it is in the head and neck region where the primary limiting toxicity of (local) radiation and infused 5-FU overlap. Both infused 5-FU and radiation can induce severe, but

Table 13.1. Quantitative effects of dose reduction ($C \times T$) during 5-FU infusions

Parameter	Amount of 5-FU reduction	Quantitative effect	Log reduction in tumor cell kill
Time	5 days to 4	24 h less 5-FU	= 1.0 log
Concentration	25 mg/kg/day to 20 mg/kg/day	300 ng to 200 ng/ml	= 1.0 log

Reference: CALABRO-JONES et al. 1982, BYFIELD et al. 1985b.

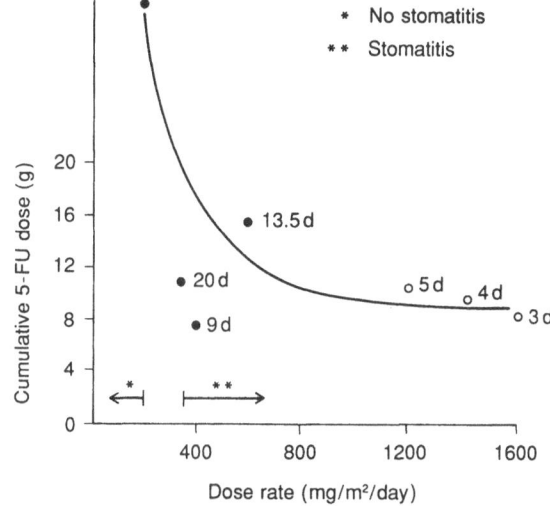

Fig. 13.3. Relationship between cumulative 5-FU dose and stomatitis in patients receiving protracted infusions (*closed circles*, LOKICH et al. 1981) or 3- to 5-day continuous 5-FU infusions (*open circles*, SIEFERT et al. 1975). The total drug dose infused is nearly independent of the infusion dose rate

Table 13.3. Results of concomitant infusional 5-FU and radiation in advanced squamous head and neck carcinoma

No. of pts.	Other drugs	CR%	Median survival	% survival 2 years	Reference
38[a]	CP	53	—	74	ADELSTEIN et al. 1986
18	None	75	>2 years	70	BYFIELD et al. 1984
41[a]	MIT	56	—	—	DOBROWSKY et al. 1989
42[a]	MIT	64	—	—	KAPLAN et al. 1985
53	CP	55	>3 years	60	TAYLOR et al. 1989
17	HU	71	>2 years	>50	VOKES et al. 1989
34	CP/FA	80	>2 years	60	WENDT et al. 1987

Abbreviations: CP, cisplatin; MIT, mitomycin C; HU, hydroxurea; FA, folinic acid

[a] Tumor-free specimen at surgery

reversible, mucositis. Mucositis appears to be due to an accumulation of the drug within the cells of the limiting tissues. This is shown in Fig. 13.3, where the total dose of 5-FU needed to develop stomatitis is plotted against the daily dose rate. The data are derived from two phase I trials that studied the toxicity to 5-day (SIEFERT et al. 1975) and long-term, continuous (protracted) infusions (LOKICH et al. 1981) of 5-FU. It can be seen that a reasonably constant plateau for the total 5-FU dose needed to achieve stomatitis was found.

The results of the existing head and neck trials of infused 5-FU and radiation are shown in Table 13.3. Our own group described the first phase I–II trial of 5-day (120-h) infused 5-FU combined with radiation in advanced squamous head and neck cancer (BYFIELD et al. 1984). We also have reported some limited data on 72-h infused 5-FU in this patient group (BYFIELD et al. 1985c). The first trial consisted of repeating cycles of 5-day infused 5-FU coupled with radiation at a constant dose rate (2.5 Gy/fraction given on each of the first 4 days of each 5-day treatment cycle). The goal of the trial was to evaluate both toxicity and response as a function of 5-FU dose rate. The 5-FU dose rate was escalated in a phase I format.

As expected, the most common toxicity (and invariably the dose-limiting toxicity) was mucositis. Since both infused 5-FU and head and neck radiation have stomatitis/pharyngitis as their major toxic manifestations, this was to be expected.

No patient could tolerate more than 25 mg/kg/day 5-FU (for each 5-day treatment cycle) for very long (two cycles was the maximum). Even at 25 mg/kg/day, about 25% of patients required dose reduction to a lower level. On the other hand, there was a clear-cut threshold for this toxicity, since only mild stomatitis was induced at the lowest dose tested (20 mg/kg/day). All 20 mg/kg/day patients completed therapy without requiring dose reduction, *despite the added radiation.* However, there also was considerably reduced patient survival seen with 20 mg/kg/day compared with higher doses, suggesting a therapeutic dose–response relationship (BYFIELD et al. 1984). In general, toxicity, response, and survival appeared linked in these results, as predicted by the theoretical basis of this treatment (BYFIELD 1989). The study showed clearly that the combination could be administered in a reasonably predictable fashion, even in head and neck cancer, with a suggestion of an improved response rate and survival benefit.

There have now been several other studies of similar combinations in head and neck cancer, each with the addition of one or more drugs. Some of these studies employed a 120-h 5-FU infusion, others used 96-h infusions. The available studies are summarized in Table 13.3 TAYLOR et al. have reported the largest group using infused 5-FU and radiation combined with platinum (MURIHY et al. 1987; TAYLOR et al 1989). They observed an interesting discordance between the clinical complete response rate (TAYLOR et al. 1989) and their clearly superior survival results, indicating that considerable residual deformity did not necessarily imply residual cancer. Their results appeared very promising (TAYLOR et al. 1989) and their group currently is conducting a randomized trial versus conventional radiation.

The data of KEANE et al. are discussed elsewhere in this volume. The Princess Margaret group added mitomycin C (MIT) following the Detroit pattern but used only one or two cycles of infused 5-FU combined with a prolonged, split-course, increased dose per fraction regimen (KEANE et al. 1985a).

KAPLAN et al. combined MIT with infused 5-FU and external beam radiation in 42 patients with advanced head and neck cancer (KAPLAN et al. 1985). Their program was a split-course treatment using 30 Gy in 3 weeks with drugs being given "up front," i.e., a bolus of MIT ($10 \, mg/m^2$) on day 1 and a 96-h infusion of 5-FU ($1.0 \, g/m^2$). Twenty-three patients had subsequent surgery with a 79% negative primary specimen and a 69% negative neck specimen. Overall, 64% of patients had a complete response.

WENDT et al. (1987) combined bolus 5-FU and cisplatin with a 4-day 5-FU plus folinic acid infusion and concomitant radiation. This program yielded an 88% regional complete remission rate, durable at 81% at 2 years. Two-year survival was 58%; however, this is slightly less than we observed with 5-FU alone (BYFIELD et al. 1984). VOKES et al. (1989) dropped the addition of any alkylating agent and added hydroxyurea with promising results. DOBROWSKY et al. (1989) included MIT in a presurgical context with promising results.

Two comments related to the chemotherapy and radiation components are relevant to these programs:

1. All of these results confirm the *lack of significant systemic effectiveness of any chemotherapy combination*. In the great majority of studies examined, death from disseminated disease predominates. Five-day infused 5-FU has a very high response rate (greater than 80%) in disseminated squamous cancer but this has a minimal effect on survival. The preliminary data recently published by JACOBS et al. (1988) shows that adding cisplatin to 4-day infused 5-FU increases the response rate from 14% to

31% but has no meaningful effect on median survival. One cannot, therefore, anticipate any "neoadjuvant" benefit from these regimens.
2. The adverse results obtained by using "split-course" radiation (AMDUR et al. 1989) do *not* apply to this form of cyclical therapy in which overall survival appears considerably better than radiation alone. Clearly, the chemotherapy component has displaced any disadvantage inherent in the necessary intratreatment rest periods.

Several of these studies used 4-day 5-FU infusions. The reduction in infusion duration from 5 days to 4 days can be seriously questioned. Unfortunately, only limited data are available comparing 4-day (96-h) with 5-day (120-h) 5-FU infusions. TAPAZOGLOU et al. (1986) reported (Table 13.2) a 100% (partial) response rate in untreated head and neck cancer patients. A much larger study recently reported by JACOBS et al. (1988) showed that the response rate in patients with advanced head and neck cancer to 4-day infused 5-FU was only 14%. Cisplatin also yielded a 14% response rate while the combination increased the response rate to 31% but had no effect on median survival. This comparison would suggest that the response rate to 5-day infused 5-FU may be much greater than either 4-day infused 5-FU (as expected) *and* even to the conventional 5-FU/cisplatin combination. Obviously, additional data on this question would be invaluable.

If the data represent the true states of affairs in the chemotherapy of head and neck cancer, the effect of the reduction of a 5-FU infusion from 5 days to 4 days *may* reduce the response rate from 100% to 14%! This would then reduce RS by an equivalent amount. The author believes that the reduction of the duration of the infusion to 4 days in order to include a second drug may have vitiated the true potential of the approach in several existing studies which have attempted to use infused 5-FU as a radiosensitizer.

The positive, uncontrolled studies in head and neck cancer (noted in Table 13.3) must be contrasted with the report by KEANE et al. (1985a), who studied the effect of split-course radiation and 4-day infused 5-FU (plus a single dose of MIT) in patients with advanced larynx and hypopharynx cancer. The radiation program included 25 Gy, a 4-week rest, followed by a second 25-Gy dose and chemotherapy. A recent update of the randomized version of this study showed no survival benefit. In

Table 13.4. Impact of 5-FU and cisplatin on tumor control in head and neck cancer (derived from TAYLOR et al. 1989) Dose versus failure rate.

Drug	Median % ideal dose delivered	<Median dose		>Median dose	
		No. of Pts.[a]	% failing	No. of Pts.[b]	% failing
5-FU	78	20	60	25	24
Cisplatin	88	20	40	25	40

[a] Number of patients receiving the planned number of cycles and getting more than or equal to the median dose delivered

[b] Number of patients receiving the planned number of cycles and getting less than the median dose delivered

KEANE et al.'s study, the radiation component was only slightly less than that reported in the other series (in NSD terms) while the chemotherapy component was dramatically less in terms of both 5-FU dose per cycle and numbers of cycles. Approximately one-third of their patients received only a single 96-h infusion cycle, i.e., less than 20% of the 5-FU dose used in the major nonsurgical pilot studies.

Interestingly, TAYLOR et al. (1989) found no effect of a reduction in cisplatin dose (Table 13.4). Since overall similar results have been obtained in the various studies cited, whether ot not cisplatin (or MIT for that matter) was included, it seems incumbent on clinicians to establish as soon as possible whether or not the very substantial additional toxicity of cisplatin is worth its inclusion. Indeed, recent studies from Yale have suggested that, if any drug is to be added to infused 5-FU, MIT may be a more logical inclusion (WEISSBERG et al. 1989).

The randomized study of full-dose radiation and full-dose infused 5-FU chemotherapy is currently being performed by TAYLOR's group, which should be helpful in resolving these questions. To date, no cooperative group has addressed these questions.

As noted above, we also studied (in a limited fashion) the tolerance of patients with various tumors to 72-h infused 5-FU (BYFIELD et al. 1985a, c). This latter study was done to see if it was possible to reduce the duration of each infusion, which would be easier on the patient and more cost-effective if equally efficacious. However, we encountered significant 5-FU CNS toxicity during these high dose, reduced duration exposures and now believe that this aspect makes such short-term

infusions less desirable than infusions lasting 5 days or more. For a different interpretation of the existing head and neck studies, the reader is referred to the excellent chapter on head and neck cancer in this volume by CUMMINGS and his colleagues (Chap. 17).

13.5.2 Esophageal Cancer

Our first trial of 5-FU used specifically as a radiosensitizer was in cancer of the esophagus, first reported in 1978 (BYFIELD et al. 1978). That trial used a dose of 20 mg/kg/day 5-FU and a 5-day infusion duration (BYFIELD et al. 1980). It also introduced the use of cyclical treatment of 5-FU as a radiosensitizer for the first time. Although primarily of an exploratory, phase I nature, the study yielded a clinical, complete response in almost all (five of six) patients, showing that the approach was both possible and useful in humans. Noteworthy is the observation that the first patient so treated lived for more than 5 years free of disease before being lost to follow-up. A second patient (two of six or 33%) remains alive and free of disease. One other patient in our initial series developed a carcinoma of the hypopharynx for which he underwent a second series of infusions with x-rays without substantial problems. This observation suggested that there is no demonstrable, cumulative toxicity with the regimen. However, the patient died of this second malignancy, as did a fourth patient of lung cancer.

Since our initial report, there have appeared numerous studies of infused 5-FU and radiation in esophageal cancer, almost all of which report enhanced local tumor control compared with radiation alone (see Table 13.5). This includes adenocarcinomas of the lower esophagus and gastroesophageal junction which appear equally responsive (COIA et al. 1988).

The existing studies *without surgery* are summarized in Table 13.5. Included in the table is the large series by Wayne State, which was, for the most part, a surgical series, i.e., patients received low dose chemotherapy/radiation therapy followed by esophagectomy (LEICHMAN et al. 1984; STEIGER et al. 1981). In most of these investigations, including the study from Wayne State, an added agent (either MIT or cisplatin) was used. In the most recent study using Wayne State data, surgery has been omitted (LEICHMAN et al. 1987).

The surgical data are of special interest since

Table 13.5. Results of infusional 5-FU and radiation in the conservative management of esophageal carcinoma

Institution	No. of pts.	CR%	Median survival	% survival 2 years	Reference
UCSD/Kern	6	83	22 mos[a]	30	BYFIELD et al. 1980
Baker Cancer Center	21	86	14 mos.	22	CHAN et al. 1989
Fox Chase Cancer Center	8	88	15 mos.	30	COIA et al. 1988
Royal Adelaide	35	69	>18 mos.	NA	DENHAM et al. 1988
Princess Margaret	35	48	12 mos.	28	KEANE et al. 1985b
Wayne State (nonop)	20	55	22 mos.	NA	LEICHMAN et al. 1987
Wayne State (preop)	21	25[b]	18 mos.	24	STEIGER et al. 1981
x-ray alone	403	—	—	12	ROBERTS 1980
Untreated	975	—	—	0.3	ROBERTS 1980

NA, no data available
[a] Survival data from author's entire experience
[b] Surgical neoadjuvant study included here for comparison

they measure histologically the effect of one or two RS cycles. Thus, the Wayne State investigators showed that about one-third of the operated patients achieved a surgically proven, complete response, if response was sufficient to render the patient operable. Median survival of the entire surgical group was 18 months while that of those whose response was sufficiently satisfactory to justify an attempt at curative surgery was 24 months. *All* of the long-term resected survivors were tumor-free at resection (including lymph nodes). Sixty percent of these pathological CR (complete response) patients lived at least 2 years. These results clearly relate tumor clearance (that is, a complete response) with long-term survival. The Wayne State authors also concluded that their results were superior to their historical control patients treated with radiation and/or surgery. CAREY et al. (1986) reported similar data. However, in both of these series, the overall pathological CR response rate was low, less than 10% when one includes those patients who remained inoperable.

The results suggest that infused 5-FU used with coincident radiation in esophageal carcinoma improves the local control compared with surgery alone. However, all long-term survivors have been tumor-free at surgery. Thus, radical surgery is probably not needed when this approach is used in esophageal cancer (POPLIN et al. 1987). As in the head and neck studies, it is unclear whether or not adding a second drug makes any difference. However, it should be noted that none of the existing studies indicate that this treatment approach has been used to maximum advantage. In none of these studies has a maximum dose of

5-FU been used in every patient or even in every cycle in any given patient. Since the RS phenomenon is clearly 5-FU dose dependent, it seems likely that a higher CR rate could be achieved with further modifications. The data of LEICHMAN et al. illustrate the relationship of a CR with survival (1984). No such relationship would be apparent if death from metastatic disease was the sole important parameter in esophageal carcinoma.

On the other hand, all of the studies show that the chemotherapy component has minimal impact on systemic disease whether manifest or occult at the time of patient treatment. Because esophageal cancer patients have a very high incidence of systemic metastases at the time of presentation (at least 70% of all patients), it seems unlikely that *median* survivorship can be used to measure treatment impact.

13.5.3 Cervix Cancer and Radiation of the Lower Bowel

There have been several trials thus far of this approach in advanced gynecological cancer. The initial study again was modeled after the anal cancer programs but omitted surgery. THOMAS et al. (1984) used split-course radiation therapy; a 72- to 96-h 5-FU infusion was added to the radiation at treatment inception and again at the resumption of radiation treatment after a midcourse break. As in the anal cancer programs, MIT was given as a single bolus each time 5-FU was started. In stage III-B patients, rapid tumor resolution was found, together with a complete response rate of 74% and a 1-year control rate of 70%, compared with an expected control rate of 43% from historical controls. Patients with recurrent disease also appeared improved. The authors have initiated a randomized trial based on these results. The program is also important because the radiation portals involved lower gastrointestinal radiation. Acute radiation toxicity did not appear much different than expected from radiation alone. Some adverse late effects on the bowel were also found but, again, at an incidence level similar to that following radiation alone.

Similar results recently have been reported by Ludgate et al. (1988). These authors used two 96-h infusions along with MIT and radiation. Enhanced responses and survival were noted in their series.

Elsewhere in this volume, additional studies in the use of 5-FU as a radiosensitizer for gynecological cancers are described in more detail (see also Kalra et al., 1985).

13.5.4 Squamous Anal Cancer

The results of the various programs used against squamous anal cancer are reviewed elsewhere (Cummings and Byfield 1988; Leichman et al. 1985; Sischy 1985) and in this volume. It is important to recognize that this approach has been quite successful in this rather uncommon squamous cancer (Nigro et al. 1974). In the series from Toronto (Cummings and Byfield 1988) and San Diego (Byfield et al. 1983a), *no* surgery was required to achieve long-term, tumor-free survival in almost all patients. These results clearly show the effectiveness of this regimen against this unique squamous malignancy when it is limited to the anal canal at presentation.

Perhaps the most useful information can be gleaned from the recent report by Sischy et al. (1989), in which a multi-institutional study was conducted using two 96-h infusions of 5-FU, a conventional "intermediate" dose of radiation (40.8 Gy at 1.7 Gy per day), and a single injection of MIT. This program led to a 97% survival rate at 1 year and 73% at 3 years. Disease-free survival at 2 years was 77% for patients with tumors smaller than 3 cm but only 53% for patients with tumors larger than 3 cm. Sixty percent of patients had tumors larger than 3 cm. These results confirm the benefit of the approach but serve to illustrate its limitations, at least as administered by the RTOG program reported by Sischy et al. (1989) One

should anticipate a locoregional failure rate for conservative tumor control (no abdominal Perineal Resection) of at least 23% in early cases (less than 3 cm lesions) and 47% with larger lesions. Given the size of tumor distribution at entry, an overall failure rate for conservative therapy of 39% can be anticipated (28% of 37% plus 33% of 66%). It is not commonly recognized that the abdominal–perineal Resection Rate (colostomy rate) in the Wayne State series was 45% (from data of Leichman et al. 1985). Because of this, their data are somewhat difficult to interpret. The clinician should, therefore, be aware that the failure rate increases with increasing tumor size and that simple transplantation of the Wayne State regimen in terms of both radiation and chemotherapy dose should be made with caution, particularly in patients with larger tumors.

The reader will recognize that these comments reflect a situation in the treatment of anal cancer analogous to head and neck and esophageal malignancies.

13.5.5 Rectal Carcinoma

Experience with infused 5-FU used as a radiosensitizer is considerably more limited in rectal cancer than in squamous anal cancer despite the more common occurrence of the former. Recently, Sischy's group updated their results of using this approach (along with MIT) in marginally operable rectal carcinoma (Haghbin et al. 1988; Sischy 1985). They found (using 1 gm^2 5-FU for 4 days) that 31% of the resected specimens contained no carcinoma while only 24% of perirectal nodes contained cancer, compared with 53% of their historical controls. Local control in patients eligible for such 5-year evaluation was 85%. The treatment proved much less effective against recurrent disease. Again, these data are reviewed in greater detail elsewhere in this volume.

Our own experience is more limited than that of Sischy and co-workers but of a similar trend. We also have been able to induce CRs but a rigorous evaluation has yet to be carried out. However, it is clear to those with experience in this cancer that the adenocarcinomas of the rectum are less responsive than their close neighbors, squamous anal carcinomas. Since these cancers originate within a few centimeters of each other, the origins of this difference is an obvious topic for future biochemical and cell kinetic investigations.

Table 13.6. Infused 5-FU and radiation in transitional bladder cancer

Authors	No. of pts.	X-ray dose (Gy)	Clearance rate (%)[a]	Cystectomy rate (%)	Death from pelvic cancer (%)
ROTMAN et al. 1987	19	4–4.5	89	11	5
RUSSELL et al. 1988	14	4	71	36	0

[a] Negative bladder biopsy or positive biopsy but negative cystectomy specimen or negative margins following transurethral resection of residual cancer

13.5.6 Bladder Carcinoma

There have been two trials of infused 5-FU and radiation in transitional cell bladder carcinoma (ROTMAN et al. 1987; RUSSELL et al. 1988). These are summarized in Table 13.6 and elsewhere in this volume. Even with modest doses of 5-FU, the majority of patients will achieve a CR avoiding cystectomy. This also has been the author's experience. More data are available in the chapter by ROTMAN et al. (Chap. 19).

13.6 Conclusions

The primary modalities of therapy in the above programs are infused 5-FU and radiation. In most cases, either MIT or cisplatin has been added but their exact role is unclear. In none of this author's studies was either MIT or cisplatin ever employed, yet seemingly equivalent results to other studies were obtained. This is true for head and neck, esophageal, and anal cancers. It is the author's belief that the critical components of this approach are the combination of the 5-FU infusion and radiation. Therefore, a full understanding of the optimal combination of 5-FU and radiation in individual tumor types appears desirable.

The application of infused 5-FU and radiation clearly appears useful in humans. Neither the ideal infusion duration nor the most appropriate radiation fractionation scheme has yet been established. Against squamous cancers, a 5-day infusion (at 25 mg/kg/day) coupled with conventional radiation (1.8–2 Gy per day for 5 days) seems suitable in most patients. The author treats debilitated patients and patients receiving more drugs than just 5-FU at 1.8 Gy per day. Patients with severe hepatic derangement, including extensive metastatic disease, need 5-FU dose reduction (FLOYD et al. 1982). At the clinical level, the induction of mild 5-FU toxicity (grade 1 to 2

stomatitis) is felt to be desirable. In the later treatment cycles, reduction of the daily 5-FU dose to 20 mg/kg/day is frequently required because of an accumulating depletion in normal tissue stem cells. Stomatitis will occur just following each period of treatment and should be (just) healed prior to resumption of therapy. *Accordingly, cyclical treatment is needed with resolution of all side-effects during each rest period* (BYFIELD 1989; BYFIELD et al. 1977, 1978, 1984). The author does not believe that the total dose of radiation need be compromised. Future clinical trials should be devoted to further defining the use of this combination in various cancers, to the development of satisfactory oral 5-FU pro-drugs (BYFIELD et al. 1982, 1985d, 1985e; TANG et al. 1984), and to the study of modulators capable of enhancing the sensitivity of tumors currently known to be resistant to 5-FU.

The properly applied use of 5-FU RS regimens appears on the verge of offering significant advances, especially in the treatment of squamous and squamous-like cancers. As has been found with bolus 5-FU, it is imperative that sufficient 5-FU be administered to achieve the expected full response rate (ANSFIELD et al. 1977). Since many forms of mutilating cancer surgery are necessitated by the

Table 13.7. Cancers sensitive to 5-FU radiosensitization[a]

Cancer	Incidence	Surgical procedure
Esophagus	9 300	Esophagectomy
Anus	2 500	Abdominal–perineal
Larynx	11 700	Larynegectomy
Vulva	4 400	Vulvectomy
Penis	1 300	Phallectomy
Bladder	40 500	Cystectomy
Rectum[b]	42 000	Abdominal–perineal
Breast	123 900	Mastectomy

[a] The total number of "radical" cancer surgical procedures performed in the United States each year is about 242 500, of which about 95% are susceptible to 5-FU radiosensitization

[b] Rectal carcinoma is moderately sensitive to 5-FU

failure of conservative therapies for squamous and other epithelial cancers, further development of this approach may have the added effect of reducing the need for radical surgery (Table 13.7). Preliminary studies already have suggested this approach may be feasible in head and neck cancer (HONG et al. 1989). It appears reasonable that the use of infused 5-FU as a radiosensitizer may assume a substantial role in the treatment of squamous and other cancers, provided clinical trials are conducted which recognize the unique requisites of this therapeutic approach.

References

Adelstein DJ, Sharea VM, Earle AS et al. (1986) Chemoradiotherapy as initial management in patients with squamous cell carcinoma of the head and neck. Cancer Treat Rep 70: 761–767

Almersjo OE, Gustavsson BG, Regardh C-G, Wahlen P (1980) Pharmacokinetic studies of 5 fluorouracil after oral and intravenous administration in man. Acta Pharmacol Toxicol 46: 329–336

Amdur RJ, Parsons JT, Mendenhall WM, Million RR, Cassisi NJ (1989) Split-course versus continuous-course irradiation in the postoperative setting for squamous cell carcinoma of the head and neck. Int J Radiat Oncol Biol Phys 17: 279–285

Ansfield FJ, Klotz J, Nealon T (1977) A phase 3 study comparing the clinical utility of four regimens of 5-fluorouracil. Cancer 39: 34–40

Ardalan B, Cooney D, MacDonald JS (1980) Physiological and pharmacological determinants of sensitivity and resistance to 5-fluorouracil in lower animals and man. Adv Pharmacol Chemother 17: 289–320

Bagshaw MA (1961) Possible role of potentiators in radiation therapy. AJR 85: 822–833

Bellamy AS, Hill BT (1984) Interactions between clinically effective antitumor drugs and radiation in experimental systems. Biochem Biophys Acta 738: 125–166

Buroker T, Nigro N, Bradley G, Pelor L, Chomchai L, Considine BG, Vaitkevicius V (1977) Combined therapy for cancer of the anal canal: a follow-up report. Dis Colon Rectum 20: 677–678

Byfield JE (1989) 5-Fluorouracil radiation sensitization – a brief review. Invest New Drugs 7: 111–116

Byfield JE, Chan PYM, Seagren SL (1977) Radiosensitization of 5-FU: molecular origins and clinical scheduling implications (abstr). Proc Am Assoc Cancer Res 18: 74

Byfield JE, Barone RM, Mendelsohn J, Seagren SL, Sharp TR, Quinol L, Frankel S (1978) Combined 5-fluorouracil and x-ray therapy in esophageal and other gastrointestinal cancers (abstr). Int J Radiat Oncol Biol Phys 4 [Suppl 2]: 136–137

Byfield JE, Barone RM, Mendelsohn J, Frankel SS, Quinol L, Sharp TR, Seagren SL (1980) Infusional 5-fluorouracil and x-ray therapy for non-resectable esophageal carcinoma. Cancer 22: 376–382

Byfield JE, Calabro-Jones P, Klisak I, Kulhanian F (1982) Pharmacologic requirements for obtaining sensitization of human tumor cells in vitro to combined 5-fluorouracil or ftorafur and x-rays. Int J Radiat Oncol Biol Phys 8: 1923–1933

Byfield JE, Barone RM, Sharp TR, Frankel SS (1983a) Conservative management of squamous anal cancer by cyclical 5-fluorouracil infusion alone and x-ray therapy. Cancer Treat Rep 67: 709–712

Byfield JE, Stanton W, Sharp TR, Frankel SS, Koziol JA (1983b) Phase I–II study of 120-hour infused 5-fluorouracil and split-course radiation therapy for localized non-small cell lung cancer. Cancer Treat Rep 67: 933–936

Byfield JE, Sharp TR, Tang S, Frankel SS, Callipari F (1984) Phase I and II trial of cyclical 5-day infused 5-fluorouracil and coincident radiation in advanced cancer of the head and neck. J Clin Oncol 2: 406–413

Byfield JE, Frankel SS, Hornbeck CL, Sharp TR, Callipari F (1985a) Phase 1 and 2 trial of cyclical 72-hour infused 5-fluorouracil and hyperfractionated radiation in man. Int J Radiat Oncol Biol Phys 11: 791–800

Byfield JE, Frankel SS, Hornbeck CL, Sharp TR, Floyd RA, Callipari F (1985b) Phase 1 and pharmacological study of 72-hour infused 5-fluorouracil. Am J Clin Oncol 8: 429–440 (CCT)

Byfield JE, Frankel SS, Sharp TR, Hornbeck CL, Callipari F (1985c) Phase I and pharmacological study of 72-hour infused 5-fluorouracil and hyperfractionated cyclical radiation. Int J Radiat Oncol Biol Phys 11: 791–800

Byfield JE, Sharp TR, Hornbeck CL, Frankel SS, Floyd RA, Griffiths J (1985d) Phase I and pharmacologic study of oral ftorafur and x-ray therapy in advanced gastrointestinal cancer. Int J Radiat Oncol Biol Phys 11: 597–602

Byfield JE, Hornbeck CL, Frankel SS, Sharp TR, Griffiths JC (1985e) Relevance of the pharmacology of oral tegafur to its use as a 5-fluorouracil pro-drug. Cancer Treat Rep 69: 645–652

Calabro-Jones PM, Byfield JE, Ward JF, Sharp TR (1982) Time-dose relationships for 5-fluorouracil cytotoxicity against human epithelial cancer cells in vitro. Cancer Res 42: 4413–4420

Carey RW, Hilgenberg AD, Wilkins EW, Choi NC, Mathisen DJ, Grillo H (1986) Preoperative chemotherapy followed by surgery with possible post operative radiotherapy in squamous cell carcinoma of the esophagus: evaluation of the chemotherapy component. J Clin Oncol 4: 697–701

Chan A, Wong A, Arthur K (1989) Concomitant 5-fluorouracil infusion, mitomycin C and radical radiation therapy in esophageal squamous cell carcinoma. Int J Radiat Oncol Biol Phys 16: 59–65

Coia LR, Paul AR, Engstrom PF (1988) Combined radiation and chemotherapy as primary management of adenocarcinoma of the esophagus and gastroesophageal junction. Cancer 61: 643–649

Collins JM, Dedrick RL, King FG, Speyer JL, Myers CE (1980) Nonlinear pharmacokinetic models for 5-fluorouracil in man: intravenous and intraperitoneal routes. Clin Pharmacol Ther 28: 235–246

Cummings BJ, Byfield JE (1988) Treatment of cancer of the anal canal. In: Withers HR, Peters LJ (eds) Innovations in radiation oncology research. Springer, Berlin Heidelberg New York, p 91

Denham JW, Gill G, Jamieson GG et al. (1988) Preliminary experience with a combined-modality approach to the management of esophageal cancer. Med J Aust 148: 9–13

Dobrowsky W, Dobrowsky E, Strassl H, Braun O, Scheiber V (1989) Response to preoperative concomitant radiochemotherapy with mitomycin C and 5 fluorouracil in advanced head and neck cancer. Eur J Cancer Clin Oncol 25: 845–849

Duschinsky R, Pleven E, Heidelberger C (1957) The synthesis of 5-fluoropyrimidines. J Am Chem Soc 79: 4559–4560

Floyd RA, Hornbeck CL, Byfield JE, Griffiths JC, Frankel SS (1982) Clearance of continuously infused 5-fluorouracil in adults having lung or gastro-intestinal carcinoma with or without hepatic metastases. Drug Intell Clin Pharm 16: 665–667

Gastrointestinal Tumor Study Group (1982) A comparison of combination chemotherapy and combined modality therapy for locally advanced gastric cancer. Cancer 49: 1771–1777

Haghbin M, Sischy B, Hinson J (1988) Combined modality preoperative therapy in poor prognostic rectal adenocarcinoma. Radiother Oncol 13: 75–81

Heidelberger C (1975) Fluorinated pyrimidines and their nucleosides. In: Sartorelli AC, Johns DG (eds) Antineoplastic and immuno-suppressive agents, vol 2. Springer, New York Berlin Heidelberg, p 193

Hong WK, Wolf GT, Fisher S et al. (1989) Laryngeal preservation with induction chemotherapy (CT) and radiotherapy (XERT) in the treatment for advanced laryngeal cancer: interim survival data of VACSP #268, VA laryngeal cancer study group (abstr). Proc Am Soc Clin Oncol 8: 167

Jacobs C, Lyman G, Velez Garcia E, Sridhar S, Schacter L, Dalton T, Rozencweig M (1988) Comparison of infusional 5-fluorouracil (5-FU) and cis-platin (CDDP) in combination and as single agents for recurrent and metastatic head and neck cancer (abstr). Am Soc Clin Oncol 7: 154

Kalra J, Cortes E, Chen S et al. (1985) Effective multimodality treatment for advanced epidermoid carcinoma of the female genital tract. J Clin Oncol 3: 917–924

Kaplan MJ, Hahn SS, Johns ME, Steward FM, Constable WC, Cantrell RW (1985) Mitomycin and fluorouracil with concomitant radiotherapy in head and neck cancer. Arch Otolaryngol 111: 220–222

Keane TJ, Harwood AR, Rider WD, Cummings BJ, Thomas GM (1984) Concomitant radiation and chemotherapy for squamous cell carcinoma (SCC) esophagus (abstr). Int J Radiat Oncol Biol Phys 10 [Suppl 2]: 89

Keane TJ, Harwood AR, Beale FA, Cummings BJ, Payne DG, Rawlinson E (1985a) A pilot study of mitomycin C and 5-fluorouracil infusion combined with split course radiation therapy for advanced carcinomas of the larynx and hypopharynx. J Otolaryngol 15: 286–288

Keane TJ, Harwood AR, Elhakim T, Rider WD, Cummings BJ, Ginsberg RJ, Cooper JC (1985b) Radical radiation therapy with 5-fluorouracil infusion and mitomycin-C for esophageal squamous carcinoma. Radiother Oncol 4: 205–210

Leichman L, Steiger Z, Seydel HG et al. (1984) Preoperative chemotherapy and radiation therapy for patients with cancer of the esophagus: a potentially curative approach. J Clin Oncol 2: 75–79

Leichman L, Nigro N, Vaitkevicius VK et al. (1985) Cancer of the anal canal. Am J Med 78: 211–215

Leichman L, Herskovic A, Leichman CG et al. (1987) Nonoperative therapy for squamous cell cancer of the esophagus. J Clin Oncol 5: 363–370

Lo TCM, Wiley AL, Ansfield FJ et al. (1976) Combined radiation therapy and 5-fluorouracil for advanced squamous cell carcinoma of the oral cavity and oropharynx: a randomized study. Radiology 126: 229–235

Lokich J, Bothe A Jr, Fine N, Perri J (1981) Phase I study of protracted venous infusion of 5-fluorouracil. Cancer 48: 2565–2568

Ludgate SM, Crandon AJ, Hudson CN, Walker Q, Langlands AO (1988) Synchronous 5-fluorouracil, mitocycin-C and radiation therapy in the treatment of locally advanced carcinoma of the cervix. Int J Radiat Oncol Biol Phys 15: 893–899

Moertel CG, Reitemeier RJ, Hahn RG (1968) Mitomycin C therapy in advanced gastrointestinal cancer. JAMA 205: 1045–1048

Moertel CG, Childs DS, Reitemeier RJ, Colby Y, Holbrook MA (1969) Combined 5-fluorouracil and supervoltage radiation therapy of locally unresctable gastrointestinal cancer. Lancet II: 865–867

Moertel CG, Schutt AJ, Reitemeier AJ, Hahn RG (1972) A comparison of 5-fluorouracil administered by slow infusion and rapid injection. Cancer Res 32: 2717–2719

Mukherjee KL, Boohar J, Wentland D, Ansfield FJ, Heidelberger C (1963) Studies of fluoropyrimidines. XIV. Metabolism of 5-fluorouracil-C-14 and 5-fluoro-2 deoxyuridine in cancer patients. Cancer Res 23: 49–66

Murthy AK, Taylor SG IV, Showel J et al. (1987) Treatment of advanced head and neck cancer with concomitant radiation and chemotherapy. Int J Radiat Oncol Biol Phys 13: 1807–1813

Myers CE (1981) The pharmacology of the fluoropyrimidines. Pharmacol Rev 33: 1–15

Nigro ND, Vaitkevicius VK, Considine B (1974) Combined therapy for cancer of the anal canal: a preliminary report. Dis Colon Rectum 17: 354–356

Pinedo HM, Peters GFJ (1988) Fluorouracil: biochemistry and pharmacology. J Clin Oncol 6: 1653–1664

Poplin E, Fleming T, Leichman L et al. (1987) Combined therapies for squamous cell carcinoma of the esophagus: a Southwest Oncology Group study (SWOG 8037). J Clin Oncol 5: 622–628

Price LA (1987) Safer cancer chemotherapy using a kinetically-based experimental approach: higher dose intensity with reduced toxicity. Cancer Treat Rev 14: 1–9

Rich TA, Lokich JJ, Chaffey JT (1985) A pilot study of protracted venous infusion of 5-fluorouracil and concomitant radiation therapy. J Clin Oncol 3: 402–406

Roberts JG (1980) Cancer of the oesophagus – How should tumor biology affect treatment? Br J Surg 67: 791–797

Rotman M, Macchia R, Silverstein M et al. (1987) Treatment of advanced bladder carcinoma with irradiation and concomitant 5-fluorouracil infusion. Cancer 59: 710–714

Russell KJ, Boileau MA, Ireon RC et al. (1988) Transitional cell carcinoma of the urinary bladder: histologic clearance with combined 5-FU chemotherapy and radiation therapy: preliminary results of a bladder-preservation study. Radiology 167: 845–848

Seifert P, Baker LH, Reed ML, Vaitkevicius VK (1975) Comparison of continuously infused 5-fluorouracil with bolus injection treatment of patients with colo-rectal adenocarcinomas. Cancer 36: 123–128

Sischy B (1985) The use of radiation therapy combined with chemotherapy in the management of squamous cell carcinoma of the anus and marginally resectable adenocarcinoma of the rectum. Int J Radiat Oncol Biol Phys 11: 1587–1593

Sischy B, Doggett RLS, Krall JM, Taylor DG, Sause WT,

Lipsett JA, Seydel HG (1989) Definitive irradiation and chemotherapy for radiosensitization in management of anal carcinoma: interim report on radiation therapy oncology group study no. 8314. JNCI 81: 850–856

Steiger Z, Franklin R, Wilson RF et al. (1981) Complete eradication of squamous cell carcinoma of the esophagus with combined chemotherapy and radiotherapy. Am Surg 47: 95–98

Szybalski W (1974) X-ray sensitization by halopyrimidines. Cancer Chemother Rep 58: 539–537

Tang SG, Hornbeck CL, Byfield JE (1984) The potential enhancement of anti-tumor effect of ftorafur by co-administration of uracil. Int J Radiat Oncol Biol Phys 10: 1697–1790

Tapazoglou E, Kish J, Ensley, Al-Sarraf M (1986) The activity of a single-agent 5-fluorouracil infusion in advanced and recurrent head and neck cancer. Cancer 57: 1105–1109

Taylor SG IV, Murthy AK, Caldarelli DD et al. (1989) Combined simultaneous cisplatin/fluorouracil chemotherapy and split course radiation in head and neck cancer. J Clin Oncol 7: 846–856

Thomas G, Dembo A, Beale F et al. (1984) Concurrent radiation, mitomycin C, and 5-fluorouracil in poor prognosis carcinoma of cervix: preliminary results of a phase I–II study. Int J Radiat Oncol Biol Phys 10: 1785–1790

Vietti T, Eggerding F, Valeriote F (1971) Combined effect of x-radiation and 5-fluorouracil on survival of transplanted leukemic cells. JNCI 47: 865–870

Vokes EE, Panje WR, Schilsky RL et al. (1989) Hydroxyurea, fluorouracil, and concomitant radiotherapy in poor-prognosis head and neck cancer: a phase I–II study. J Clin Oncol 7: 761–768

Weissberg JB, Son YH, Papac RJ et al. (1989) Randomized clinical trial of mitomycin C as an adjunct to radiotherapy in head and neck cancer. Int J Radiat Oncol 17: 3–9

Wendt TG, Wustrow TPU, Hartenstein RC, Rohloff R, Trott KR (1987) Accelerated split-course radiotherapy and simultaneous cis-dichlorodiammine platinum and 5-fluorouracil chemotherapy with folinic acid enhancement for unresectable carcinoma of the head and neck. Radiother Oncol 10: 277–284

14 Efficacy of 5-Fluorouracil by Continuous Infusion as a Radiopotentiator – Anal and Rectal Carcinoma

BEN SISCHY

CONTENTS

14.1 Introduction

The conventional treatment for both rectal and anal carcinomas remains surgery, with a characteristic 5-year survival rate of approximately 50% at each disease site (ENBALD and ADAMI 1988). The role of radiation therapy in the management of these diseases was not recognized until fairly recently; initially radiation therapy played a palliative role but was not regarded with favor as either a definitive or an adjunct modality. Early suboptimal equipment and poor quality of delivery, coupled with disappointing results and significant morbidity, caused surgeons to remain antagonistic. Once supervoltage irradiation became available, results improved and it was possible to treat patients to tumoricidal doses within normal tissue tolerance dose levels.

In 1974 a report (NIGRO et al. 1974) was published on the use of chemotherapeutic agents [5-fluorouracil (5-FU)] administered by continuous infusion for radiopotentiation in the management of anal carcinoma. A similar pilot study was designed at Highland Hospital for patients with both rectal and anal cancers. Twelve patients were treated with continuous infusional 5-FU and eight were treated by bolus 5-FU. Within a relatively short time span it became apparent that clinical responses to therapy were enhanced when 5-FU was administered by continuous infusion and this method of delivery continues to the present time. A number of modifications have taken place in the treatment regimen, including the addition of mitomycin C.

Subsequent to this work, a variety of reports indicated that combined radiation therapy and 5-FU significantly increases tumor growth delay over the additive effect of the two modalities given independently, for schedules in which irradiation was given prior to the 5-FU. Maximum tumor growth delay occurred when radiation therapy was given prior to 5-FU, being 2.5 times the additive effect of each modality (LOONEY et al. 1979). A report (LOKICH 1985) on the optimal schedule for 5-FU therapy discussed that theoretically cancer chemotherapy should be administered continually, based on the fact that the pharmacology of most of the active chemotherapeutic agents is characterized by a short plasma half-life (10–20 min) (BYFIELD et al. 1985). It has also be demonstrated that chemotherapy toxicity is substantially reduced by a continuous infusion schedule (LOONEY et al. 1979; VOGELZANG 1984).

Two factors have emerged since combined modality therapy was instituted for patients with rectal and anal cancers. Firstly, the response of adenocarcinoma of the rectum to irradiation is much slower compared with squamous cell carcinoma of the anal canal and may continue for several months. Secondly, the time–dose relationship is not as critical in the management of squamous cell carcinoma of the anus as it is in the treatment of rectal cancer. This allows for split-course therapy if the local skin reaction necessitates a break in the treatment.

14.2 Adenocarcinoma of the Rectum

In spite of the improvements in surgery, the 5-year survival rate remains fairly static following both

BEN SISCHY, MD, Clinical Professor of Radiation Oncology, University of Rochester School of Medicine and Dentistry, and the Daisy Marquis Jones Radiation Oncology Center, at Highland Hospital, 1000 South Avenue, Rochester, NY 14620, USA

abdominoperineal (AP) and low anterior resections (BUTCHER 1971; RAO et al. 1981; BETHUNE 1987). Since the first trial which studied the effectiveness of preoperative irradiation at the Memorial Hospital (LEAMING et al. 1961) there has been a lasting interest in the role of adjuvant irradiation. The well-known study from the Veteran's Administration Surgical Oncology Group (ROSWIT et al. 1975) provided the first indication of benefit from adjuvant radiation therapy. Despite reports (FRIEDMANN et al. 1985; VIGILOTTI et al. 1987) of its efficacy, no clear-cut randomized controlled study has been available to document statistically the effectiveness of the modality and this has led surgeons to question the value of adjuvant therapy.

Recent reports are at last showing evidence of favorable and encouraging results. The final results of a randomized study by the European Organization for Research and Treatment of Cancer (EORTC) (GÉRARD et al. 1988) comparing preoperative irradiation versus surgery alone showed that the incidence of local recurrence following 34.5 Gy in 15 fractions was twice as high in the control group as in the group receiving adjuvant therapy (30% vs 15% respectively). This observed benefit was statistically significant. Following curative resection, the 5-year survival rates were 59% for patients in the control group and 69% for those in the radiation therapy group. While this difference was not statistically significant, a benefit in terms of life expectancy cannot be discounted.

A further issue has been the relative effectiveness of pre- versus postoperative radiation therapy. A report on a Swedish trial (PÅHMAN et al. 1986) with a minimum follow-up interval of 30 months showed that 13% of patients (28/217) in the preoperative group suffered local recurrence compared with 22% of patients (47/215) in the postoperative group. This difference was statistically significant. No difference in survival rates was seen between the two groups. Postoperative irradiation was less well tolerated than preoperative therapy and it was concluded that preoperative treatment may be the optimal adjunct in rectal carcinoma. In a randomized multicenter Danish trial (BALSLEV et al. 1986), 49 patients with carcinoma of the rectum and rectosigmoid were treated by postoperative irradiation or surgery alone. The probability of disease-free survival was significantly higher after radiation therapy in patients with Dukes' C tumors; the time to local failure was delayed by 1 year.

The National Surgical Project for Breast and Bowel cancers (NSABP) initiated a randomized protocol (R-01) (FISHER et al. 1988) to evaluate postoperative chemotherapy and radiation therapy in patients with Dukes' B and C lesions who had undergone a "curative" resection. One hundred and eighty-four patients were accrued to the control arm (no further therapy). An additional 184 patients received a midpelvic dose of 46 Gy (51–53 Gy maximum to the perineum), and 187 patients received chemotherapy which consisted of 5-FU, semustine, and vincristine (MOF). Radiation therapy was shown to reduce the local–regional recurrence rate, (15% vs 25%) but did not appear to influence the overall survival or disease-free survival rates.

The Gastrointestinal Tumor Study Group (GITSG) trial (1985) accrued a total of 227 patients on a four-arm study comparing postoperative irradiation, chemotherapy, postoperative irradiation combined with chemotherapy, and a control (no treatment) arm. At 5 years the group of patients who received radiation therapy and chemotherapy demonstrated the lowest recurrence rate and the control arm the highest recurrence rate. The disease-free interval for patients treated by radiation therapy and chemotherapy was significantly greater than for patients on the control arm and differed significantly between all four arms. An update of this study (DOUGLASS and MOERTEL 1986) demonstrated a survival advantage of 24% for patients on the combined treatment arm at 7 years.

The use of chemotherapeutic agents for radiosensitization is a subject that attracted considerable interest for a number of years (NIGRO et al. 1974; HEIDELBERGER et al. 1958; VIETTI et al. 1971; BYFIELD et al. 1980; NAKAJIMA et al. 1979; ROCKWELL 1982; SPREMULLI et al. 1983). Work continues in order to identify the most effective chemotherapy agents for this task, the sequencing of the two modalities, and the optimal method of administration. It is shown (HEIDELBERGER et al. 1958) that irradiation produces enhanced cell kill when tumor cells are exposed to 5-FU, and the majority of published series use a regime containing this agent, very often combined with either mitomycin C or semustine (methyl-CCNU). At this time there is no objective evidence to suggest whether bolus or continuously infused 5-FU produces the maximal enhancement of irradiation although in clinical experience (SISCHY 1985) it appears that a protracted infusion is effective. In vitro studies (BYFIELD et al. 1985; MYERS et al.

1976) indicate that the phenomenon of radiosensitization is time rather than dose dependent. A current intergroup study which is seeking to compare the effectiveness of bolus versus infusional 5-FU has been selected as one of the National Cancer Institute's high priority clinical trails. This study is examining whether adjuvant chemotherapy plus radiation can prevent relapse and also whether the administration of 5-FU by a bolus injection is as effective as by continuous infusion. The trial is being conducted jointly by the North Central Cancer Treatment Group, the Eastern Cooperative Oncology Group, the Radiation Therapy Oncology Group, the Southwestern Oncology Group, and the Cancer and Leukemia Group B.

Commencing in 1976 a series of patients with adenocarcinoma of the rectum were treated at Highland Hospital by preoperative irradiation in conjunction with chemotherapy (HAGHBIN et al. 1988). The treatment regime was designed for patients with locally advanced tumors at high risk for local recurrence. All patients had ulcerated rectal lesions at least 4 cm in size which were either partially or completely fixed. Nineteen patients had histologically well-differentiated tumors, 40 had moderately differentiated lesions, and five had poorly differentiated lesions. Sixteen lesions were judged to be initially unresectable. Between 1976 and 1986 47 males and 17 females received therapy.

All patients received a total tumor dose of 40 Gy in 4½ weeks by parallel opposed fields on an 8-MeV linear accelerator. The inferior border of the target volume was at the anal sphincter or mid-obturator foramina, depending on the location of the tumor, allowing a 2- to 5-cm margin from the distal edge of the tumor. The superior border of the treatment field was the L5–S1 interspace. The lateral margins extended to the lateral pelvic side walls with superior and inferior bilateral corners blocked obliquely (elongated diamond-shaped field). On the 2nd day of irradiation, a 96-h infusion of 5-FU at a dose schedule of $1000 \, mg/m^2/24 \, h$ was commenced. Patients also received a bolus injection of mitomycin C at a dose of 10 mg/m^2. The infusion of 5-FU was repeated, starting on day 28 of therapy. Between 4 and 6 weeks following completion of the irradiation, surgical resection was performed.

All patients achieved a response following therapy. In 12.5% of patients no residual tumor cells were identified in the operative specimen and no nodal involvement was evident in 73.5% of patients. Historically, over 50% of patients have positive nodes at surgery (GUNDERSON and SOSIN 1974). The projected disease-free survival at 5 years was 64%, with an actuarial survival of 68%. Although the small number of patients in this study prohibits subset analysis, there is a trend towards a lower rate of pelvic recurrences among those patients with no residual, or Dukes' A disease at surgery.

Since 1986 a further 11 patients have been similarly treated. This subsequent group consists of six males and five females. All lesions were greater than 4 cm in size; seven were partially fixed and four were totally fixed. Tumors in five of the patients had been declared unresectable by the referring surgeon and the remainder were marginally resectable. All these patients received between 40 and 45.9 Gy in 4.5–5 weeks, i.e., slightly higher doses than previously. The radiation fields were placed as in the original group and sensitizers were administered in an identical manner. Following therapy, three patients in this group had no residual tumor at surgery; two had perirectal lymph node involvement. One patient had an incomplete resection and received an additional postoperative irradiation boost dose of 21.98 Gy to the presacral space. Following a disease-free interval of 17 months this patient died of disease. The other ten patients remain alive and well with a follow-up period of between 4 and 29 months.

14.3 Squamous Cell Carcinoma of the Anal Canal

Squamous cell carcinoma of the anal canal is less common than adenocarcinoma of the rectum (2%–4% of rectal lesions) and relatively few patients are seen by any one physician over a period of time. It appears, however, that carcinoma of the anus is becoming more common and a greater number of cases are being referred for radiation therapy. There seems to be a relationship between squamous cell carcinoma of the anus and immune deficiency diseases (SLATER et al. 1984; PETERS et al. 1984).

The use of radiation therapy in the management of anal canal carcinoma can be traced back 70 years. The early experience, however, was limited and only small series of patients were reported. The characteristics of the x-ray equipment dictated suboptimal treatment, and complications, undesirable side-effects, and failures were often encountered. The dose-limiting factor at that time was the radiotolerance of the skin; in particular, perineal reactions were very poorly tolerated, especially by elderly patients. For this reason surgery was the treatment of choice for many years. Due to the dosimetric factors of orthovoltage therapy, interstitial irradiation was commonly used for distally situated tumors. The morbidity rate, however, remained high due to the limited experience of each operator and the lack of understanding of accurate dosimetry at that time. Most of the patients who were referred for radiation therapy in those days were medically inoperable.

A report from the Institute Curie published in 1948 (ROUXBERGER and ENNUYER 1948) discussed a series of patients who had been treated by various radiation therapy techniques and this encouraged the use of the modality. COURTAIL and FENADEZ COLMEIRO (1960) reported on 183 patients treated between 1941 and 1953 by orthovoltage irradiation and a 37% overall survival rate was achieved. It is interesting to note that the slight improvements in survival over the years bore a direct relationship to the increase in the kilovoltage used.

The problem of the inadequate depth dose was resolved in the 1950s with the advent of cobalt 60 and supervoltage equipment. As high energy radiation beams (1 MeV and higher) became available, more patients with anal carcinomas were treated by irradiation, less morbidity was experienced, and the results improved. Surgeons, however, remained reluctant to refer patients for radiotherapy and the modality was used for large inoperable lesions only. In recent years great interest has arisen in sphincter-preserving techniques and an increasing number of patients are now referred for definitive irradiation. Optimal radiation therapy techniques include the use of radiation fields to the pelvis in addition to a direct field to the perineum. The use of an *en face* electron beam to the anus as a major component of the treatment is not to the advocated, as fibrosis leading to sphincter incompetence may result. The results that may be obtained with modern radiation therapy techniques suggest that there is ample evidence to confirm Sweet's belief that anal canal carcinoma responds favorably to radiation therapy (SWEET 1947).

Although it is possible to achieve local control of primary anal canal carcinoma with definitive irradiation, total doses to the anus in the realm of 45.25–75.5 Gy are required for total tumor era-

dication. In a series of 35 patients thus treated, local control was achieved in 27 patients (77%) (DOGGETT et al. 1988). Seven patients (20%) lost sphincteric function; two of the seven required a permanent colostomy and five underwent an AP resection for either persistent or recurrent disease. Significant local morbidity may be anticipated during and following the delivery of doses of this magnitude to the perineal area.

It has become important to attempt to increase the effectiveness of irradiation biologically, particularly in areas such as the perineum where a reduction in the optimal total dose could lower the morbidity considerably. If the therapeutic gain could be enhanced, patients could be offered definitive treatment with a reasonable chance of cure while still maintaining sphincter function and sexual potency.

The radiation therapy technique that is used for any particular patient is governed by the stage of the disease and the philosophy of the radiation therapist. The status of the inguinal nodes at presentation also dictates the appropriate technique. Many patients present with a fairly long history, and because the pattern of spread is such that local and regional nodes may be involved when the primary disease is locally advanced, it is wise to treat the inguinal and pelvic nodes in all patients. The conventional field arrangement is two parallel-opposed anterior and posterior fields; great care must be taken during simulation; lead markers may be used to ensure that the anal orifice and the soft tissue of the perineum are included in the field as the position of these structures in relation to the bony landmarks is often deceptive in obese patients. The superior border of the pelvic field should extend to the L5–S1 interspace and the lateral borders of the field should extend 1 cm onto the bony pelvis. The anterior field should be approximately 3 cm greater in width than the posterior field and have approximately 1.5 cm shielded from each side in such a manner that the inguinal nodes remain in the field (inverted T) while keeping the amount of bowel exposed to the radiation to a minimum. Following delivery of the pelvic irradiation, a direct perineal field may be used to augment the radiation dose delivered to the anal canal.

Between June 1976 and August 1977, four patients with squamous cell carcinoma of the anus were treated by combined therapy at Highland Hospital (SISCHY et al. 1980). Treatment consisted of a total tumor dose of 40 Gy combined with a concurrent continuous 96-h infusion of 5-FU ($1000 \text{ mg/m}^2/24 \text{ h}$ on days 2–5 and days 28–32. A bolus injection of mitomycin C (10 mg/m^2) was also administered on day 2. Because of the accepted clinical practice at that time, each patient underwent an AP resection 4 weeks after the completion of irradiation; no tumor was identified in any of the operative specimens. Following this initial experience, 39 subsequent patients have been treated definitively by similar combined modality therapy. The dose of irradiation in this group varied from 45 to 60 Gy. The total dose was tailored to the size of the tumor and the response during therapy. If residual nodularity remained at 40 Gy an interstitial implant was performed, but the maximum dose to the anal canal never exceeded 60 Gy. Twenty-seven patients in the series were treated following superficial biopsies only. Of this number, seven patients had T_1 and T_2 lesions and 20 patients had more advanced lesions (T_3 and T_4 lesions). Twelve patients were treated following a local excision; six patients immediately postexcision and six patients at the time of tumor recurrence. The follow-up period for this group of patients is between 1 and 11 years. In those patients treated following biopsy only, the size of the lesion did not affect the immediate response rate. This may be accounted for by the fact that higher doses of irradiation were delivered to the larger lesions. However, a higher percentage of the larger lesions recurred. In the group of patients with T_1 and T_2 lesions, five of seven patients had complete clinical responses. One complete responder died of other disease. Of the two partial responders, one was salvaged by surgery and the other died of disease.

In the group of patients with T_3 and T_4 disease, 18 of 20 patients were complete clinical responders. Recurrences occurred in five of these patients, and one of them was surgically salvaged. The two partial responders both eventually died of disease.

Of these patients treated either following excision or recurrence, five patients in each category responded completely. Four patients are alive in each group but only two patients in each group remain free of disease.

Subsequent to documented evidence of the synergism of 5-FU and radiation therapy and an additive effect with mitomycin C, the Radiation Therapy Oncology Group opened a nonrandomized study (SISCHY et al. 1989) to demonstrate the effect of combined therapy for patients with anal canal

carcinomas. Following informed consent, 83 patients were entered into the study. Of 79 eligible patients there were 28 males and 51 females. Twenty-four patients (30%) had $T_1N_0M_0$ lesions, 18 (23%) had $T_2N_0M_0$ lesions, 30 (38%) had $T_3N_0M_0$ lesions, and seven (9%) had $T_4N_0M_0$ lesions. Eleven lesions (14%) were well differentiated histologically, 33 (42%) were moderately differentiate, 21 (27%) were poorly differentiated, and in 14 (18%) patients the differentiation was not stated.

All patients received 40 Gy to the pelvis combined with 5-FU and mitomycin C. Between 6 and 8 weeks following the completion of irradiation, a full-thickness biopsy of the anal canal at the site of the original lesion was performed. If the biopsy specimen was positive for tumor cells, the patient underwent an AP resection.

Of the 83 patients accrued to the study from 1983 to 1987, 79 were eligible and evaluable. Eight (10%) patients had persistent disease at the completion of therapy and underwent an AP resection; five patients received curative resection and residual disease remained in three patients. Two of these latter patients died with local disease and the third died with liver metastases, having received postoperative irradiation which achieved local control. All patients who underwent a curative resection remain well. The overall estimated survival for the group of 79 patients was 97% at 1 year, 87% at 2 years, and 73% at 3 years. The overall estimated local–regional control rate was 73% at 1 year and 71% at both 2 and 3 years. the overall estimated disease-free survival was 70% at 1 year, 63% at 2 years, and 61% at 3 years. Sixty-six patients (84%) are alive. Twelve patients (15%) are dead; nine died of anal cancer and three of intercurrent disease, including one patient who tested positive for HIV following protocol therapy.

At 3 years maximum follow-up, a statistical trend became apparent between the survival, local–regional control, and disease-free survival of patients treated strictly according to protocol guidelines compared with those patients whose treatment was not in compliance. The principal reason for noncompliance was that 5-FU was given on days during which the patient did not receive irradiation.

The Eastern Cooperative Oncology Group sponsored a trial similar to that run by the RTOG, except that following 40 Gy pelvic irradiation a boost dose of 10–12 Gy was added to the perineum (unpublished data). The median age was 59 years and there were twice as many females as males. Sixty-two percent of lesions were $T_3N_0M_0$ and extra-anal spread was present in 76% of patients. The study accrued 52 patients, of whom 50 were eligible and 45 were eligible and evaluable. Posttreatment biopsies were performed on 37 of 45 patients. The complete response rate among all 45 patients was 76%, and 81% among patients with full pathological data. The complete response rate in patients with a treatment variation was 71%. The 1-year survival of all patients in the study was 90% and the 3-year survival rate was 69%. The disease-free survival of the 45 evaluable patients was 93% at 1 year and 76% at 3 years. Three of the 45 patients have relapsed to date. In one additional patient the disease has progressed. This patient was eligible for the protocol but could not be evaluated for response because of lack of adequate data. Age, stage, and cell type did not appear to affect response or survival.

14.4 Conclusion

In spite of the fact that the optimal sequencing of surgery and irradiation has yet to be determined in the management of adenocarcinoma of the rectum, it does appear that the addition of concurrent 5-FU and mitomycin C for radiosensitization can produce a significant effect which may be translated into downstaging prior to surgery and improved survival rates.

When used in the management of squamous cell carcinoma of the anus, radiosensitizers have allowed sphincter preservation in many patients and moderate doses of irradiation may be delivered to the perineum with acceptable morbidity. At a time of heightened consumer advocacy, combined therapy is making an important contribution to the management of patients who might otherwise undergo radical surgery.

"The question is" said Alice, "whether you *can* make words mean so many different things."

References

Balslev IB, Pederson M, Teglbjaerg PS et al. (1986) Postoperative radiotherapy in Dukes' B and C carcinoma of the rectum and rectosigmoid: a randomized study. Cancer 58: 22–28

Bethune WA (1987) Carcinoma of the rectum: 508 patients with failure analysis and implication of adjuvant therapy. J Can Assoc Radiol 38: 209–216

Butcher HR Jr (1971) Carcinoma of the rectum — a choice between an anterior resection and abdomino-perineal resection of the rectum. Cancer 28: 204–207

Byfield JE, Barone R, Medelson J et al. (1980) Infusional 5-fluorouracil and x-ray therapy for non-resectable esophageal cancer. Cancer 45: 703–708

Byfield JE, Frankel SS, Hornbeck CL et al. (1985) Phase 1 and pharmacologic study of 72-hour infused 5-fluorouracil in man. Am J Clin Oncol 8: 429–440

Courtail J, Fenadez Colmeiro JM (1960) Les indications et les resultats de la roentgentherapie et al curie dans le cancer du canal anal. Arch Mal Appar Dig Suppl 49: 43–54

Doggett SW, Green JP, Cantril ST (1988) Efficacy of radiation therapy alone for limited squamous cell carcinoma of the anal canal. Int J Radiat Oncol Biol Phys 15: 1069–1072

Douglass HO Jr, Moertel CG (1986) Survival after postoperative combination treatment of rectal cancer. N Engl J Med 315: 1294

Enbald P, Adami HO (1988) Improved survival of patients with cancers of the colon and rectum? JNCI 80: 586–591

Fisher B, Woolmark N, Rockette H et al. (1988) Postoperative adjuvant chemotherapy or radiation therapy for rectal cancer: results from NSABP protocol R-01. JNCI 80: 21–29

Friedmann P, Garb JL, Park WC et al. (1985) Survival following moderate-dose preoperative radiation therapy of carcinoma of the rectum. Cancer 55: 967–973

Gastrointestinal Tumor Study Group (1985) Prolongation of the disease-free interval in surgically treated rectal carcinoma. N Engl J Med 312: 1465–1472

Gérard A, Buyse M, Nordlinger B et al. (1988) Preoperative radiotherapy as adjuvant treatment in rectal cancer. Final results of a randomized study of the European Organization of Research and Treatment of Cancer (EORTC). Ann Surg 208: 60–64

Gunderson LL, Sosin H (1974) Areas of failure found at reoperation (second or symptomatic look) following "curative surgery" for adenocarcinoma of the rectum. Clinicopathologic correlation and implications for adjuvant therapy. Cancer 34: 1278–1292

Haghbin M, Sischy B, Hinson EJ (1988) Combined modality preoperative therapy in poor prognostic rectal adenocarcinoma. Radiother Oncol 13: 75–81

Heidelberger C, Griesbach L, Montago BJ et al. (1958) Studies on fluorinated pyrimidines. 11. Effects on transplanted tumors. Cancer Res 18: 305–317

Leaming RH, Stearns MW Jr, Deddish MR (1961) Preoperative irradiation in rectal carcinoma. Radiology 77: 257–263

Lokich JJ (1985) Optimal schedule for 5-fluorouracil chemotherapy. Intermittent bolus of continuous infusion? Am J Clin Oncol 8: 445–448

Looney WB, Hopkins HA, MacLeod MS et al. (1979) Solid tumor models for the assessment of different treatment modalities. XII. Combined chemotherapy-radiotherapy: variation of time interval between time of administration of 5-fluorouracil and radiation and its effect on the control of tumor growth. Cancer 44: 437–445

Myers CE, Diasio R, Elliot HM et al. (1976) Pharmacokinetics of the fluoropyrimidines: implication for their use. Cancer Treat Rev 3: 175–183

Nakajima Y, Miyamoto T, Tanake M et al. (1979) Enhancement of mammalian cell killing by 5-fluorouracil in combination with x-rays. Cancer Res 39: 3736–3637

Nigro N, Vaitkevicius VK, Considine B Jr (1974) Combined therapy for cancer of the anal canal: a preliminary report. Dis Colon Rectum 17: 354–356

Påhman L, Glimelius B, Graffman S (1986) Pre- versus postoperative radiotherapy in rectal carcinoma: an interim report from a randomized multicentre trial. Br J Surg 72: 961–966

Peters RK, Mack TM, Berstein L (1984) Parallels in the epidemiology of selected anogenital carcinomas. JNCI 72: 609–615

Rao AR, Dagan AR, Chan PM et al. (1981) Patterns of recurrence following curative resection alone for adenocarcinoma of the rectum and sigmoid colon. Cancer 48: 1492–1495

Rockwell S (1982) Cytotoxicities of mitomycin C and x-rays to aerobic and hypoxic cells in vitro. Int J Radiat Oncol Biol Phys 8: 1035–1039

Roswit B, Higgins CA, Park WC et al. (1975) Preoperative radiation for carcinoma of the rectum and rectosigmoid. Cancer 35: 1597–1602

Roux-Berger JL, Ennuyer A (1948) Carcinoma of the anal canal; Statistic Foundation Curie. AJR 60: 807–815

Sischy B (1985) The use of radiation therapy combined with chemotherapy in the management of squamous cell carcinoma of the anus and marginally resectable adenocarcinoma of the rectum. Int J Radiat Oncol Biol Phys 11: 1587–1593

Sishcy B, Remington JH, Sobel SH et al. (1980) Treatment of carcinoma of the rectum and squamous cell carcinoma of the anus by combination chemotherapy, radiotherapy and operation. Surg Gynecol Obstet 151: 369–371

Sischy B, Doggett RLS, Krall JM et al. (1989) JNCI 81: 850–856

Slater G, Greenstein A, Aufses AH Jr (1984) Anal carcinoma in patients with Crohn's disease. Ann Surg 199: 348–350

Spremullt EN, Leith JT, Bliven SF et al. (1983) Response of a human colon adenocarcinoma (DLD-I) to x-irradiation and mitomycin C in vitro. Int J Radiat Oncol Biol Phys 9: 1209–1212

Sweet RH (1947) Results of treatment of epidermoid carcinoma of the anus and rectum. Surg Gynecol Obstet 84: 967–972

Vietti T, Enggerding R, Valeriote F (1971) Combined effect of x-radiation and 5-fluorouracil on survival of transplanted leukemic cells. JNCI 47: 865–870

Vigilotti A, Rich TA, Romsdahl MM et al. (1987) Postoperative adjuvant radiotherapy for adenocarcinoma of the rectum and recto-sigmoid. Int J Radiat Oncol Biol Phys 13: 999–1006

Vogelzang NJ (1984) Continuous infusion chemotherapy: a critical review. J Clin Oncol 2: 1289–1304

15 Hepatic Metastases from Gastrointestinal Malignancies and Hepatocellular Carcinoma

Marvin Rotman, Hassan Aziz, Seth Reiner, Jean-Philippe Austin, Richard Stark, and C. Julian Rosenthal

CONTENTS

15.1 Hepatic Metastases

The liver is the primary site of distant metastases of colorectal carcinoma and as such becomes of significant concern to the oncologist in not only advanced local disease but also the planning of early stage adjuvant therapy. WELCH and DONALDSON (1979), through a study of autopsy series, estimated that more than 80% of patients with metastatic colorectal cancer had tumor involvement of the liver. It was also estimated that in more than half of those dying of metastatic disease, the liver was the only site of involvement with the disease. This finding prompted the surgical resection of solitary metastases which yielded a relatively high 5-year survival rate of up to 33% (ADSON et al. 1984; CADY and McDERMOTT

MARVIN ROTMAN, MD, Professor and Chairman, Department of Radiation Oncology,

HASSAN AZIZ, MD, Associate Professor, Radiation Oncology,

SETH REINER, MD, Department of Radiation Oncology,

C. JULIAN ROSENTHAL, MD, Professor of Medicine and Oncology, SUNY Health Science Center at Brooklyn, 450 Clarkson Avenue, Brooklyn, NY 11203, USA

JEAN-PHILIPPE AUSTIN, MD, Department of Radiation Oncology, Charity Hospital of New Orleans, 1532 Tulane Ave., New Orleans, LA 70140, USA

RICHARD S. STARK, MD, Director Medical Oncology, Interfaith Medical Center, 555 Prospect Place, Brooklyn, NY 11238, USA

1985). Untreated patients, however, have a poor prognosis. JAFFE et al. (1968) studied the natural history of 390 patients with untreated liver metastases and estimated that the median survival of such patients was only 75 days. Later, WOODS et al. (1976) also showed a poor survival of 6–20 weeks for patients with liver metastases secondary to colorectal cancer if the liver remains untreated.

Considering the extent of the disease, the aim of treatment is twofold. For those patients in whom the liver is the only site of involvement, treatmet is aimed at prolonging survival as well as palliation. In the second group of patients in whom disease is not confined to the liver, the primary aim of treatment is palliation of pain, and the relief of conditions such as hepatic enlargement with bowel encroachment, abdominal distention, and jaundice. Prolonging symptom-free survival is an additional bonus.

15.2 Toxicity

Since the early 1920s radiotherapeutic efforts have been mainly directed toward palliating pain caused by enlargement of the liver and jaundice. Due to uncertainties about the radiation tolerance of the liver, the availability of only rudimentary ortho-voltage equipment, and the absence of medicines to relieve or prevent symptoms, hepatic irradiation was not practiced widely. More recently, with the advent of supravoltage equipment and with the development of experience gained from irradiation of the liver in patients with lymphomas and ovarian cancer, the time–dose requirements of the liver for radiation have become well established. In 1965, INGOLD et al. outlined the effect of radiation on the liver by describing the syndrome of radiation hepatitis with hepatomegaly, ascitis, jaundice, and abnormal liver chemistries. These authors stated that doses of 25–30 Gy given over 3 weeks to the entire liver are relatively safe and well tolerated. While these doses may be safe, they are also regarded as the threshhold dose range for radiation-induced hepatitis. PHILLIPS et al. (1954), who delivered doses up to 37.5 Gy in eight fractions in a series of 17 patients, reported one case of radiation hepatitis, two cases of gastrointestinal damage, and one case of radiation nephritis. An RTOG trial (BORGELT et al. 1981) in which 109 patients received a variety of doses ranging from 20 Gy in ten fractions for multiple metastases to 50 Gy in 25 fractions, including the boost dose, for solitary metastases, reported no cases of radiation hepatitis, nephritis, or pneumonitis.

In acute radiation hepatitis, the pathological changes which occur include intimal proliferation and sclerosis of central and sublobular veins. If these changes are progressive due to higher doses of radiation, partial or complete luminal obstruction will result. Vascular changes lead to sinusoidal congestion and atrophy of centrolobular liver cells (LEIBEL 1985; LEWIN and MILLIS 1973). Thus, veno-occlusive changes in the liver are the end result of acute radiation hepatitis. At this stage, some patients may recover with reversal of the histological changes described before, or these changes may lead to rapid liver failure and death. Some patients may also progress to chronic changes, which include not only the histological findings of acute changes but also portal fibrosis and lobular distortion; clinically the latter changes are accompanied by portal hypertension, development of ascites, and splenomegaly.

15.3 Survival

Radiation alone, although producing excellent palliation rates, fails to achieve any worthwhile survival rates. In 1977, PARASAD et al. reported on a series of 27 patients who were treated with radiation alone, receiving doses of up to 31 Gy in 2–5 weeks. Fifty percent of these patients showed a reduction in the size of the liver as demonstrated by physical examination and liver scan, and 70% achieved symptomatic relief with improvement of liver function tests. However, the average survival was only 4 months. SHERMAN et al. (1978) reported on a group of 55 patients who had received 24 Gy to the entire liver in eight fractions. Of these 55 patients, 24 had received radiation alone and the

rest also received chemotherapy. Analysis of the results of the entire group showed that 90% of the patients experienced symptomatic relief with a reduction in liver size. Twenty-one patients who had an excellent response had a median survival of 9 months. However, the median survival of the entire group was only 4.5 months. The RTOG (BORGELT et al. 1981) reported on a series of 109 patients with multiple or solitary liver metastases who were treated with doses ranging from 20 Gy in ten fractions to 50 Gy in 25 fractions according to whether the patient had multiple or solitary metastases. Pain was relieved in 55%, while palpable liver mass was reduced in 49%. There was no relationship between dose received and response. The median survival of patients who had died was only 11 weeks.

In an effort to improve the results of radiation alone, RTOG (LEIBEL et al. 1985) tried using misonidazole as a radiosensitizer along with irradiation of the liver. Adding misonidazole only slightly improved the results, with a median survival of 29 weeks as compared to 25 weeks without misonidazole. The failure of misonidazole to produce any substantial response led to increased use of other radiosensitizers such as 5-fluorouracil (5-FU) and halogenated pyrimidine. LOKICH et al. (1981) reported on a series of 16 patients treated with a radiation dose of 25–30 Gy in 10–12 fractions along with concomitant intra-arterial infusion of 5-FU or 5-fluorouracil deoxyribonucleoside (FUdR) given at the rate of 1 g/day and 0.5 mg/kg/day, respectively, through a hepatic catheter. A response rate of 62% was obtained and could be mostly monitored with carcinoembryonic antigen levels and liver scan. Of the 16 patients, however, eight developed thrombosis at the catheter site, which was nevertheless not life threatening. BYFIELD et al. (1984) reported on a series of 28 patients who were treated for liver metastases secondary to carcinoma of the colon, with a protracted continuous intra-arterial infusion achieved with external and internal pumps and a split course of radiation. 5-FUdR was given at 0.2 mg/kg/day and the total dose of radiation was up to 30 Gy given at 2.5 Gy/fraction for 4 days in a week followed by 10 days' rest between these cycles. Survival was analyzed according to liver function and the dose of radiation received. Patients with significant liver function impairment showed a poor median survival of only 240 days as compared to 770 days for the group with better liver function tests. Patients who received a total dose of up to

30 Gy were the longest survivors. Complications were moderate: eight patients developed severe gastrointestinal toxicity, and one patient died of radiation hepatitis.

Rotman et al. (1986) studied the use of split-course liver irradiation with continuous systemic infusion of 5-FU for the treatment of colorectal hepatic metastases. They reported on 23 patients (13 females and 10 males) with ages ranging from 41 to 84 and a median age of 62 years, all with histologically proven colorectal primaries with liver metastases.

Prior to treatment, 61% of the patients had a Karnofsky performance score of less than 60 and more than three-quarters demonstrated abnormal pretreatment liver function indices. Thirty-five percent of the patients had evidence of only hepatic metastatic disease whereas the remaining 65% had multiple organs involved with metastatic disease. Twenty patients demonstrated multiple metastases with both hepatic lobes involved while only three patients had clinically unilateral solitary lesions.

Patients were treated with external beam hepatic radiation employing a 4-MeV linear accelerator or ^{60}Co using anterior and posterior parallel opposed ports. The kidneys were localized radiographically and blocked posteriorly if indicated. Hepatic irradiation was administered with concomitant intravenous 5-FU, 25 mg/kg/24 h, over 5 days during weeks 1, 3, and 5 (Fig. 15.1). Patients were not treated during weeks 2 and 4. Radiation was given in 1.5–2 Gy fractions 5 days a week with an average radiation dose of 27.25 ± 5 Gy.

The mean and median survival for patients completing therapy was 46.21 and 30 weeks respectively. Palliation was observed in 83% (19 patients) in terms of improved performance status, reduction in pain, increased appetite, weight gain, and/or a sense of well-being. Anorexia and lassitude improved in more than 80% of the patients. No patients obtained a complete response although 15 who demonstrated an objective partial response had a mean and median survival of 62.39 and 45 weeks (Table 15.1), whereas nonrespon-

Table 15.1. Treatment of hepatic metastases with radiation and concomitant 5-FU infusion: response and survival

Objective response PR only		Median survival (weeks)
Overall		
Responders	15/13	45
Nonresponders	8/23	17
Liver involvement only	—	49
Multiple organ involvement	—	25
Karnofsky > 60	—	49
Karnofsky < 60	—	27

ders had a mean and median survival of 15.87 and 17 weeks respectively. The investigators' analysis of these data suggests that treatment-induced response was responsible for the prolonged survival.

This study also demonstrated that patients with metastases involving the liver alone had a mean and median survival of 72.56 and 49 weeks, which was significantly better than the survival of 25.07 and 25 weeks, respectively, of those patients with multiple organ involvement. Patients with a Karnofsky score of greater than 60 also demonstrated improved survival (mean and median survival of 70.11 and 49 weeks respectively) compared with those with a Karnofsky score of less than 60 (mean and median survival of 26.64 and 27 weeks respectively).

It was noted that no severe complications were encountered with the combined modality treatment. Five patients complained of nausea and one vomited during treatment. In addition, seven patients developed oral mucositis, while, as demonstrated by endoscopy, five developed superficial ulcerations of the gastrointestinal tract. Hematological toxicity also remained mild as only three patients had a WBC count lower than 2000, and only one patient had thrombocytopenia of 30 000. No patients had treatment interrupted due to hematological toxicity.

The investigators conclude that with appropriate prospective randomized studies, future elective treatment may be aimed toward combined adjunctive hepatic radiation and radiosensitization

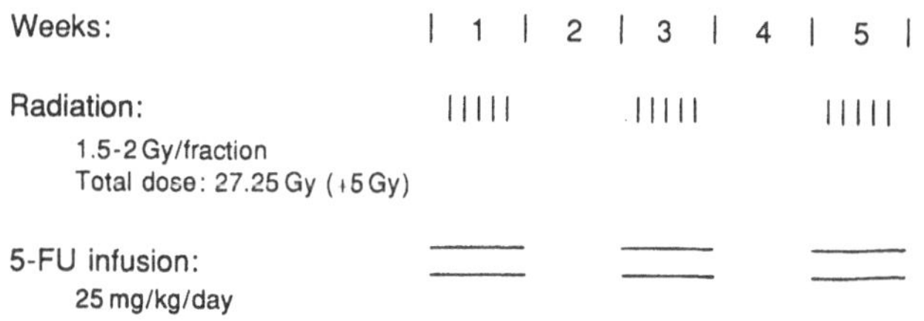

Weeks: | 1 | 2 | 3 | 4 | 5 |

Radiation: ||||| ||||| |||||
1.5-2 Gy/fraction
Total dose: 27.25 Gy (±5 Gy)

5-FU infusion: —— —— ——
25 mg/kg/day

Fig. 15.1. Treatment schema of radiation and concomitant 5-FU infusion in cases of hepatic metastases from colorectal carcinoma

with 5-FU for patients with subclinical hepatic involvement. The hope with this new approach is for eventual long-term survival and cure.

15.4 Hepatocellular Carcinoma

Surgical resection is the best mode of therapy for patients with hepatocellular carcinoma. The best 5-year survival with this form of treatment has been reported in the range of 20%–46% (IWATSU-KI et al. 1983;LEE et al. 1982). However, only a small number of patients, up to 24%–30%, can benefit from such an approach (EL-DOMEIRI et al. 1971; The Liver Study Group of Japan 1987), as the majority of patients may have extensive locoregional or distant disease. In addition, some of these patients are high surgical risks because of associated cirrhotic disease of the liver. The range of survival of patients who are not surgical candidates and remain untreated is only 2–6 months (DOCI et al. 1988; EL-DOMEIRI et al. 1971). In view of this, an alternative method of treatment has been sought for several decades.

PHILIPS and MURIKAMI at Memorial Hospital in 1960 reported the results of treatment of 26 hepatocellular carcinoma patients with radiation alone, using an average dose of 30 Gy. Since these patients belonged to a prognostically favorable group, results were correspondingly better. Of 22 patients who had received more than 20 Gy, nine exhibited marked regression of the tumor, while 11 of all 26 patients experienced excellent relief of symptoms. However, a later report from Memorial Hospital (EL-DOMEIRI et al. 1971) indicated that 30 patients receiving radiation therapy alone had very poor survival, 70% dying within a 6-month period. Eleven patients who had both radiation and sequential chemotherapy had slightly better survival, but none survived more than a year.

Regional infusion via the hepatic artery of drugs like Adriamycin, mitomycin C, 5-FU, and FUdR has also been tried. DOCI et al. (1988) recently reported the results of treatment with intra-arterial infusion of Adriamycin and 5-FU. The overall response rate with Adriamycin was 42% and with 5-FU, 22%. The overall median survival of both groups was only 3.2 months. Responders, however, had a better median survival of 13 months. FRIEDMAN et al. (1979) reported on the use of intra-arterial 5-FU infusion and hepatic radiation together with Adriamycin being given as bolus. Of 13 patients, six achieved tumor regression for a period of 4–15 months, while the majority, 11, achieved symptomatic improvement. Later FRIEDMAN (1985), through a randomized trial, showed that patients who received intravenous Adriamycin, 5-FU, and mitomycin C with radiation had a better response rate of 42% as compared with patients receiving intra-arterial Adriamycin, 5-FU, and mitomycin C with radiation, among whom there was only one responder. In this trial, all patients who received radiation alone showed no response. A further problem with intra-arterial regional infusion is that toxicity may be significant. DOCI et al. (1988), using this approach, reported that treatment-related hepatic failure occurred in 66% of cirrhotic patients and in 19% of noncirrhotic patients. The incidence of catheter-related complication was 15%. In addition, the use of intra-arterial chemotherapy is impractical, with no proven superiority over that of systemic chemotherapy.

A unique method of treatment is in use at Johns Hopkins, where ORDER et al. (1985) are delivering radiation to a dose of 21 Gy in seven fractions with simultaneous bolus injection of 5-FU and Adriamycin. A month later these patients are treated with ^{131}I antiferritin antibodies. So far, more than 100 patients have been treated. Of 79 patients evaluated for response, seven showed complete response and 43% partial response. Patients with initial low levels of α-fetoprotein had a median survival of 10.5 months.

Recently, at SUNY-Health Science Center at Brooklyn a study was initiated (ROSENTHAL et al. 1986) utilizing radiation of the liver and concomitant systemic infusion of Adriamycin in the treatment of hepatocellular carcinoma. In this study, the liver received three split courses of radiation of 1 week each. A rest period of 3 weeks was allowed between each course of radiation and Adriamycin infusion in view of the anticipated bone marrow suppression. Each course of radiation consisted of 9 Gy given at 1.8 Gy/fraction. Thus the dose of radiation achieved in three courses was 27 Gy (Fig. 15.2). Each course of radiation was accompanied by concomitant infusion of Adriamycin for 5 days given at 12 mg/m^2/day.

A total of 12 patients – seven new patients and five patients who had progressed on other treatments – were included in this study. Due to the inclusion of patients who had already failed on radiation alone or radiation together with sequen-

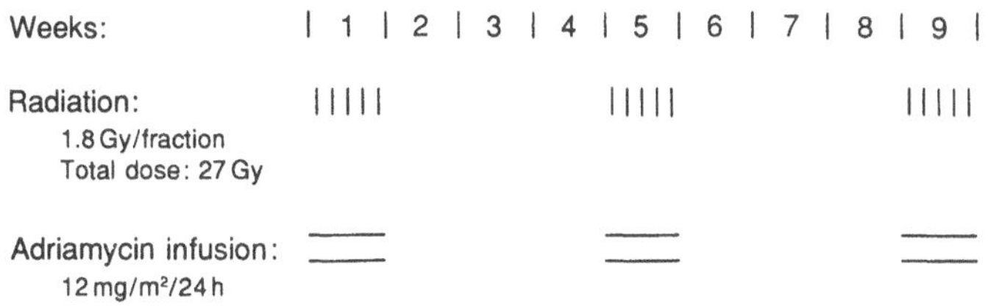

Fig. 15.2. Treatment schema of radiation and concomitant Adriamycin infusion in cases of hepatocellular carcinoma

Weeks: | 1 | 2 | 3 | 4 | 5 | 6 | 7 | 8 | 9 |

Radiation: ||||| ||||| |||||
1.8 Gy/fraction
Total dose: 27 Gy

Adriamycin infusion: ═══   ═══   ═══
12 mg/m²/24 h

tial bolus Adriamycin therapy, tolerance was only moderate. For this reason, only six of the 12 patients completed all three cycles of therapy, receiving a mean dose of 25.5 Gy and 160 mg/m^2 Adriamycin. Three patients from this group achieved partial response and one patient had his disease stabilized, while one patient progressed. Among four of the 12 patients who received only two cycles with a mean dose of 14.6 Gy and 120 mg/m^2 Adriamycin, there was one partial responder, while the other three patients progressed. The treatment of the remaining two patients was stopped due to progression of the disease. Considering all patients, four of the 12 had a partial response, with a mean survival time of 40 weeks (Table 15.2). The longest survival was 72 weeks and the shortest was 24 weeks. One patient with stable disease was lost to follow-up after 32 weeks of survival.

Assessment of toxicity was difficult due to the inclusion of patients, as discussed above, who already had failed on hepatic radiation or hepatic radiation and bolus Adriamycin therapy. However, all patients demonstrated leukopenia with a range of 0.7–3.7, with one patient developing sepsis. The platelet range was between 28 000 and 214 000. Gastrointestinal toxicity was moderate: five patients experienced nausea and vomiting, while two patients had mucositis. Hepatic toxicity was demonstrated in three patients: two patients

had a transient rise of bilirubin and one patient, at 72 weeks, developed intrahepatic cholestasis. Deterioration of liver function, which was noted in most of the patients, could not be conclusively attributed to either the treatment or the disease.

15.5 Conclusion

Successful treatment of hepatic metastases is still evolving. Considerable experience has been gained with hepatic artery infusion with 5-FU or 5-FUdR with or without radiation. However, in a randomized study, systemic continuous infusion chemotherapy and radiation has been shown to be a superior method of treatment. The use of a split-course of radiation with the concomitant use of i.v. 5-FU as a radiosensitizer not only has enhanced the therapeutic ratio, reducing the complication rates experienced with intra-arterial infusion, but also has proven to be more practical. The results of an ongoing RTOG trial (RTOG Protocol 84–05) using accelerated fractionation are also awaited.

Similarly, in hepatocellular carcinoma, radiation of the liver combined with systemic chemotherapy can produce a response rate of 40%–50%. These results approach those obtained by regional intra-arterial infusion and radiation. Although antiferritin antibody ^{131}I treatment appears better in terms of response and survival, its availability and usage is more limited. The split course of radiation and concomitant use of infusion of Adriamycin is well tolerated, and clinically does not produce significant hepatocellular dysfunction except for mildly elevated liver function tests. The response rate and survival in our series were poor becasue of inclusion of patients who already had failed other therapies. With careful selection of patients with better prognostic features, the treatment with a split course of radiation to the liver together with infusion of Adriamycin may represent an optimal therapy.

Table 15.2. Treatment of hepatocellular carcinoma with radiation and concomitant Adriamycin infusion: response and survival

	Objective response PR only	Median survival (weeks)
Overall	4/12	40 (range 24–72 weeks)
Pts completing 3 cyles of therapy	3/6	—
Pts with 2 cycles of therapy	1/4	—
Pts with 1 cycle of therapy only	0/2	—

References

Adson MA, Van Heerden JA, Adsen M (1984) Resection of hepatic metastases from colorectal cancer. Arch Surg 119: 647

Borgelt BB, Gelber R, Brady LW, Griffin T, Hendrickson R (1981) The palliation of hepatic metastases: results of the Radiation Therapy Oncology Group pilot study. Int J Radiat Oncol Biol Phys 7: 587–590

Byfield JE, Barone RM, Frankel SS, Sharp TR (1984) Treatment with combined arterial 5-FUDR infusion and whole liver radiation for colon carcinoma metastatic to liver. Am J Clin Oncol 7: 319–325

Cady B, McDermott W (1985) Major hepatic resection for metachronous metastases from colon cancer. Ann Surg 201–204

Case TJ, Warthin AS (1924) The occurrence of hepatic lesions in patients treated by intensive deep roentgen irradiation. AJR 12: 27–46

Doci R, Bignami P, Bozzetti F, Bonfanti G, Audiso R, Colombo M, Gennari L (1988) Intrahepatic chemotherapy for unresectable hepatocellular carcinoma. Cancer 61: 1983

El-Domeiri AA, Huvos AG, Goldsmith HS, Foot W (1971) Primary neoplasm of the liver: results of radiation therapy. Cancer 27: 7–11

Friedman MA (1985) Combination chemotherapy and whole liver irradiation for hepatic tumors. In: Bottino JC, Opfell RW, Muggia FM (eds) Liver cancer. Martinus Nijhoff, Boston, p 315

Friedman MA, Volberding PA, Cassidy MJ, Resser KJ, Wasserman TH, Philips TL (1979) Therapy for hepatocellular cancer with intrahepatic intra-arterial Adriamycin and 5-fluorouracil combined with whole liver radiation: an NCOG study. Cancer Treat Rep 63: 1885–1888

Ingold JA, Reed GB, Kaplan HS, Bagshaw MA (1965) Radiation hepatitis. AJR 93: 200–208

Iwatsuki S, Shaw BWI, Starzl TE (1983) Experience with 150 liver resections. Ann Surg 2: 247–253

Jaffe BM, Donegan WL, Watson F, Spratt JS Jr (1968) Factors influencing survival in patients with untreated hepatic metastases. Surg Gynecol Obstet 127: 1–11

Lee NW, Wong J, Ong GB (1982) The surgical management of primary cancer of the liver. World J Surg 6: 66–75

Leibel SA (1985) Radiation therapy of hepatobiliary tumors. In: Bottino JC, Opfell RW, Muggia FM (eds) Liver cancer. Martinus Nijhoff, Boston, pp 297–312

Leibel SA, Pajak TF, Order SE et al. (1985) Hepatic metastases: results of treatment and identification of prognostic factors (Radiation Therapy Oncology Group report) (abstr). Int J Radiat Oncol Biol Phys II [Suppl I]: 116–117

Lewin K, Millis RR (1973) Human radiation hepatitis. A morphologic study with emphasis on the late changes. Arch Pathol 96: 21–26

Lokich J, Kinsella T, Perri J, Malcolm A, Clouse M (1981) Concomitant hepatic radiation and intraarterial fluorinated pyrimidine therapy. Correlation of liver scan, liver function tests and plasma CEA with tumor response. Cancer 48: 2569–2574

Order SE, Stillwagon GB, Klein JL et al. (1985) Iodine[131] antiferritin: a new treatment modality in hepatoma. A Radiation Therapy Oncology Group study. J Clin Oncol 3: 1573–1582

Parasad B, Lee MS, Hendrickson FR (1977) Radiation of hepatic metastases. Int J Radiat Oncol Biol Phys 2: 129–132

Phillips R, Murakami F (1960) Primary neoplasm of the liver: results of radiation therapy. Cancer 13: 714–720

Phillips R, Karnofsky DA, Hamilton LD, Nickson JJ (1954) Roentgen therapy of hepatic metastases. AJR 71: 826–834

Rosenthal CJ, Rotman M, Bhutiani I (1986) Concomitant radiation therapy and doxirubicin by continuous infusion in advanced malignancies – a phase II study. Evidence of synergistic effect in soft tissue sarcomas and hepatomas. In: Rosenthal CJ, Rotman M (eds) Clinical applications of continuous infusion chemotherapy and concomitant radiation therapy. Plenum, New York, p 159

Rotman M, Kuruvilla A, Choi K et al. (1986) Response of colorectal metastases to concomitant radiotherapy and intravenous infusion 5-fluorouracil. Int J Radiat Oncol Biol Phys 12: 2179–2187

RTOG Protocol 84–05. Phase I/II dose-escalating trial of accelerated fractionation in palliative irradiation of hepatic metastases.

Sherman DM, Weichselbaum R, Order SE, Cloud L, Trey C, Piro AJ (1978) Palliation of hepatic metastases. Cancer 41: 2013–2017

The Liver Study Group of Japan (1987) Primary liver cancer in Japan. Sixth report. Cancer 60: 1400–1411

Welch JP, Donaldson GA (1979) The clinical correlation of an autopsy study of recurrent colorectal cancer. Ann Surg 189: 496

Woods CR, Gillis CR, Blumgart LH (1976) A retrospective study of the natural history of patients with liver metastases from colorectal cancer. Clin Oncol 2: 285–288

16 The Use of Infusional 5-Fluorouracil, Mitomycin C, and Radiation as the Primary Management of Esophageal Cancer

LAWRENCE R. COIA, PATRICK STAFFORD, PAUL F. ENGSTROM, ANTHONY R. PAUL, and GERALD E. HANKS

CONTENTS

The results of surgery or radiation therapy as primary management of esophageal cancer have been dismal, with median survivals generally less than 1 year and 5-year survivals under 10% (EAR-LAN and CUNHA-MELO 1980; LANGER et al. 1986). There have been several reports which indicate that the use of concurrent chemotherapy and radiation therapy in the management of esophageal cancer may offer an alternative to the standard approaches (COIA et al. 1987; JOHN et al. 1987; KEANE et al. 1989). These studies demon-strate that excellent local control and palliation with a chance for long-term survival can be obtained.

In 1980, investigators at the Fox Chase Cancer Center began a pilot study which involved the use of conventional radiation to 60 Gy with two 4-day infusions of 5-fluorouracil (5-FU) (1 g/m^2 days 2–5 and 29–32) and bolus mitomycin C (10 mg/m^2 day 2). All patients, regardless of age, tumor location, tumor size, or presence of distant metastases, were eligible for this study if they had biopsy-proven cancer of the esophagus, ECOG performance of 0, 1, or 2, and adequate renal, hepatic, and hemato-logical function. Less than 10% of patients evalu-ated were excluded because of failure to meet these eligibility criteria. Between 1980 and 1989, 95 patients have been treated in this protocol. The results of 90 patients treated through September 1989, which have been published in full detail elsewhere, form the basis of this report (COIA et al. 1990).

There have been 57 patients with clinical stage I or II disease, that is, disease limited to the esopha-gus, who have been treated with curative intent. Thirty-three patients with clinical or pathological evidence of extraesophageal extension or distant metastases or who had recurrent tumor or multiple primary tumors were treated with palliative intent. The treatment of the palliative patients differed from the definitive ones in that the dose of radia-tion was generally decreased to 50 Gy and che-motherapy, i.e., 5-FU, was continued following the initial treatment regimen until the time of disease progression.

LAWRENCE R. COIA, MD, Fox Chase Cancer Center, Associate Professor Radiation Oncology, University of Pennsylvania School of Medicine, Central & Shelmire Aves., Philadelphia, PA 19111, USA

PATRICK STAFFORD, PhD, Fox Chase Cancer Center, Assis-tant Professor Dept. of Radiation Oncology, University of Pennsylvania School of Medicine, Central & Shelmire Aves., Philadelphia, PA 19111, USA

PAUL F. ENGSTROM, MD, Vice President, Population Sci-ence, Department of Medical Oncology, Fox Chase Cancer Center, Central & Shelmire Aves., Philadelphia, PA 19111, USA

ANTHONY R. PAUL, MD, Department of Radiation Oncol-ogy, Fox Chase Cancer Center, Central & Shelmire Aves., Philadelphia, PA 19111, USA

GERALD E. HANKS, MD, Chairman, Dept. of Radiation Oncology, Fox Chase Cancer Center, Professor and Vice-Chairman, Dept. of Radiation Oncology, University of Pennsylvania, School of Medicine, Central & Shelmire Aves., Philadelphia, PA 19111, USA

16.1 Radiation Treatment Technique

All patients underwent simulation of radiation treatment fields prior to treatment. Treatments were given at 2 Gy/day with 10 MeV or higher energy photons and there was no correction for lung inhomogeneity. Custom fabricated blocks were used to block lung, stomach, heart, or liver when appropriate. Compensating filters were also used where appropriate. The initial target volume included a minimum of 5 cm above and below the tumor with lateral borders at least 2 cm beyond the tumor. Tumor extent was defined by endoscopic examination, esophagogram, and CT scan. The periesophageal nodes were always included, as was the mediastinum. The supraclavicular nodes were included for tumors located above the carina while the celiac nodes were included with distal esophageal disease. The initial target volume received 40 Gy. The first 30 Gy was given AP-PA with patients in either supine or prone position. The next 10 Gy was given with a three-field technique – one anterior field and two posterior obliques. The patient was treated in the prone position after 30 Gy in order to displace the esophagus from the spinal cord. During the reduced field treatment of 20 Gy (definitive) or 10 Gy (palliative) the patient was treated in the prone position using a target volume 2 cm beyond the tumor in superior, inferior, and radial extent. The boost field for distal lesions generally excluded at least one-half of the stomach. The spinal cord dose never exceeded 46 Gy even including the contribution from the oblique fields. All fields were treated daily.

16.2 Chemotherapy

Although it is feasible to deliver infusional 5-FU at home, most patients received infusional chemotherapy as inpatients. Patients received two 4-day infusions of 5-FU starting days 2 and 29 at 1 g/m^2/24 h with a maximum daily dose of 1900 g. Mitomycin C was given at 10 mg/m^2 as a single bolus on day 2 only, with a maximum single dose of 19 mg. Full calculated doses were administered unless there were concerns related to the patient's ability to tolerate a full dose, e.g., age >75 years. A dose reduction of 10%–20% was made under such circumstances. Weekly or more frequent blood counts were monitored and a 25% dose reduction in 5-FU was administered if the WBC was 3000–5000 or the platelet count was 75 000 to 100 000 on day 29.

Table 16.1. Staging of esophageal cancer

Stage I	Tumor ≤5 cm, no obstruction, not circumferential, no extraesophageal spread[a]
Stage II	Tumor >5 cm, obstructing or circumferential, but no extraesophageal spread[a]
Stage III	Tumor with extraesophageal spread
Stage IV	Tumor with distant metastases

[a] Extraesophageal spread defined by: recurrent laryngeal, phrenic, or sympathetic nerve involvement; fistula formation; involvement of trachea or bronchial tree; vena caval obstruction; malignant effusion; biopsy-proven supraclavicular, mediastinal, or celiac nodal involvement

16.3 Staging

Patients were staged using a modification of the 1978 AJC staging system (shown in Table 16.1). This was a clinical staging system and not based on post-surgical results as is the present system. The results of the CT scan had no bearing on patient stage unless the CT scan documented distant metastases (liver, lung, brain). A stage IV was added to differentiate patients with distant metastases from those with local extraesophageal spread (stage III).

16.4 Definitive Treatment Results

The patient characteristics in the definitive (curative) group are shown in Table 16.2. Note that even patients 92 years of age have been treated with this aggressive regimen. Although most patients had squamous cell carcinoma there were a large number of patients with adenocarcinoma. There were only three cervical esophageal cancers, and the majority of thoracic esophageal cancers were in the distal thoracic esophagus, i.e., the last 10 cm. Although nearly half the tumors were less than 5 cm in length, most were obstructing. There were 13 stage I tumors and 44 stage II.

The disease-specific actuarial survival in the definitive group of 57 patients was 51% at 2 years, while with 14 patients at risk for 5 years the actuarial 5-year survival was 39%. As illustrated in Figure 16.1, patients with Stage I cancer had a significantly better survival than patients with Stage II cancer (p = .03). The 2-year actuarial survival for patients with Stage I cancer was 91% compared to 33% for patients with Stage II can-

Table 16.2. Patient and tumor characteristics for definitively treated patients

No. of patients	57
Age	
Median	66
Range	45–92
Sex	
Male	41
Female	16
Location	
Cervical	3
Thoracic – upper 2/3	18
Thoracic – lower 1/3	36
Histology	
Squamous	39
Adenocarcinoma	16
Undifferentiated	2
Length	
≤5 cm	25
>5 cm	28
>10 cm	4
Stage	
(definitive)	
I	13
II	44

cer. Examining survival by histology, a better outcome for patients with squamous cell carcinoma than adenocarcinoma was found although these differences did not reach statistical significance. The 2-year actuarial survival for squamous cell carcinoma was 57%, compared with 38% for adenocarcinoma. In addition, the median survival for patients with squamous cell cancer was 33 months, compared with 15 months for adenocarcinoma.

The actuarial local relapse-free survival in the definitive group is shown in Fig. 16.2. At 2 years and beyond the local relapse-free survival was 70%. Again patients with stage I cancer had a significantly better local relapse free survival than patients with stage II cancer. The local relapse free survival at 3 years was 100% for stage I cancer vs 60% for Stage II (p = .04). When examining the local relapse-free survival by histology a modest improvement for squamous cell cancers over adenocarcinomas was seen although again statistical significance was not reached. At 1 year there was an 82% local relapse-free survival for squamous cell cancers versus 69% for adenocarcinomas.

Of the 57 patients treated definitively there were only five who had local only failure. Twenty-seven have had a recurrence. Twelve of the 27 had local failure as some component of failure, whereas 22 have had a distant component of failure. The subsequent management of patients with local only recurrence has occasionally been successful, as shown in Table 16.3. Patient #1 failed more than 6 years after diagnosis and because of his advanced age and debilitated condition was not able to undergo esophagectomy. Patient #2, with a recurrent adenocarcinoma of the esophagus, underwent esophagectomy at 10 months and is still disease-free more than 5 years following initial diagnosis. Patient #3 developed a local only recurrence 2 years following diagnosis and still has local only disease nearly 4 years after initial treatment. She has refused esophagectomy and has been managed with brachytherapy and laser treatments. Patients #4 and #5 have had persistent local disease or early recurrence and have both died.

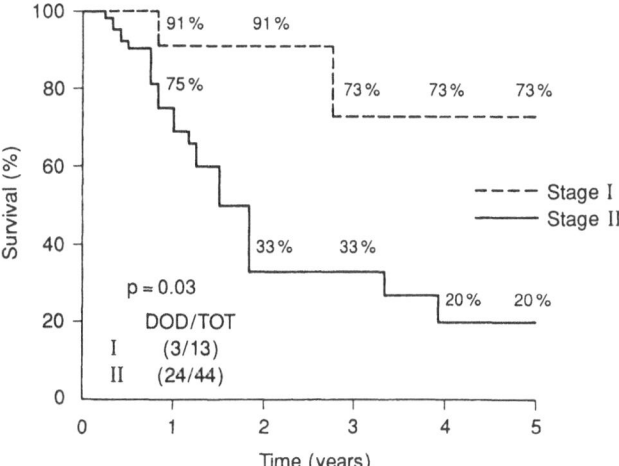

Fig. 16.1. Disease-specific actuarial survival of 57 definitively treated patients with esophageal cancer: stage I vs stage II

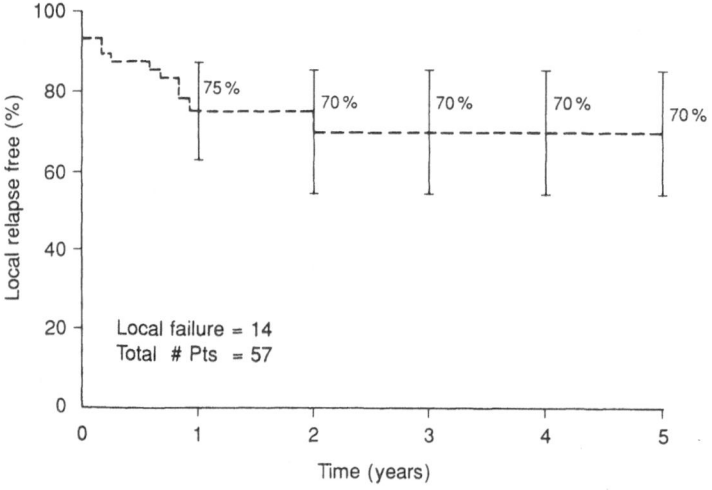

Fig. 16.2. Actuarial local relapse-free survival of 57 definitively treated patients with esophageal cancer. *Error bars* represent ± 2 standard errors

Table 16.3. Management and outcome of patients with local only failure

Patient No.	Histology	Time to local failure	Salvage	Outcome
1	Adenocarcinoma	75 mo	None	Dead 81 mo
2	Adenocarcinoma	10 mo	Resection	NED 64 mo
3	Squamous	24 mo	Laser/brachy therapy	Persistence 45 mo
4	Adenocarcinoma	2 mo	Resection	Lung mets., 5 mo
5	Squamous	0 mo	–	Died 1 mo post Rx

NED, no evidence of disease

16.5 Palliative Treatment Results

There were 33 patients treated palliatively and their characteristics are listed in Table 16.4. Again, there was a relatively high proportion of patients with adenocarcinoma compared to the literature. This treatment provides a high degree of palliation even in patients with advanced disease, as shown in Table 16.5. Palliation, defined as the ability to swallow at least soft solid foods, was obtained in 23 of the 30 evaluable patients (77%). Lasting palliation was obtained in 18 of the 30 patients (60%). The median survival was 8 months and there are two patients surviving more than 2 years following treatment. Figure 16.3 shows the overall survival of this palliative group of patients. The median survival for patients with stage III disease was 7 months while for patients with stage IV disease it was 9 months.

Table 16.4. Patient and tumor characteristics for palliatively treated patients

No. of patients	33
Age	
Median	64
Range	45–81
Sex	
Male	28
Female	5
Location	
Cervical	1
Thoracic – upper 2/3	14
Thoracic – lower 1/3	18
Histology	
Squamous	19
Adenocarcinoma	12
Undifferentiated	2
Length	
≤5 cm	3
>5 cm	21
>10 cm	9
Stage (palliative)	
III	12
IV	13
Other	8

16.6 Overall Morbidity

The acute toxicities of treatment include esophagitis, stomatitis, candidiasis, and nausea as well as hematological problems including leukopenia and thrombocytopenia. About 10% of the patients developed severe acute esophagitis or hematological problems which required more than 10 days' treatment break or hospitalization for manage-

Table 16.5. Freedom from dysphagia in the palliative group

No. of patients	No. with dysphagia pre-Rx	No. free of dysphagia post-Rx	No. without dysphagia until death	Median dysphagia-free duration
33	30	23 (77%)	18 (60%)	5 months

ment. There have been two treatment-related deaths. One patient had a perforated esophagus and mediastinitis with no tumor seen at autopsy. Another patient died of a myocardial infarction 1 month posttreatment.

Late complications are moderate in severity and include stricture, gastritis, pneumonitis, and pericarditis. There have been only two patients with pneumonitis and one patient with pericarditis. Most of the patients with gastritis had distal lesions with substantial portions of the gastric mucosa included in the field. The gastritis generally has resolved with conservative outpatient management. The most significant late complication is symptomatic stricture, which has occurred in about 11% of the patients. There has been no patient with radiation-related symptomatic stricture who has not achieved relief in dysphagia symptoms through the use of esophageal dilatation.

16.7 Conclusions

This treatment regimen of 5-FU, mitomycin C, and radiation is an effective and well-tolerated regimen that provides a preferred alternative to surgery in the definitive and palliative management in most patients with esophageal cancer. The results of selected studies employing concurrent radiation and chemotherapy as primary therapy indicate that a local relapse-free rate of 70% or more is achievable (COIA et al. 1987; JOHN et al. 1987; KEANE et al. 1989). These nonsurgical regimens have also demonstrated the potential for long-term survival in patients with clinical stage I and II disease, with approximately half such patients living at least 2 years. Long-term palliation is achievable in nearly two-thirds of patients with clinical evidence of extra-esophageal extension. Treatment mortality from this regimen is less than 5%.

These results are also superior to most studies utilizing preoperative chemotherapy and concurrent radiation to 30 Gy (FRANKLIN et al. 1983; LEICHMAN et al. 1984; POPLIN et al. 1987). The median survival in three such studies ranged from 12 to 19 months and treatment-related mortality was 11%–13%. About one-quarter to one-third of the patients had no evidence of cancer in the resected specimens in these studies; however, it was only that group of patients that had any chance for long-term survival. These preoperative studies question the need for esophagectomy and would lend support to the use of high dose radiation with concurrent chemotherapy to improve local response. The most promising results of combined radiation and chemotherapy prior to surgery have been reported by FORASTIERE et al. (1990). Using an aggressive combined modality approach they obtained a median survival of 21 months for patients with squamous cell cancer while the median survival for patients with adenocarcinoma has

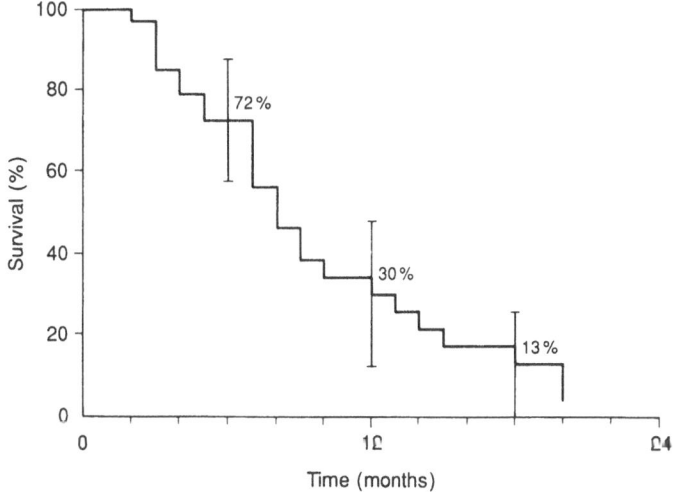

Fig. 16.3. Actuarial survival of patients treated with palliative intent (stage III and IV). Survival at 6, 12, and 18 months is shown along with ± 2 standard errors

not been reached. However, the median follow-up was only 26 months and there was considerable toxicity with a minimum hospitalization of 3 weeks prior to surgery as well as the postoperative recovery period.

Our results indicate that significant local control and palliation can be obtained with concurrent high dose radiation and chemotherapy. Preliminary results from a recent randomized study by the Eastern Cooperative Oncology Group indicate improved survival in patients with esophageal squamous cell cancer who received a similar chemoradiation treatment regimen when compared with radiation alone controls. These results and those of other randomized studies are needed to establish the superiority of chemoradiation over radiation alone.

References

Coia LR, Engstrom PF, Paul AR (1987) Nonsurgical management of esophageal cancer: report of a study of combined radiotherapy and chemotherapy. J Clin Oncol 5: 1783–1790

Earlan R, Cunha-Melo JR (1980) Esophageal squamous cell carcinoma: a critical review of surgery. Br J Surg 67: 381–390

Franklin R, Steiger Z, Vaishnampayan G et al. (1983) Combined modality therapy for esophageal squamous cell carcinoma. Cancer 51: 1062–1071

John M, Flan M, Wittlinger P (1987) Inoperable esophageal carcinoma: results of aggressive synchronous radiotherapy and chemotherapy. Am J Clin Oncol (CCT) 10: 310–316

Keane TJ, Harwood AR, Elhakin T et al. (1989) Radical radiation therapy with 5-fluorouracil infusion and mitomycin C for esophageal squamous carcinoma. Rad Ther Oncol 4: 205–210

Langer M, Choi NC, Orlow E et al. (1986) Radiation therapy alone or in combination with surgery in the treatment of carcinoma of the esophagus. Cancer 58: 1208–1213

Leichman L, Steiger Z, Seydel HG et al. (1984) Preoperative chemotherapy and radiation therapy for patients with cancer of the esophagus: a potentially curative approach. J Clin Oncol 2: 75–79

Poplin E, Fleming T, Leichman L et al. (1987) Combined therapies for squamous cell carcinoma of the esophagus: a SWOG study. J Clin Oncol 5: 622–628

Forastiere A, Orringer M, Perez-Tanayo C, Urba S, Husted S, Takasugi B, Zaharak M (1990) Concurrent chemotherapy and radiation followed by transhiatal esophagectomy for local-regional cancer of the esophagus. J Clin Oncol 8: 119–127

Coia L, Engstrom P, Paul A, Stafford P, Hanks G (1990) Long-term results of infusional 5-FU, mitomycin-C and radiation as primary management of esophageal carcinoma. Int J Radiat Oncol Biol Phys (in press)

17 Concomitant Radiation and 5-Fluorouracil for Head and Neck Cancer

Bernard J. Cummings, Thomas J. Keane, and A. Michael Rauth

CONTENTS

17.1 Introduction

One of the first trials of concomitant radiation and chemotherapy to show any improvement in survival rates included the administration of 5-fluorouracil (5-FU) during the course of radiation treatment of oral and oropharyngeal cancers (Lo et al. 1976). Nevertheless, while the premise that the cure rates for squamous cell cancers of the head and neck can be increased by the addition of chemotherapy to radiotherapeutic and surgical protocols is attractive, any clear demonstration of benefit from such combinations remains elusive. If a cytotoxic drug has demonstrable activity against the cancer being treated, combining such a drug with radiation might improve local control rates and reduce the incidence of distant metastases. If there is any synergistic interaction between the drug and radiation, a greater level of control might be achieved in tissues exposed to both agents than would result from the additive cytotoxic effects of the combination (Steel and Peckham 1979). However, if synergistic or additive effects also increase damage to normal tissues, the therapeutic ratio could be adversely affected by combined

Bernard J. Cummings, MBChB, FRCPC, Thomas J. Keane, MBChB, MRCPI, FRCPC, Department of Radiation Oncology, A. Michael Rauth, PhD, Division of Physics, Ontario Cancer Institute, 500 Sherbourne Street – Princess Margaret Hospital, Toronto, M4X 1K9, Canada

modality therapy. The many difficulties in interpreting the literature relating to laboratory studies and to clinical trials of combinations of radiation and cytotoxic drugs have been reviewed recently (Fu 1985; Iscoe 1987; Steel 1988; Tannock 1989).

Radiation produces response rates close to 100% in primary squamous cell cancers of the head and neck, but whereas such response rates are associated with high cure rates in early stage cancers, more advanced disease frequently relapses even when radiation is combined with radical resection. Treatment with 5-FU results in overall response rates of about 15% in recurrent and metastatic squamous cell cancers of the head and neck (Carter 1977), but there are virtually no data on the response rate to 5-FU as a single agent in previously untreated head and neck cancer. The interaction of 5-FU and radiation has been studied in the laboratory and in the clinic since the synthesis of 5-FU in 1957. In this chapter the results of studies of concomitant radiation and 5-FU as they apply to the treatment of squamous cell cancers of the head and neck are surveyed.

17.2 Laboratory Studies

5-Fluorouracil is a fluorinated pyrimidine which is anticipated to demonstrate activity only in cycling cells. The anabolic products of 5-FU may interfere with DNA production by inhibiting the enzyme thymidylate synthetase, be incorporated into RNA via a ribose nucleotide, or be incorporated into DNA as a deoxyribose nucleotide, and cause other changes such as membrane effects and alterations of mitochondrial function (see reviews by Valeriote and Santelli 1984; Pinedo and Peters 1988) Radiation induces a variety of physically and chemically mediated perturbations in cell metabolism and growth. Which of these effects, if any, might lead to synergistic potentiation of radiation damage, or conversely to radiation enhancement of drug action, in cells exposed to both 5-FU and radiation is not known.

Despite 30 years of study there is still considerable dispute over whether 5-FU acts additively with radiation, or whether there is synergistic interaction or "potentiation." Different conclusions may be drawn according to the experimental system used and the endpoints studied (WEINBERG and RAUTH 1987; STEEL 1988). WEINBERG and RAUTH (1987) have summarized the conclusions from the various laboratory studies as follows: in in vitro experiments any increased effect of combined 5-FU and radiation over radiation alone (a) has occurred only when 5-FU is itself toxic to the cells under study, (b) is greater when 5-FU is present for extended durations, and (c) is not apparently due to inhibition of repair of the sublethal or potentially lethal damage induced by radiation. WEINBERG and RAUTH (1987) consider that most results from in vitro studies can be interpreted as favoring additive rather than synergistic interaction. Most in vivo experiments have been conducted in mice and have used intraperitoneal bolus injections of 5-FU and single large doses of radiation, or continuous drug infusions and continuous low dose-rate irradiation, and do not simulate clinical practice. Although some studies have suggested a time-dependent increase in response to combinations of radiation and 5-FU, the mode of interaction and the optimum sequencing of drug and radiation have not been clarified (WEINBERG and RAUTH 1987; STEEL 1988). WEINBERG and RAUTH's (1987) experiments were based on a tumor regrowth delay assay in a murine squamous cell tumor (SCC VII/SF), continuous infusion 5-FU, and multiple radiation fractions. They found that infusions of 5-FU produced greater effects than intraperitoneal bolus injections, and that tumor responses were dependent on total 5-FU dose, but independent of time of drug administration with respect to radiation when 5-FU was given shortly before or after radiation. The efficacy of high dose, extended duration 5-FU infusion and radiation combinations was limited, probably because of overlapping radiation and drug-sensitive cell populations in the tumor. Isobologram analysis suggested additive, and in some situations subadditive, effects rather than any synergistic interaction between 5-FU and radiation. These results differed from the observations of BYFIELD et al. (1982), who found synergistic potentiation when cells were subjected in vitro to prolonged 5-FU exposure after irradiation, and

WEINBERG and RAUTH (1987) speculated that this difference might be due to the types of cells used in the different experiments, because only in the HeLa and HT29 adenocarcinoma cell lines studied by BYFIELD has a change in the slope of the radiation dose–response curve been observed after exposure to combined 5-FU and radiation. Thus the mode of interaction of 5-FU and radiation may be dependent on the cells used and/or the level within the cell at which 5-FU expresses its critical effects, such as the incorporation of metabolites into DNA or RNA or the blockade of thymidylate synthetase.

The effects of combining radiation and 5-FU have been evaluated principally in tumors and in other acute-reacting tissues, and it is possible that different conclusions on interactions between drug and radiation might be drawn from studies based on late-reacting tissues. In one such experiment, VON DER MAASE et al. (1986) found no enhancement of late lung damage in mice treated with single doses of intraperitoneal 5-FU 15 min before single dose total lung irradiation. In a wide-ranging review of in vivo studies in which radiation and cytotoxic drugs were combined, STEEL (1988) emphasized the potential for increased normal tissue toxicity from concurrent radiation and chemotherapy. The issue of therapeutic ratio has not been addressed in most in vivo laboratory studies although Fu et al. (1984) observed a small therapeutic gain in an experiment in which mouse intestinal crypt cells were used as the reference normal tissue.

The relevance of many of these laboratory studies to clinical practice is not yet clear. In some instances, clinical treatment protocols have been designed on the basis of observations made in the laboratory. In other cases, experimental evidence has been invoked in efforts to explain the results of empirically developed clinical programs.

17.3 Clinical Studies

17.3.1 5-Fluorouracil Alone Combined with Radiation Therapy

One of the earliest randomized studies which combined 5-FU and radiation in head and neck cancer was conducted at the MD Anderson Hospital (FLETCHER et al. 1963, 1967) (Table 17.1). Twelve patients with pharyngeal wall carcinomas received

Table 17.1 Radiation and concurrent 5-FU

Reference	Treatment, dose and schedule	5-FU timing	Toxicity	Patients	Tumor sites	Outcome
FLETCHER et al. 1963, 1967 (randomized)	5-FU 12 mg/kg/dx5, IVB; RT 60 Gy/6 wk (2 Gy/d); (Control RT 60–74 Gy/6–8 wk)	Second week of RT	Increased acute Increased late fibrosis	28	Pharyngeal walls	No benefit
Lo et al. 1976 (randomized)	5-FU 10 mg/kg/d D1–3, IVB; 5-FU 5 mg/kg/d Mon, Wed, Fri during RT, IVB; RT 60–70 Gy/7–10 wk (2 Gy/d);	1–3 h before RT	Increased acute Increased late	66	Oral cavity	Improved 5-yr survival 40% vs 15%, $P < 0.05$
Lo et al. 1976 (randomized)	As above	As above	Increased acute Increased late	70	Oropharynx	Improved 5-yr survival, P not significant
Lo et al. 1976 (randomized)	As above	As above	Not stated	45	Nasopharynx, hypopharynx, larynx	No benefit
BYFIELD et al. 1984	5-FU 20–30 mg/kg/24 hr, D1–5, CVI; RT 10 Gy/4 d (2.5 Gy/d) D1–4; Cycles repeated each 2 wk × 5	Concurrent with RT	Tolerable mucositis Increased late fibrosis	12	Various	9/12 local control 70% 2-yr survival
HODSON, personal communication, 1989 (randomized)	5-FU 1200 mg/m²/24 hr, D1–3 and D14–16, CVI; RT 66 Gy/ 6.5 wk (2 Gy/d); (Control RT same)	Concurrent with RT	–		Oral cavity, oropharynx, hypopharynx, larynx	In progress
SHIGEMATSU et al. 1971 (randomized)	5-FU 2–10 mg/kg/d, IAI, up to 4 wk; RT 50–80 Gy/5–8 wk (2 Gy/d); (Control RT same)	Concurrent with RT	Increased acute skin and mucosal reaction. Late toxicity not described	63	Paranasal sinuses	No survival benefit
NITZE et al. 1971	5-Fu 1000 mg/12 hr, CVI, twice a wk; RT 5 Gy twice a wk to 40–60 Gy	Stop 8 h before RT	Not described	13	Various	"Tumor regression"

IVB = intravenous bolus injection, CVI = continuous venous infusion, IAI = intraarterial infusion

five daily bolus intravenous injections of 5-FU 12 mg/kg/day given either immediately prior to the commencement of radiation therapy or during the 2nd week of treatment, and 16 patients received radiation plus a placebo drug. Radiation therapy was tolerated when delivered at the rate of 10 Gy each week to a total dose of 60 Gy. Bone marrow depression, pulmonary infections, and gastrointestinal reactions were considered to be the most significant acute side-effects, and severe late tissue fibrosis was more common than after radiation alone. The authors did not consider the combination produced better local control or survival than radical radiation alone, and no details were given to suggest any difference in outcome in those patients who received 5-FU during the course of radiation rather than before radiation.

A trial generally considered to have shown benefit from combining 5-FU with radiation was started at the University of Wisconsin in 1961. In an analysis of 136 patients with advanced cancers arising in the oral cavity (66 patients) or oropharynx (70 patients) treated by either radiation or by radiation plus 5-FU, Lo et al. (1976) concluded that local control and survival were better in the combined treatment group than in patients who received radiation alone. In patients with oral cavity cancer, the difference in 5-year survival was statistically significant ($P < 0.05$, 40% vs 15%), whereas although an advantage was also seen from combined treatment in those with oropharyngeal cancers, the difference was not significant (25% vs 15%). The addition of 5-FU improved the probability of locoregional control but did not alter the incidence of distant metastases. Patients in the combined treatment group developed more severe acute mucosal reactions, and major late complications such as bone necrosis or fistula formation were seen only in those who had received 5-FU and radiation. In this study 5-FU was given by intravenous bolus injection about 1–3 h prior to radiation. The dose was 10 mg/kg/day on the first 3 days of treatment, followed by 5 mg/kg on day 4, and then continued at 5 mg/kg/day each Monday, Wednesday, and Friday until the completion of radiation treatment unless severe toxicity developed. The minimum radiation dose to the primary tumor was 60–70 Gy in 6–10 weeks. Smaller numbers of patients with cancers of the hypopharynx, nasopharynx, or larynx were treated with a similar protocol without any apparent benefit (ANSFIELD et al. 1970).

BYFIELD et al. (1984) described a treatment protocol based on their in vitro studies which indicated that synergistic interaction of 5-FU and radiation would be most likely if 5-FU was present for 48 h after radiation, and in doses sufficient to produce a primary cytotoxic effect from 5-FU. Peripheral intravenous infusions of 5-FU lasting 120 h were delivered, with concurrent radiation in four sequential daily fractions of 2.5 Gy on days 1 through 4 of each 5-day infusion cycle. An interval of at least 9 days or longer was allowed after each cycle so that local mucositis could resolve. A total of five radiation–drug cycles was given, followed usually by further radiation alone to a total dose of about 70 Gy. Doses of 5-FU between 20 and 30 mg/kg/24 h were evaluated. The maximum tolerated dose, based on the occurrence of confluent mucositis and the ability to take only fluids by mouth, was 25 mg/kg/24 h [34 of 47 (72%) cycles completed]. Skin reactions and systemic toxicity were mild and did not limit treatment. Late fibrosis in the irradiated areas was thought to be greater than that expected after radiation alone. Nine of 12 evaluable patients with stage IV cancers at a variety of sites achieved a complete response with a 2-year survival rate of 70%. In a related study, SHARP et al. (1983) found that 72-h infusions of 5-FU 40 mg/kg/24 h could be combined with four radiation fractions of 2.5 Gy, two fractions each day for 2 days, and delivered in a similar cyclical fashion. The limiting toxicity was mucositis in the irradiated volume, and neurological toxicity was also somewhat more common with the shorter higher dose 5-FU infusions. There was no comment on the response to treatment in the few patients mentioned in this report. There are no completed randomized trials of radiation and concurrent intravenous infusional 5-FU given as a single drug, although such studies are in progress. HODSON (personal communication, 1989) is conducting a randomized trial in which radical radiation (66 Gy in 33 fractions in 6½ weeks) is compared with similar radiation combined with two 72-h infusions of 5-FU 1200 mg/m²/24 h (1000 mg/m² is equivalent to approximately

20–25 mg/kg) given during the 1st and 3rd week of treatment.

Several studies have been reported in which intravenous infusions of 5-FU have been given on the same day as radiation but have been deliberately terminated several hours prior to radiation (NITZE et al. 1971; MARZECKI et al. 1980; WILL et al. 1983). The objective of these schedules has been to induce some degree of cell synchrony by exposure to 5-FU, and then to irradiate about 8 h later when tumor cells are considered likely to have progressed to a more radiosensitive phase of the cell cycle. These studies have not been randomized, and no convincing evidence of benefit has been presented.

Several investigators, particularly in Japan, have studied the role of intra-arterial infusions of 5-FU and radiation in the treatment of paranasal sinus cancers. None of these studies has been randomized, and opinion is mixed on the value of such treatment (SATO et al. 1970; SHIGEMATSU et al. 1971; GOEPFERT et al. 1973; TSUJII et al. 1986). In one center in which treatment was allocated on the basis of odd and even case record numbers, SHIGEMATSU et al. (1971) found improved local control from combined treatment in the 1st year after therapy, but no survival advantage. In these treatment protocols the usual dose of 5-FU was 250 mg (about 5 mg/kg) delivered over 1–24 h either immediately prior to or concurrently with radiation via a catheter inserted into an artery feeding the sinus cancer. Total doses of 5-FU ranged from about 2000 mg to 5000 mg in 4–5 weeks. Radiation was usually delivered at the rate of 10 Gy each week to total doses of about 50–80 Gy. Systemic effects such as leukopenia and gastrointestinal reactions were infrequent, but skin and mucosal reactions were often severe and dose limiting (SATO et al. 1970; SHIGEMATSU et al. 1971; TSUJII et al. 1986). No detailed information has been published on late normal tissue damage following these treatment programs.

17.3.2 Multiple Drug Therapy Including 5-FU Combined with Radiation Therapy

Because 5-FU as a single agent has relatively limited activity against squamous cell cancers arising in the head and neck, it is not surprising that it has been combined with other drugs, often of similarly limited effectiveness, in efforts to improve clinical results. The interpretation of the results of such studies, and the identification of the mechanism of any interactions in these multiple agent protocols, is very difficult.

The combination of radiation, 5-FU, and mitomycin C has received wide attention because of its apparent effectiveness in producing responses in squamous cell cancers in a variety of sites (CUMMINGS et al. 1986) (Table 17.2). Nonrandomized studies of this combination for advanced head and neck cancers produced high response rates (KAPLAN et al. 1985; KEANE et al. 1985; MAGUIRE et al. 1987; DOBROWSKY et al. 1989). It was thus disappointing to find in a large randomized trial for patients with advanced cancers of the larynx or hypopharynx that the combination of 5-FU and mitomycin C with split-course radiotherapy produced results that were no better than those of standard uninterrupted radiation alone (KEANE and HARWOOD, unpublished data). One hundred and six patients were treated by radical radiation therapy (50 Gy in 20 fractions in 28 days), and 103 received split-course radiation (25 Gy in 10 fractions in 14 days, repeated after a 28-day interval) with a continuous peripheral intravenous infusion over 96 h of 5-FU 1000 mg/m²/24 h on the first 4 days of each course, and mitomycin C 10 mg/m² by intravenous bolus injection on the 1st day of each course. In both groups, surgery was reserved for the management of residual or recurrent cancer. There were no differences in overall survival between the treatment arms (3-year actuarial rate, 45%), or in survival or local control rates in the laryngeal and pharyngeal subsets. Acute toxicity, the morbidity following salvage surgery, and late normal tissue changes were similar following both treatment schedules. Mucositis was apparent in the irradiated volume after about 15 Gy in patients who received radiation combined with chemotherapy, compared with about 20–25 Gy in those treated by radiation alone. Split-course radiation was adopted for this trial after an earlier pilot study had shown that this chemotherapy protocol caused intolerable mucositis when combined with uninterrupted radical radiation as given in the control arm of the trial (KEANE et al. 1985).

The combination of 5-FU, mitomycin C, and radiation has also been evaluated as preoperative adjuvant therapy. KAPLAN et al. (1985) gave 5-FU 1000 mg/m²/24 h by continuous intravenous infusion on days 1 through 4, and mitomycin C 10 mg/m² by intravenous bolus injection on day 1. Radiation was begun on day 1 and was given in a split-course, 30 Gy in 15 treatments in 3 weeks, followed by a 2-week rest, and a further 20 Gy in ten treatments without concomitant chemotherapy. Surgery followed 4–6 weeks after the completion of radiotherapy. DOBROWSKY et al. (1989) used an uninterrupted schedule of 50 Gy in 25 treatments in 5 weeks, with concurrent 5-FU 750 mg/m²/24 h by continuous intravenous infusion over the first 5 days of treatment, coupled with a

Table 17.2 Radiation and concurrent 5-FU and mitomycin C (MTC)

Reference	Treatment, dose and schedule	5-FU timing	Toxicity	Patients	Tumor sites	Outcome
KEANE and HARWOOD (unpublished) (randomized)	5 FU 1000 mg/m²/24 hr D1–4 and D49–52, CVI; MTC 10 mg/m² D1 and D49, IVB; RT 25 Gy/2 wk (2.5 Gy/d) starting D1 and D49; (Control RT 50 Gy/4 wk)	Concurrent with RT	Tolerable acute No increase in late	209	Larynx, hypopharynx	No benefit in survival or in locoregional control
KAPLAN et al. 1985	5-FU 1000 mg/m²/24 hr D1–4, CVI; MTC 10 mg/m² D1, IVB; RT 30 Gy/3 wk (2 Gy/d); 2 wk interval; 20 Gy/ 2 wk ± 10 Gy/ wk; Surgery 4–6 wk after RT	Concurrent with RT	Severe mucositis 5/ 31 No increase in surgical complications	31	Various	61% CR rate clinical 52% CR rate histopath. No survival data
DOBROWSKY et al. 1989	5-FU 750 mg/m²/24 hr D1–5, CVI; MTC 15 mg/m² D1, IVB; RT 50 Gy/5 wk (2 Gy/d); Surgery 3–5 wk after RT	Concurrent with RT	Mucositis tolerable	41	Oral cavity, oropharynx	56% CR rate histopath. 63% 18 to 30 month survival
MAGUIRE et al. 1987	5-FU 20 mg/kg/24 hr D1–5, and D22–26, CVI; MTC 7.5 mg/kg D1, IVB; RT 10 GY/2 wk (2 Gy/d); 1 wk interval; 20 Gy/2 wk; Cycle of drugs and RT repeated after 2 wk	Concurrent with RT	Tolerable acute	24	Various	88% CR rate clinical

single bolus dose of mitomycin C 15 mg/m² on day 1. In this protocol surgery was performed 3–5 weeks after radiation. DOBROWSKY et al. (1989) noted that while pronounced mucositis generally appeared at about 20 Gy, interruption of the treatment was rarely required. Both DOBROWSKY and KAPLAN observed clinical and histopathological response rates of about 90% (complete plus partial response rates) although it is noteworthy that both also found microscopic residual cancer, of unknown viability, in about 40% of the patients in whom response was considered complete clinically. A randomized trial comparing preoperative radiation with preoperative radiation and concomitant 5-FU and mitomycin C is in progress (CONSTABLE, personal communication, 1989).

One of the most popular current cytotoxic drug regimens for head and neck cancer is cisplatin combined with infusional 5-FU. This combination has achieved a response rate of about 90% in previously untreated patients in several series

(ISCOE 1987). Both cisplatin and 5-FU have produced radiosensitization in some laboratory studies (see also Chap. 27) (Table 17.3). MURTHY et al. (1987) adopted a similar philosophy to that followed by BYFIELD et al. (1984) and developed a cyclical protocol in which high doses of chemotherapy were combined with multiple short courses of radiation. They described a protocol in which each treatment cycle consisted of cisplatin 60 mg/m² on day 1, 5-FU continuous peripheral intravenous infusion 800 mg/m²/24 h for 5 days, and radiation 2 Gy each day for days 1 through 5. The treatment cycle was repeated every 2 weeks for seven cycles over a total of 13 weeks. In this regimen mucositis was not found to be dose limiting in 34 patients with advanced cancers at various sites who were treated with curative intent. Fifty percent had a complete response and 41% a partial response. Including those patients who underwent surgery after chemotherapy and radiation, locoregional control was maintained in 87%, and

Table 17.3. Radiation and concurrent 5-FU and cisplatin (CP)

Reference	Treatment, dose and schedule	5-FU timing	Toxicity	Patients	Tumor sites	Outcome
MURTHY et al. 1987	5-FU 800 mg/m²/24 hr D1–5, CVI; CP 60 mg/m² D1, IVB; RT 10 Gy/5 d (2 Gy/d) D1–5; Cycle repeated alternate wk to 70 Gy/13 wk	Concurrent with RT	4 deaths attributed in part to chemotherapy. Mucositis tolerable. Late toxicity not described	34	Various	59% CR rate clinical; Locoregional control 27/31 53% 2-yr survival
ADELSTEIN et al. 1986	5-FU 1000 mg/m²/24 hr D1–4, CVI; CP 75 mg/m² D1, IVB; RT 30 Gy/3 wk (2 Gy/d); Surgery 5–9 wk after RT; Cycle repeated postoperatively	Concurrent with RT	Severe myelosuppression 42%; Weight loss average 12%; Severe mucositis 21%	38	Oral cavity, oropharynx, hypopharynx, larynx	74% disease-free at 2 years
WENDT et al. 1987	5-FU 350 mg/m² D1, IVB; FA 50 mg/m² D1, IVB; 5-FU 350 mg/m²/24 hr D1–4, CVI; FA 100 mg/m²/24 hr D1–4, CVI; CP 60 mg/m² D1, IVB; RT 23.4 Gy/9 d (1.8 Gy 2x/d); Cycle repeated D1 and D44 to 70.2 Gy/51 d	Concurrent with RT	Mucositis tolerable	34	Oral cavity, oropharynx, hypopharynx, larynx	87% CR rate clinical; Local control 81% 2 yr 58% 2-yr; survival
BOLLA et al. 1988	5-FU 400 mg/m² D1–6, 2 hr CVI; CP 20 mg/m² D1,2,5,6 20 min CVI; RT 3 Gy D3 and D4; Cycle repeated 3x at 3 wk intervals; Then 60 Gy/6 wk (2 Gy/d) without chemotherapy	After RT on D3 and D4	Mucositis tolerable Late toxicity not described	36	Various	11% CR rate clinical after 3 courses drugs and RT; 30% CR rate clinical after definitive RT

FA = Folinic Acid

actuarial survival at 2 years was 66%. Four deaths occurred during treatment which were considered to be due, at least in part, to chemotherapy-related toxicity. ADELSTEIN et al. (1986) treated patients with advanced cancers with concurrent multimodality therapy preoperatively, and again postoperatively. Their schedule was designed to deliver a total of four 4-day infusions of 5-FU, four bolus injections of cisplatin, and two courses of radiation, each of 30 Gy in 3 weeks. The protocol was considered relatively toxic, but tolerable. Thirty-five of 38 (92%) patients were rendered disease-free, and the projected 2-year disease-free survival rate was 74%. In efforts to exploit several currently popular treatment strategies, WENDT et al. (1987) treated patients with cancers arising in various head and neck sites with a program of cyclical twice daily radiation together with concurrent cisplatin by bolus intravenous injection, combined with 5-FU and folinic acid, which were each given as both bolus injections and infusions. Overall acute toxicity levels were considered acceptable, and a 2-year local control rate of about 80% and survival rate of about 60% were obtained. Based on laboratory experiments with L1210 ascitic tumor and a fibrosarcoma in the mouse, a group at Grenoble developed a clinical treatment program in which they delivered three courses of chemotherapy and low doses of radiation, followed after 3 weeks by definitive radiation (BOLLA et al. 1988; DIONET et al. 1988). Each course was repeated every 3 weeks according to a relatively complicated protocol. Cisplatin (20 mg/m^2) was given in a 20-min infusion, followed by a 2-h infusion of 5-FU (400 mg/m^2) on days 1, 2, 5, and 6. Radiation in doses of 3 Gy each day was given on days 3 and 4, followed by a 2-h infusion of 5-FU (400 mg/m^2). Definitive irradiation was given in a dose of 60 Gy in 30 fractions in 6 weeks. Thirty-six patients with advanced cancers were treated, and a complete response rate of 30% and a partial response rate of 30% were achieved. This program is currently being compared in a randomized trial with radical radiation, 76 Gy in 38 fractions in 52 days (BOLLA et al. 1988).

Several other drug and radiation combinations have been evaluated in nonrandomized studies, including intravenous bolus 5-FU–adriamycin–bleomycin (SMITH et al. 1980), intravenous bolus 5-FU and intramuscular retinol palmitate (KOMIYAMA et al. 1985), and intravenous infusions of 5-FU and hydroxyurea (see Chap. 18). As with all of the pilot studies mentioned in this survey, high response rates are reported but are difficult to evaluate in the absence of concurrent and randomized control groups.

17.4 Discussion

It would seem that any benefits from administering 5-FU concurrently with radiation therapy for squamous cell cancers of the head and neck are marginal, at least in the schedules and patient groups so far reported. However, the myriad variations in scheduling and patient selection have made interpretation of the published studies difficult and require further clarification.

It is often assumed, on the basis of that laboratory evidence which does suggest synergistic interaction between 5-FU and radiation (BYFIELD et al. 1982), that any potentiating effect requires prolonged exposure to 5-FU during radiation therapy, but the most appropriate duration of that exposure and the means of attaining it are unclear. Most recent studies have adopted the 4- or 5-day continuous infusion and dosage schedules developed for the treatment of colorectal cancer (LOKICH 1985), but there are no studies which address the ideal schedule for the use of 5-FU against head and neck cancer. These short infusion schedules were developed to deliver as much 5-FU as possible with tolerable acute normal tissue toxicity. While there is evidence that response rates, and therefore by inference tumor cytotoxicity, are higher with short course infusions of 5-FU than with repeated bolus injections (LOKICH 1985), there is no evidence that maximum cytotoxicity from 5-FU is associated with maximum sensitization. In view of the short half-life of 5-FU, continuous infusion may be desirable if the presence of the intact 5-FU molecule during radiation is necessary, but the half-lives of the various metabolites of 5-FU may be more relevant, and effective drug–radiation interactions may be achievable by multiple intravenous bolus injections such as those given by Lo et al. (1976). If interaction is desirable throughout the radiation schedule, should infusions of 5-FU be prolonged over full 4- to 7-week courses of radical radiation? There may be an upper limit to the optimum duration of 5-FU infusion for it to be active as a single agent with radiation (WEINBERG and RAUTH 1987). Prolonged low dose infusions of 5-FU may not provide the drug-mediated tumor cytotoxicity which some laboratory studies suggest is necessary for potentiating interaction (see also Chap. 21), and higher dose prolonged infusions of 5-FU may cause unwanted toxicity because of the saturable clearance process (PINEDO and PETERS 1988).

The limiting acute toxicity of high-dose infusional 5-FU includes oral and gastrointestinal mucositis. FU (1979) noted that enhancement of normal tissue damage from concurrent radiation and chemotherapy is likely to be more severe when the cytotoxic drug in question is also toxic to the tissue irradiated. When given concurrently with radiation, intravenous and intra-arterial infusions of 5-FU, and even repeated bolus injections of 5-FU, have all produced significant and at times dose-limiting oral and pharyngeal mucositis. It is impossible to determine from the published reports whether this is due simply to the additive effects of overlapping spectra of normal tissue toxicity, or whether there is a true synergistic interaction between radiation and drug in the normal mucosa. Similarly, the increase in late fibrosis described in some series may be due to simple additive normal tissue damage.

The severe acute mucositis produced by radiation and concurrent high dose 5-FU has often forced investigators to adopt unconventional, split-course radiation protocols. BYFIELD et al. (1984) have shown that a recovery period of about 9 days is generally required to allow further treatment after four daily radiation doses each of 2.5 Gy with concurrent 120-h infusions of 5-FU at dose levels of up to 25 mg/kg/24 h. After ten treatments each of 2.5 Gy in 12 days with concurrent 5-FU infusions (1000 mg/m^2/24 h for 4 days) and mitomycin C, the Princess Margaret Hospital group found that recovery of the mucosa took about 3 weeks (KEANE et al. 1985). However, DOBROWSKY et al. (1989) were able to deliver both mitomycin C and infusional 5-FU (750 mg/m^2/24 h for 5 days) with uninterrupted radiation up to 50 Gy at 2 Gy each day, and HODSON (personal communication, 1989) has found that two 72-h infusions of 5-FU 1200 mg/m^2/24 h can be given 2 weeks apart during an uninterrupted course of 66 Gy in daily fractions of 2 Gy. The development and intensity of mucositis thus seems to be a function of both the size of the daily radiation fractions, and the dose and duration of the 5-FU infusion, and may be further affected by any other cytotoxic drugs given concurrently with the radia-

tion. Another variable which may have an effect on the extent and severity and tolerability of mucositis, but on which there is no information in the published reports, is the volume of the various mucosal regions irradiated and the location of the reaction within the air and food passages of the head and neck. While split-course or multiple short cycles of radiation will diminish acute tissue reactions, the prolongation of treatment in this way does not protect against late normal tissue damage, and may also be inferior treatment if accelerated tumor growth occurs during the extended treatment period (WITHERS et al. 1988). Furthermore, split-course radiation generally controls fewer cancers than uninterrupted radiation delivered to a similar total dose, and attempts to compensate for extended overall treatment times by increasing the radiation dose may greatly increase the incidence of late normal tissue toxicity (OVERGAARD et al. 1988). It is important to resolve the issue of whether chemotherapy schedules should be adjusted in order to be compatible with conventional uninterrupted radiation schedules, or whether multiple cycles of radiation should be adopted, each coupled with concurrent chemotherapy as favored by BYFIELD et al. (1984) and others. Radiation oncologists are reluctant to interfere with established uninterrupted radiation protocols, and these will presumably remain the standard against which programs of radiation and concurrent chemotherapy will be tested. The critical endpoints for establishing whether there has been an improvement in therapeutic ratio will depend not so much on acute toxicity levels, which have determined the design of so many of the protocols, as on sustained tumor control rates and late normal tissue toxicity. There has been too little attention given to the assessment and reporting of late normal tissue damage in most of the studies published.

When 5-FU is delivered concurrently with radiation, the intention is principally to exploit any sensitizing interaction between radiation and 5-FU on the primary tumor and the regional lymph nodes. Although there is a high incidence of distant metastases from advanced head and neck cancers – up to 50% in some series (PAPAC 1984) – the limited doses of 5-FU used in most of the protocols can be expected to have only a minor therapeutic influence on distant metastases. The multiple courses of concurrent radiation and chemotherapy in schedules such as those developed by BYFIELD et al. (1984) and MURTHY et al. (1987)

may have greater effect against systemic metastases, but similar doses of chemotherapy can be delivered without concurrent radiation. There is some evidence from in vitro studies that 5-FU can increase the risk of distant metastases from irradiated tumor cells (VAN PUTTEN et al. 1975), but the relevance of these experiments to clinical practice is unknown and the clinical studies which have included 5-FU have not suggested any adverse effects of this kind.

Many of the more recently published protocols include the concurrent use of more than one cytotoxic agent. Drugs may be combined to take advantage of differing normal tissue toxicities, or for their effects on different target cell populations in the tumor. For example, mitomycin C in the concentrations used in clinical practice has no demonstrable value in the laboratory as a radiosensitizer, but may be of value because of its relatively greater toxicity for hypoxic cells (ROCKWELL 1982; MARSHALL and RAUTH 1988). However, caution is required in combining cytotoxic drugs, since there may be unanticipated alterations in pharmacokinetics, as has been demonstrated with mitomycin C (VERWEIJ et al. 1986), or unexpected increases in damage to normal tissues (STEEL 1988).

Only five of the many clinical studies reviewed have been randomized in any way (FLETCHER et al. 1963; ANSFIELD et al. 1970; SHIGEMATSU et al. 1971; Lo et al. 1976; KEANE and HARWOOD, unpublished). Of these only one has used high dose infusional intravenous 5-FU and in that trial mitomycin C was also given (KEANE and HARWOOD, unpublished) (Tables 17.1–17.3). The single positive result was for patients with oral cavity cancers who received multiple bolus injections of 5-FU during the course of radiation (Lo et al. 1976), and it is disappointing to note that this study has never been repeated. The design of the Wisconsin trial (Lo et al. 1976) does not permit any conclusion as to whether 5-FU and radiation had additive or synergistic effects. As discussed previously, until the mechanisms of potentiating interactions are clarified, the relative merits of multiple daily intravenous bolus injections and of continuous infusions will remain unknown. Although survival and control rates were not improved in the Toronto randomized trial of split-course radiation, 5-FU, and mitomycin C, there may be an exploitable benefit to be realized from this drug combination, particularly if it can be integrated into a conventional course of uninter-

rupted radical radiation. Since split-course radiation alone is inferior to a similar total dose of uninterrupted radiation (OVERGAARD et al. 1988), it appears that the two courses of 5-FU and mitomycin C given in this study compensated for any tumor regrowth during the additional 4-week duration of the protocol. It is also of interest that there has so far been no apparent increase in late normal tissue toxicity following the split-course radiation and 5-FU and mitomycin C, whereas increased toxicity would have been anticipated if the radiation dose had been increased to compensate for the extended overall treatment time (OVERGAARD et al. 1988). There are no completed randomized trials of other multiple drug combinations and radiation.

The empirical nature of most of the studies, and the relative infrequency of head and neck cancer, has frequently led to the aggregation of patients with cancers in many different sites. The variable natural histories of cancers arising in different sites, even in restricted regions such as the larynx or hypopharynx, are well known. Many of the studies which have grouped together all advanced head and neck cancers may have been capable of detecting only a very large effect from the combinations of radiation and chemotherapy. Since the benefits of combination therapy may be marginal against large cancers, it may be more useful to test combinations such as 5-FU and radiation against more limited early stage cancers, in patient groups stratified by the site of origin of the cancer.

One of the disappointments in most of the randomized trials which have employed concurrent and cytotoxic drugs has been the failure to produce the improvements in tumor control and survival anticipated from laboratory experiments or from the response rates seen in pilot clinical studies. Possible explanations for this failure have been discussed by TANNOCK (1989), and include the often relatively limited tumor cell kill achieved by cytotoxic drugs, subpopulations of tumor cells resistant to both radiation and chemotherapy, and stimulation of tumor cell proliferation by cytotoxic drugs. Whatever the reasons, infusions of 5-FU given concurrently with radiation have as yet no place as standard therapy for head and neck cancers, but there are many possibilities for further studies. The greatest priorities are for randomized clinical studies in which radiation protocols use identical fractionation schedules, and in which preferably only one variable, for example an infusion of 5-FU, is evaluated in each trial. Such studies may be relatively tedious, and progress slow, but they will avoid many of the problems of interpretation present in more complex protocols and allow a firm basis to be laid for studies of concurrent cytotoxic drug and radiation combinations.

References

Adelstein DJ, Sharan VM, Earle AS et al. (1986) Chemoradiotherapy as initial management in patients with squamous cell carcinoma of the head and neck. Cancer Treat Rep 70: 761–767

Ansfield FJ, Ramirez G, Davis HL, Korbitz BC, Vermund H, Gollin FF (1970) Treatment of advanced cancer of the head and neck. Cancer 25: 78–82

Bolla M, Borgel J, Guenon A, Junien-Lavillauroy C, Dionet C, Vrousos C (1988) Chemotherapy with low doses of radiation followed by definitive radiotherapy for advanced unresectable carcinoma of the head and neck. NCI Monogr 6: 357–359

Byfield JE, Calabro-Jones PM, Klisak I, Kulhanian F (1982) Pharmacologic requirements for obtaining sensitization of human tumor cells in vitro to combined 5-fluorouracil or ftorafur and x-rays. Int J Radiat Oncol Biol Phys 8: 1923–1933

Byfield JE, Sharp TR, Frankel SS, Tang SG, Callipari FB (1984) Phase I and II trial of five-day infused 5-fluorouracil and radiation in advanced cancer of the head and neck. J Clin Oncol 2: 406–413

Carter SK (1977) The chemotherapy of head and neck cancer. Semin Oncol 4: 413–424

Cummings BJ, Keane TJ, Harwood AR, Thomas GM (1986) Combined modality therapy with 5-fluorouracil, mitomycin C and radiation therapy for squamous cell cancer. In: Rosenthal CJ, Rotman M (eds) Clinical applications of continuous infusion chemotherapy and concomitant radiation therapy. Plenum, New York, pp 133–147

Dionet C, Rozan R, Achard JL et al. (1988) Sequential combination of 5-fluorouracil, cis-platinum and irradiation. 1. Advanced head and neck cancers. Radiother Oncol 11: 123–131

Dobrowsky W, Dobrowsky E, Strassl H, Braun O, Scheiber V (1989) Response to preoperative concomitant radiochemotherapy with mitomycin C and 5-fluorouracil in advanced head and neck cancer. Eur J Cancer Clin Oncol 25: 845–849

Fletcher GH, Suit HD, Howe CD, Samuels M, Jesse RH, Villareal RU (1963) Clinical method of testing radiation-sensitizing agents in squamous cell carcinoma. Cancer 16: 355–363

Fletcher GH, Suit HD, Lindberg RD, Howe CD, Samuels ML, Jesse RH, Smith JP (1967) Chemotherapy as an adjuvant to surgery and radiation therapy. Proceedings 9th International Cancer Congress. UICC Monograph vol 10. Springer, Berlin Heidelberg New York, pp 177–184

Fu KK (1979) Normal tissue effects of combined radiotherapy and chemotherapy for head and neck cancer. Front Radiat Ther Oncol 13: 113–132

Fu KK (1985) Biological basis for the interaction of chemotherapeutic agents and radiation therapy. Cancer 55: 2123–2130

Fu KK, Raynes BS, Lam KN (1984) Modification of the effects of continuous low dose rate irradiation by concurrent chemotherapy infusion. Int J Radiat Oncol Biol Phys 10: 1473–1478

Goepfert H, Jesse RH, Lindberg RD (1973) Arterial infusion and radiation therapy in the treatment of advanced cancer of the nasal cavity and paranasal sinuses. Am J Surg 16: 464–468

Iscoe N (1987) Chemotherapy of head and neck cancer. Clin Oncol 5: 575–593

Kaplan MJ, Hahn SS, Johns ME, Stewart FM, Constable WC, Cantrell RW (1985) Mitomycin and fluorouracil with concomitant radiotherapy in head and neck cancer. Arch Otolaryngol 111: 220–222

Keane TJ, Harwood AR, Beale FA, Cummings BJ, Payne DG, Rawlinson E (1985) A pilot study of mitomycin C and 5-fluorouracil infusion combined with split course radiation therapy for advanced carcinomas of the larynx and hypopharynx. J Otolaryngol 15: 286–288

Komiyama S, Kudoh S, Yanagita, T, Kuwano M (1985) Synergistic combination therapy of 5-fluorouracil, vitamin A, and cobalt-60 radiation for head and neck tumors – antitumor combination therapy with Vitamin A. Auris Nasus Larynx 12 [Suppl II]: S239–S243

Lo TCM, Wiley AL, Ansfield FJ et al. (1976) Combined radiation therapy and 5-fluorouracil for advanced squamous cell carcinoma of the oral cavity and oropharynx: a randomized study. AJR 126: 229–235

Lokich JJ (1985) Optimal schedule for 5-fluorouracil chemotherapy. Am J Clin Oncol 8: 445–448

Maguire LC, Mendiondo OA, Medina WD, Cronin JD, Wheeler BM, Bartmas S (1987) Improved disease free survival in advanced head and neck carcinoma. Head and Neck Oncology Research. Kugler, Amsterdam, pp 271–274

Marshall RS, Rauth AM (1988) Oxygen and exposure kinetics as factors influencing the cytotoxicity of porfiromycin, a mitomycin C analogue, in Chinese hamster ovary cells. Cancer Res 48: 5655–5659

Marzecki Z, Krygier-Stojalowska A, Zaborek B, Mietkiewski J, Meyer A, Mazuryk R, Torbe Z (1980) Early clinical experience with radiation therapy of the advanced tumors following synchronization of the cell cycle with 5-fluorouracil. Radiobiol Radiother 21: 417–423

Murthy AK, Taylor SG, Showel J et al. (1987) Treatment of advanced head and neck cancer with concomitant radiation and chemotherapy. Int J Radiat Oncol Biol Phys 13: 1807–1813

Nitze HR, Vosteen KH, Ganzer U (1971) Radiation treatment of human tumors following the in vivo synchronization of the cell cycle. Acta Otolaryngol 71: 227–231

Overgaard J, Hjelm-Hanesen M, Vendelbo-Johansen L, Andersen AP (1988) Comparison of conventional and split course radiotherapy as primary treatment in carcinoma of the larynx. Acta Oncol 27: 147–152

Papac RJ (1984) Distant metastases from head and neck cancer. Cancer 53: 342–345

Pinedo HM, Peters GJ (1988) Fluorouracil: biochemistry and pharmacology. J Clin Oncol 6: 1653–1664

Rockwell S (1982) Cytotoxicities of mitomycin C and x-rays to aerobic and hypoxic cells in vitro. Int J Radiat Oncol Biol Phys 8: 1035–1039

Sato Y, Morita M, Takahashi H, Watanabe N, Kirikae I (1970) Combined surgery, radiotherapy, and regional chemotherapy in carcinoma of the paranasal sinuses. Cancer 25: 571–579

Sharp TR, Frankel SS, Byfield JE, Callipari F, Hornbeck CL (1983) Combined infusional 5-FU and x-ray therapy for advanced head and neck cancer – scheduling of radiosensitizing programs. Proc Am Soc Clin Oncol 2: 168

Shigematsu Y, Sakai S, Fuchihata H (1971) Recent trials in the treatment of maxillary sinus carcinoma, with special reference to the chemical potentiation of radiation therapy. Acta Otolaryngol 71: 63–70

Smith BL, Franz JL, Mira JG, Gates GA, Sapp J, Cruz AB (1980) Simultaneous combination radiotherapy and multidrug chemotherapy for stage III and stage IV squamous cell carcinoma of the head and neck. J Surg Oncol 15: 91–98

Steel GG (1988) The search for therapeutic gain in the combination of radiotherapy and chemotherapy. Radiother Oncol 11: 31–53

Steel GG, Peckham MJ (1979) Exploitable mechanisms in combined radiotherapy-chemotherapy: the concept of additivity. Int J Radiat Oncol Biol Phys 5: 85–91

Tannock IF (1989) Combined modality treatment with radiotherapy and chemotherapy. Radiother Oncol 16: 83–101

Tsujii H, Kamada T, Arimoto T, Mizoe J, Shirato H, Matsuoka Y, Irie G (1986) The role of radiotherapy in the management of maxillary sinus carcinoma. Cancer 57: 2261–2266

Valeriote F, Santelli G (1984) 5-Fluorouracil (FUra). Pharmacol Ther 24: 107–132

Van Putten LM, Kram LK, van Dierendonck HH, Smink T, Fuzy M (1975) Enhancement by drugs of metastatic lung nodule formation after intravenous tumor cell injection. Int J Cancer 15: 588–595

Verweij J, Stuurman M, De Vries J, Pinedo HM (1986) The difference in pharmacokinetics of mitomycin C, given either as a single agent or as part of a combination chemotherapy. J Cancer Res Clinic Oncol 112: 283–285

von der Maase H, Overgaard J, Vaeth M (1986) Effect of cancer chemotherapeutic drugs on radiation-induced lung damage in mice. Radiother Oncol 5: 245–257

Weinberg MJ, Rauth AM (1987) 5-Fluorouracil infusions and fractionated doses of radiation: studies with a murine squamous cell carcinoma. Int J Radiat Oncol Biol Phys 13: 1691–1699

Wendt TG, Wustrow TPU, Hartenstein RC, Rohloff R, Trott KR (1987) Accelerated split-course radiotherapy and simultaneous cis-dichlorodiammine-platinum and 5-fluorouracil chemotherapy with folinic acid enhancement for unresectable carcinoma of the head and neck. Radiother Oncol 10: 277–284

Will CH, Hering KG, Dieckmann J (1983) Combination of 5-fluorouracil and Co-60 irradiation in the treatment of carcinoma of the oro-facial region. Int J Oral Surg 12: 141–146

Withers HR, Taylor JMG, Maciejewski B (1988) The hazard of accelerated tumor clonogen repopulation during radiotherapy. Acta Oncol 27: 131–146

18 Continuous Intravenous 5-Fluorouracil with Hydroxyurea and Concomitant Radiotherapy for Advanced Head and Neck Cancer

Everett E. Vokes

CONTENTS

18.1 Introduction

Head and neck cancer affects approximately 40 000 patients each year in the United States (Cancer Statistics 1988). About one-third of these will present with early stage disease that can usually be cured with surgery or radiotherapy used as single treatment modalities. However, the majority of patients will present with regionally advanced disease. These patients can also be treated with curative intent; however, most will experience disease recurrence despite aggressive treatment combining surgery and radiotherapy.

Chemotherapy remains an investigational tool in patients with head and neck cancer (Hong and Bromer 1983; Mead and Jacobs 1982; Tannock and Browman 1986). It is frequently used with palliative therapeutic intent in patients with recurrent and/or metastatic head and neck cancer. In this setting, drugs such as methotrexate or cisplatin will result in overall response rates of 30% – 60% (Hong and Bromer 1983; Hong et al. 1983; Mead and Jacobs 1982). However, these responses are partial in extent and brief in duration. For previously untreated patients with regionally advanced head and neck cancer, chemotherapy is frequently used in combination with surgery and/ or radiotherapy, e.g., as neoadjuvant chemotherapy. While higher response rates, including complete responses, have consistently been reported in those patients (Ervin et al. 1987; Rooney et al. 1985; Vokes et al. 1989a, and 1990a), a survival advantage for patients treated in this manner occurring as a direct result of the use of chemotherapy has not yet been shown (Al-Sarraf 1988; Chokski et al. 1988; Tannock and Browman 1986).

Head and neck cancer remains regionally confined throughout most of its natural history. Therefore, efforts at improving the survival of patients with head and neck cancer need to focus on increasing the locoregional efficacy of therapy. These efforts have frequently concentrated on the simultaneous use of radiotherapy and chemotherapy (Fu 1985, Vokes and Weichselbaum 1990). Here the chemotherapy is administered with the hope of enhancing the activity of radiotherapy locally, while also being active systemically, e.g., against clinically undetectable micrometastatic tumor deposits. Earlier studies using simultaneous chemoradiotherapy consistently reported increased toxicity (Fu 1985; Fu et al. 1987; Kramer 1969). Therefore, more recently, treatment schemes have been developed that use chemoradiotherapy with regularly scheduled treatment breaks analogous to the administration of chemotherapy in cycles (Adelstein et al. 1986; Byfield et al. 1984; Murthy et al. 1987).

At the University of Chicago we have studied the use of infusional 5-fluorouracil (5-FU) and oral hydroxyurea with concomitant radiotherapy. Both hydroxyurea and 5-FU have single agent cytotoxic activity in this disease (Hong and Bromer 1983; Mead and Jacobs 1982). In addition, both drugs have been shown to be synergistic in vitro (Moran et al. 1982). Finally, randomized studies in patients with head and neck cancer have suggested that the radiosensitizing potential of 5-FU (Lo et al. 1976) and hydroxyurea (Richard and Chambers 1969) may be clinically significant. Similar studies have been published for hydroxyurea in patients with cervical cancer (Piver et al. 1983)

Everett E. Vokes, MD, Assistant Professor of Medicine and Radiation Oncology, The University of Chicago Medical Center, 5841 S. Maryland Ave., Box 420, Chicago, IL 60637, USA

and malignant brain tumors (LEVIN et al. 1979) and for 5-FU in patients with pancreatic tumors (MOERTEL et al. 1969).

18.2 Patients and Methods

Our goal in this study was to identify the optimal doses of drugs to use when combining hydroxyurea with 5-FU and radiotherapy, and to define the pattern of toxicities in a phase I format. Patients were eligible for this study if they had biopsy-proven inoperable squamous cell or mucoepidermoid carcinoma originating in the head and neck, a performance status of ≤3 (ECOG), and signed informed consent.

There was no limitation on prior therapy, including prior radiotherapy. Both patients who had failed previous curative intent local therapy (group 1) and those who had not received prior local therapy with surgery and/or radiotherapy (group 2) were eligible. In group 2 eligible patients were judged to have a dismal prognosis with standard therapy; this included patients with metastatic disease in need of local palliation, patients who had been treated with neoadjuvant chemotherapy and had either failed to respond or had refused local therapy following completion of chemotherapy, and patients with stage IV disease who had poor pulmonary and renal function.

Staging procedures prior to starting therapy included a history and physical examination, standard blood tests, and radiographic studies including a CT scan of the head and neck and other clinically involved areas. Local tumor extent was also documented by triple endoscopy. Prior to initiating therapy, patient eligibility was deter-mined at a multidisciplinary patient management conference.

The treatment regimen called for patients to receive hydroxyurea, continuous infusion 5-FU, and radiotherapy every other week (Fig. 18.1). The starting dose of hydroxyurea was 500 mg p.o. on day 1, repeated 2 h prior to radiotherapy on days 2–6. This dose of hydroxyurea was increased in 500-mg increments until definition of its max-imally tolerated dose (MTD). This was defined as the dose at which >33% of patients developed a WBC count of <2000/µl or a platelet count of <75 000/µl. At daily doses of hydroxyurea ranging from 1000 to 3000 mg, the total daily dose was split to allow for its administration every 12 h. One dose of hydroxyurea always preceded daily radiotherapy by 2 h. A continuous intravenous infusion of 5-FU was administered at $800 \, mg/m^2$ on days 2–6. Radiotherapy was delivered on days 2–6 at daily fractions of 1.8–2 Gy by a 4-MeV or 6-MeV linear accelerator. This week of treatment was followed by a week of rest (one cycle). Treat-ment cycles were repeated until a planned course of radiotherapy was completed. For previously irradiated patients total radiotherapy doses to the tumor were in the range of 40–60 Gy to keep the maximal cumulative spinal cord dose below 50 Gy and the maximal cumulative soft tissue dose below 110 Gy. For previously unirradiated patients radiotherapy consisted of 66–80 Gy to areas of gross disease and 45–50 Gy to areas of potential microscopic disease. Electron boosts were used when appropriate. An interstitial implant was used in one patient.

The dose of 5-FU was decreased to $600 \, mg/m^2/$ day for moderate mucositis during the preceding cycle, and to $400 \, mg/m^2/day$ for severe or life-threatening mucositis. For severe or life-threatening mucositis persisting on day 14 of a

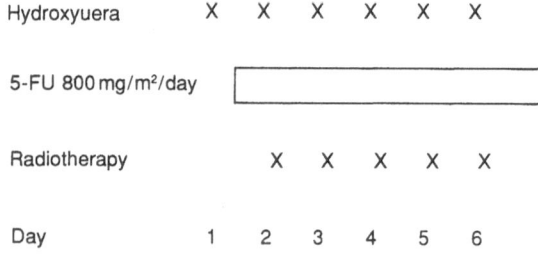

Hydroxyuera   X   X   X   X   X   X

5-FU 800 mg/m²/day

Radiotherapy   X   X   X   X   X

Day   1   2   3   4   5   6

Cycle length: 2 weeks

Hydroxyuera dose levels: 500, 1000, 1500, 2000, 2500, 3000 mg daily   **Fig. 18.1.** The treatment regimen

cycle, the next cycle was postponed by 1 week. The dose of hydroxyurea was not reduced for mucositis. Patients who developed a WBC count nadir of $<2.0 \times 10^3/\mu l$ generally continued their therapy at 50% of the previous dose of hydroxyurea to prevent further episodes of neutropenia. Patients receiving an initial total daily dose of 2500 or 3000 mg hydroxyurea continued their therapy at 2000 mg hydroxyurea daily.

Standard response criteria were used. The duration of response was measured from the date of first documentation of maximal tumor response to the date of disease progression, death, or last patient contact. Survival was calculated from the date of starting the first cycle of therapy until the date of death or last patient contact. Survival and response duration were estimated according to Kaplan and Meier (1958).

18.3 Results

Thirty-nine patients were treated on this study between April 1986 and January 1988. Twenty of these had failed prior local therapy (group 1) and 19 had not received prior surgery or radiotherapy (group 2). The patient characteristics for both groups are shown in Table 18.1.

The toxicities encountered in this phase I study have been described in detail (Vokes et al., 1989b) Patients were treated at six dose levels of hydroxyurea ranging from 500 mg daily to 3000 mg daily. In the majority of patients treated with 2500 or 3000 mg daily, severe myelosuppression (a WBC count $<2000/\mu l$) occurred, usually manifesting early in the course of treatment.

Mucositis was a frequent side-effect that affected patients treated at all dose levels of hydroxyurea. Only the dose of 5-FU was adjusted for mucositis in this study; i.e., the dose of hydroxyurea was not decreased for mucositis. In order to evaluate whether mucositis was more severe at higher hydroxyurea dose levels, we calculated the 5-FU dose intensity for each hydroxyurea level (Vokes et al. 1989b). This showed that in patients treated at hydroxyurea doses exceeding 2000 mg/day, the actual median 5-FU dose administered was less than 60% of the intended dose of 5-FU while in patients treated at equal to or less than 2000 mg/day of hydroxyurea, greater than 80% of the intended 5-FU dose could be administered. This indicated that at lower doses of hydroxyurea mucositis was less severe. Additional acute toxicities were seen in individual patients and included cardiac arrhythmia and hand-foot syndrome.

When evaluating the antitumor efficacy of this regimen one must consider that the patient cohort in this study was very heterogeneous in regard to prior therapy, the sites of disease, and patient performance status. In addition, due to the phase I design of this study, patients were treated at six different dose levels of hydroxyurea. We have, therefore, divided out patient cohort into two groups for the response and survival analysis.

Group 1 consists of 20 patients who had received prior local therapy with surgery (17 patients) and/or radiotherapy (17 patients). In addition, nine patients had also received combination chemotherapy, usually for recurrent disease. The disease was localized to the head and neck area in 19 patients, while one patient also had lung metastases. Five patients were not evaluable for response because of cardiac toxicity during cycles 1 and 2 (one patient) or lack of measurable disease (four patients). Of 15 evaluable patients six and a clinical complete response and eight had a partial response. Only one patient failed to respond (Table 18.2).

At a median follow-up of 18 months, the median survival for all patients in this group is 8

Table 18.1. Patient characteristics

	Group 1	Group 2
Number of patients	20	19
Sex		
Male	15	13
Female	5	6
Performance status		
0	1	2
1	7	14
2	9	1
3	3	2
Age, median (years)	59	63
(range)	(37–82)	(37–82)

Table 18.2. Response

	Group 1 ($n = 20$)	Group 2 ($n = 19$)
Evaluable	15	17
CR	6	12
PR	8	5
NR	1	0

CR, complete, response; PR, partial response; NR, no response

months. Overall, 15 patients in this group have developed disease progression. This occurred locoregionally in ten patients, distantly in two patients, and both locoregionally and distantly in three patients. Fourteen patients have died of their head and neck cancer, four have died of other causes, one is alive with disease, and one is alive with no evidence of disease.

Group 2 consisted of 19 patients with locoregionally advanced disease who had not previously received local therapy with surgery and/or radiotherapy; six patients in this group also had biopsy-proven distant metastases. Two patients in this group received two cycles of this regimen only and then refused further therapy. These two patients could not be evaluated for response. Twelve patients had a clinical complete response in the irradiated field and five had a partial response (Table 18.2).

At a median follow-up time of 22 months, the median survival for all 19 patients in group 2 is 14 months. Overall, ten patients have developed progressive disease: the site of disease progression was within the irradiated field in four patients (including the two nonevaluable patients and two partial responders) and outside of the irradiated field in six patients (including two partial responders and four patients with complete response in the irradiated field). Progression occurred in previously known sites of metastatic disease in five patients, while only one patient developed new liver metastases, this within 2 weeks of completing local therapy for nasopharyngeal carcinoma. At present, seven patients are alive (including one partial responder with known local disease), nine have died of their head and neck cancer, and three have died of other causes (one patient each of sudden death, respiratory insufficiency, and secondary non-small cell lung cancer). Eight of 11 patients who had locoregionally advanced disease only and completed their planned course of therapy had a clinical complete response to this regimen. Six of these remain alive with no evidence of disease, while two have died of other causes with no clinical evidence of tumor recurrence at the time of their death.

18.4 Discussion

Our goal in this study was the definition of the MTD of hydroxyurea when administered with 5-FU and concomitant radiotherapy every other week. Our toxicity analysis as well as the analysis of the 5-FU dose intensity for each hydroxyurea dose level supports a hydroxyurea dose of 2000 mg daily. At that dose, only mild to moderate myelosuppression will be observed. In our experience, the dose of 5-FU will need to be reduced to $<800 \, mg/m^2/day$ in most patients at some time during their therapy because of mucositis. However, at a daily hydroxyurea dose not exceeding 2000 mg, it should be possible to administer $\geq 80\%$ of the intended 5-FU dose.

The activity of this regimen was impressive. All evaluable patients but one had at least a partial response. In group 1, these responses were usually of short duration. Extensive prior therapy and the fact that less than an optimal total radiotherapy dose could be administered to most patients may have contributed to this fact. However, reasonable temporary palliation was achieved in most patients. Responses in group 2 were generally of longer duration. It is of interest that most patients experienced disease progression outside of the irradiated field, usually in sites of previously known metastatic disease. This indicates a high local activity of this regimen, which is also supported by the fact that none of the patients with locoregional disease achieving a complete response to this regimen have had documented disease recurrence. It is based on these results that we have further investigated this regimen in previously untreated patients with stage III and IV locally advanced disease (VOKES et al. 1990, b). These patients initially received two cycles of neoadjuvant chemotherapy aiming at decreasing their local tumor burden and eradicating distant micrometastases. This was followed by local therapy consisting of surgery and/or concomitant chemotherapy with hydroxyurea and 5-FU. For this trial we also added oral leucovorin to the chemoradiotherapy portion in an attempt to increase further the efficacy of 5-FU in this combination (DANENBERG et al. 1974; ERLICHMAN et al. 1988). We are hopeful that in this follow-up trial the high local control rate achieved in our initial study may translate into improved survival for these previously untreated patients with locally advanced disease.

Acknowledgments. I wish to thank Drs. RALPH R. WEICH-SELBAUM, WILLIAM R. PANJE, and RICHARD L. SCHILSKY and ROSEMARIE MICK for their contributions to this work, and Ms. DORA CURRIN for preparation of the manuscript.

References

Adelstein DJ, Sharah VM, Earle AS et al. (1986) Chemoradiotherapy as initial management in patients with squamous cell carcinoma of the head and neck. Cancer Treat Rep 70: 761–767

Al-Sarraf M (1988) Head and neck cancer: chemotherapy concepts. Semin Oncol 15: 70–85

Byfield JE, Sharp TR, Frankel SS et al. (1984) Phase I and II trial of five-day infused 5-fluorouracil and radiation in advanced cancer of the head and neck. J Clin Oncol 2: 406–413

Cancer Statistics (1988) American Cancer Society, New York

Choksi AJ, Dimery IW, Hong WK (1988) Adjuvant chemotherapy of head and neck cancer: the past, the present, and the future. Semin Oncol 15: 45–59

Danenberg PV, Langenbach RJ, Heidelberger C (1974) Structures of irreversible complexes of thymidylate synthetase and fluorinated pyrimidine nucleotides. Biochemistry 13; 926–933

Erlichman C, Fine S, Wong A, Elhakim T (1988) A randomized trial of fluorouracil and folinic acid in patients with metastatic colorectal carcinoma. J Clin Oncol 6: 469–475

Ervin TJ, Clark JR, Weichselbaum RR et al. (1987) An analysis of induction and adjuvant chemotherapy in the multidisciplinary treatment of squamous-cell carcinoma of the head and neck. J Clin Oncol 5: 10–20

Fu KK (1985) Concurrent radiotherapy and chemotherapy. In: Wittes RE (ed) Head and neck cancer. John Wiley, London, pp 221–248

Fu KK, Phillips TL, Silverberg IY et al. (1987) Combined radiotherapy and chemotherapy with bleomycin and methotrexate for advanced inoperable head and neck cancer: Update of a Northern California Oncology Group randomized trial. J Clin Oncol 5: 1410–1418

Hong WK, Bromer R (1983) Chemotherapy in head and neck cancer. N Engl J Med 308: 75–79

Hong WK, Schaefer S, Issell B et al. (1983) A prospective randomized trial of methotrexate versus cisplatin in the treatment of recurrent squamous cell carcinoma of the head and neck. Cancer 52: 206–210

Kaplan EL, Meier P (1958) Nonparametric estimation from incomplete observations. J Am Stat Assoc 53: 457–481

Kramer S (1969) Use of methotrexate and radiation therapy for advanced cancer of the head and neck. Front Radiat Ther Oncol 4: 116–125

Levin VA, Wilson CB, Davis R et al. (1979) A phase III comparison of BCNU, hydroxyurea and radiation therapy to BCNU and radiation therapy for treatment of primary malignant gliomas. J Neurosurg 51: 526–532

Lo TC, Wiley AL Jr, Ainsfield FJ et al. (1976) Combined radiation therapy and 5-fluorouracil for advanced squamous cell carcinoma of the oral cavity and oropharynx: a randomized study. AJR 126: 229–235

Mead GM, Jacobs C (1982) Changing role of chemotherapy in treatment of head and neck cancer. Am J Med 73: 582–595

Moertel CT, Childs DS Jr, Reitemeir FJ et al. (1969) Combined 5-fluorouracil and super voltage radiation therapy of locally unresectable gastrointestinal cancer. Lancet II: 865–867

Moran RG, Danenberg PV, Heidelberger C (1982) Therapeutic response of leukemic mice treated with fluorinated pyrimidines and inhibitors of deoxyuridylate synthesis. Biochem Pharmacol 31: 2929–2935

Murthy AK, Taylor SG, Showel J et al. (1987) Treatment of advanced head and neck cancer with concomitant radiation and chemotherapy. Int J Radiat Oncol Biol Phys 13: 1807–1813

Piver MS, Barlow JJ, Vongtama V, Blumenson L (1983) Hydroxyurea: a radiation potentiator in carcinoma of the uterine cervix. Am J Obstet Gynecol 147: 803–808

Richard GJ, Chambers RG (1969) Hydroxyurea: a radiosensitizer in the treatment of neoplasms of the head and neck. Am J Roentgenol Radium Nucl Med 55: 555–565

Rooney M, Kish J, Jacobs J et al. (1985) Improved complete response rate and survival in advanced head and neck cancer after three course induction therapy with 120-hour 5-FU infusion and cisplatin. Cancer 55; 1123–1128

Tannock IF, Browman G (1986) Lack of evidence for a role of chemotherapy in the routine management of locally advanced head and neck cancer. J Clin Oncol 4: 1121–1126

Vokes EE, Moran WJ, Mick R et al. 1989a, Neoadjuvant and adjuvant methotrexate, cisplatin, and fluorouracil in multimodal therapy of head and neck cancer. J Clin Oncol 7: 838–845

Vokes EE, Panje WR, Schilsky RL et al. 1989b, Hydroxyurea, 5-fluorouracil and concomitant radiotherapy in poor prognosis head and neck cancer: a phase I-II study. J Clin Oncol 7: 761–768

Vokes EE, Schilsky RL, Weichselbaum RR et al. Induction chemotherapy with cisplatin, fluorouracil and high-dose leucovorin for locally advanced head and neck cancer: a clinical and pharmacologic analysis. J Clin Oncol 8: 241–247, 1990, a

Vokes EE, Panje WR, Mick R et al. (1990b): Neoadjuvant chemotherapy, surgery and concomitant chemoradiotherapy for locally advanced head and neck cancer. Proc Am Soc Clin Oncol 9: 174 (Abstr.)

Vokes EE, Weichselbaum RR (1990): Concomitant chemoradiotherapy: rationale and clinical experience in patients with solid tumors. J Clin Oncol 8: 911–934

19 Treatment of Advanced Carcinoma of the Bladder with Concomitant 5-Fluorouracil Infusion and Radiation

Marvin Rotman, Hassan Aziz, Louis Potters, and Kwang Choi

CONTENTS

19.1 Introduction

It is estimated that in the United States during 1989, a total of 47 100 patients will be diagnosed with bladder carcinoma (Silowberg and Lubera 1989). During this same year, a sizeable number of patients (approximately 10 200) are expected to die from this disease. Unfortunately, despite recent advances in surgical and radiotherapeutic techniques, the percentage of patients dying from this disease has not changed since 1930. For superficial bladder carcinomas (stage 0, A, B_1), acceptable locoregional control rates and 5-year survivals have been obtained with transurethral resection of the bladder, partial cystectomy, interstitial implants, and intravesicular chemotherapy. With deeply infiltrating tumors, a high incidence of lymphatic involvement significantly worsens the prognosis, whatever treatment modality is attempted. In the best reported series, surgery or definitive radiotherapy for invasive bladder carcinoma achieved only a 25%–30% survival rate (Pearse

et al. 1978; Prout 1976; Richie et al. 1975). When surgery was combined with radiation, the survival increased to 40%–45% (Batata et al. 1981; Bloom et al. 1982; Miller and Johnson 1972; Sagerman et al. 1968; Scanlon et al. 1983; van der Werf-Messing et al. 1982). Even when patients with more favorable tumors are selected for radical surgery, either with or without radiation, the survival, clearly, is still poor. In addition, the surgery is mutilating, and leaves the patient with a permanent ileal conduit, loss of sexual potency, and psychosocial stress.

However, when definitive radiotherapy was used (Blandy et al. 1980; Coffinet et al. 1975), or preoperative radiation (Bloom et al. 1982; Miller and Johnson 1972; Sagerman et al. 1968; Scanlon et al. 1983), those patients who achieved a complete response to the radiation had a better overall survival. Therefore, various techniques were tried to enhance the complete response rate as a means of improving overall survival rates. Electronofluence compounds (RTOG 81-05 1981), high LET radiation (RTOG 77-05/81-10 1981), hyperbaric oxygen (Cade and McEwen 1978), and altered fractionation schemes were all tried, but with little if any success.

An alternative approach to improving the complete response rate has been to bring chemotherapeutic agents into the radiotherapy regimen. In recent years, there has been growing evidence of the effectiveness of certain drugs as radiosensitizers in the treatment of epithelial tumors, with improved tumor clearance and survival. The use of continuous infusion 5-fluorouracil (5-FU) and concomitant radiation has achieved improved local and regional control and survival in epithelial cancers of the anus (Cummings et al. 1982), esophagus (John et al. 1987), and head and neck (Morthy et al. 1987). Since July 1980, we have, therefore, attempted to improve survival in 22 patients with advanced bladder cancer by treating them with concomitant continuous infusion 5-FU and radiation. An additional benefit of this ap-

---

Marvin Rotman, MD, Professor and Chairman
Hassan Aziz, MD, Associate Professor
Louis Potters, MD, Kwang Choi, MD, Associate Professor, Radiation Oncology, SUNY-Health Science Center at Brooklyn, 450 Clarkson Avenue, Brooklyn, NY 11203, USA

proach is that it avoids the need to sacrifice the bladder.

19.2 Methods and Materials

A total of 22 patients, 20 with transitional cell and 2 with squamous cell carcinoma, were included in this study. The patients referred to us for treatment either had refused surgery or had medical contraindications to surgery or had locally advanced disease. All patients underwent full staging work-up, such as blood chemistries, chest x-ray, intravenous pyelogram (IVP), bone scan, CT scan, and liver function tests. At the start of treatment, the disease was confined to the pelvis. However, two patients were found to have metastatic disease during their treatment and were staged as D_2. All patients had a Karnofsky performance status of 50 or above, adequate renal function (blood urea nitrogen level <4.0 mg/ml), hemoglobin level >10 g/100 ml, and platelet count $>100\,000/m^2$. Tumor volume was estimated at cystoscopy and the size of the intravesical tumor was available at the time of treatment.

There were 17 male and 5 female patients and their ages ranged between 45 and 95 years (Median 72 years). Using the Jewett-Marshall staging system (STEIN and KAUFMAN 1968), one patient was thought to have stage A disease but had a clinically suspicious bony metastatic focus, which had become painful 3 weeks after completing treatment. This patient, however, is still included in our analysis for response and survival. Five

Table 19.1. Patient characteristics

Characteristics	No. of patients
Total	22
Age	
Range	45–95 years
Median	72 years
Sex (male:female)	3:1
Clinical stage (Jewett-Marshall system)	
A[a]	1
B_1	5
B_2	8
C	4
D_1	2
D_2[b]	2

[a] Suspicious of D_2 pretreatment – confirmed 6 weeks later
[b] included for assessment of response but excluded for determination of survival

Table 19.2. Tumor pathology, grade, and volume

	No. of patients
Grade 1–2	3
Grade 3–4	17
Pathology	
Transitional cell	20
Squamous cell	2
IVP (intravenous pyelogram)	
Normal	15
Abnormal	7
Bladder tumor volume	
$>50\%$	7
25%–50%	6
$<25\%$	9

patients had stage B_1, eight had stage B_2, four had stage C, two had stage D_1, and two had stage D_2 disease (Tables 19.1, 19.2). Three patients with transitional cell carcinomas had grade 1 and 2 tumor, while 17 patients had grade 3 and 4 disease. Seven patients had more than 50% of the bladder involved, six had 25%–50% of the bladder involved, and nine had less than 25% of the bladder involved. Seven patients had an abnormal IVP that indicated hydronephrosis.

All patients were treated on a 4-MeV linear accelerator with four field box technique to include the whole pelvis initially. Shaped portals were used, receiving 40–50 Gy using five 1.8-Gy fractions per week for 4.5–5 weeks. This was followed by a boost dose to the bladder of 20–25 Gy in 2.5–3 weeks, using arc rotation technique. One patient with extensive ulcerated tumor was given a 30-Gy boost using an iridium implant. Thus, total tumor doses of 60–65 Gy in 33–35 fractions were delivered to the bladder.

All patients received concomitant continuous infusion of 5-FU (CCIC) with the radiation. 5-FU was delivered intravenously over 120 h at a concentration of 25 mg/kg/day on weeks 1, 4, and 7 of treatments (Fig. 19.1). All patients received a minimum of two complete cycles of concomitant infusion of 5-FU. Five patients also received mitomycin C at 10 mg/m² as i.v. bolus on day 1 of radiation therapy.

Initial assessment of tumor response with cystoscopy and biopsy was scheduled at 3 months after completion of therapy. Subsequently, all patients were assessed by serial cystoscopy and biopsy. In addition, urine cytology was obtained at 3- to 6-month intervals, and an IVP was repeated once yearly. A complete response was defined as total visual and histological clearance on cystoscopy

Fig. 19.1. Schema of combined infusion 5-FU and mitomycin C with radiation for bladder

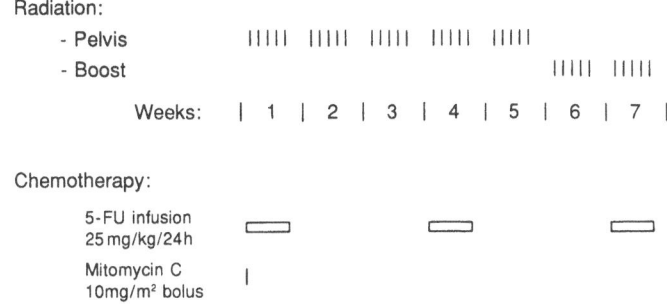

19.3 Results

19.3.1 Response

Twenty-one of 22 patients were available for evaluation of local response (one patient refused cystoscopy) within 6 months of treatment (Table 19.3). Five of six patients with stage A and B_1 disease achieved a complete local response, as did 10 of 15 patients with stage B_2, C, D_1, and D_2 disease. This resulted in an initial complete response in 15 of 21 (71.5%) patients. An additional three patients achieved complete response after transurethral resection of persistent superficial tumor followed by intravesicular mitomycin C therapy. Therefore, a total complete response was achieved in 18 of 21 (85%) patients. This also included one patient with residual carcinoma in situ. The complete response rates for superficially infiltrating tumors (A and B_1) and deeply invasive tumors were 83% and 86%, respectively. In only one patient was there local recurrence after treat-

ment. The presence of residual disease at the start of therapy did not influence ultimate local response rate.

Two patients with transitional cell carcinoma and one patient with squamous cell carcinoma failed to achieve a complete response. One of the patients with transitional cell carcinoma had persistent abnormal urinary cytology that was discovered to be secondary to an infiltrative tumor in the renal pelvis as well as a small focus of superficial tumor remaining in the bladder. This patient underwent nephroureterocystectomy and is alive and without disease after 5½ years. The second patient with transitional cell carcinoma developed distant metastases and died. The third patient, who had squamous cell carcinoma, underwent salvage cystectomy at 6 months. Therefore, with the exception of the two patients undergoing salvage cystectomy, all patients retained their bladders.

The use of routine serial urinary cytology is of paramount importance for the detection of either recurrent disease or a new urothelial tract neoplasm. Five patients in our series ultimately were found to have a positive cytology. One patient who had extensive carcinoma in situ of the bladder was successfully treated with intravesicular mitomycin C and BCG. He died 5½ years later of a myocardial infarction. A second patient was found to have a carcinoma in the distal ureter and underwent nephroureterectomy. The third patient, already discussed above, was found to have lesions in the renal pelvis and bladder, and is alive 5½ years later. Two patients had a bladder recurrence and residual disease and died of metastases at 9 and 12 months.

19.3.2 Survival

Of the original 22 patients, two were found to be stage D_2 at the start of therapy and were excluded

Table 19.3. Results of patients evaluated for local response[a]

Stage	CR	CR + add. Modalities	Total CR
A, B_1	5/6 (83%)	0/6 (0%)	5/6 (83%)
B_2, C, D_1, D_2	10/15 (66%)	3/15 (20%)	3/21 (14%)
All patients	15/21 (71%)	3/21 (14%)	18/21 (86%)

CR, complete response
[a] One patient refused cystoscopy (21/22 patients evaluated)

from analysis for survival. Of the 20 remaining patients with stages A through D_1, 12 have died. Eight patients died of distant metastases, one died with regional disease only, and three died of intercurrent disease at 50, 51, and 78 months. Eight patients are alive without disease from 51 to 78 months. The adjusted overall 5-year survival, as calculated by the Life Table Method, was 53.6%. For stages A_2 and B_1, the 5-year survival was 80%, while for stages B_2, C, and D_1 it was 40%. Metastatic disease was the main cause of death in the latter group. It is interesting to note that all patients who died of their bladder carcinoma did so within 2 years of completing therapy.

19.4 Complications

19.4.1 Acute

The most common symptoms were gastrointestinal. Almost all patients (81%) developed diarrhea by the 2nd week of treatment. Oral mucositis was the second most common side-effect, occurring in 4 of 22 (18%) patients. Another 4 of 22 (18%) patients complained of anorexia. None of these side-effects were severe enough to require discontinuation of therapy or reduction in the doses of either radiation or chemotherapy. None of the patients developed hematological toxicity (Table 19.4).

19.4.2 Chronic

One patient, aged 80, developed proctitis and rectal bleeding, requiring a colostomy. Three of 22 (13%) patients had persistent diarrhea for more than 1 year. Late urinary complications included chronic dysuria and cystitis in two patients, hemorrhagic cystitis in one patient, and increased frequency due to an irritable bladder in two patients (Table 19.4).

19.5 Discussion

In bladder carcinoma, a strong correlation exists between complete local response and survival when patients are treated with either curative (BLANDY et al. 1980; COFFINET et al. 1975) or

Table 19.4. Complications

Complications	No. of patients (%)
Acute	
Diarrhea	18/22 (81%)
Anorexia	4/22 (18%)
Mucositis	4/22 (18%)
Hematological	0/22 (0%)
Late	
Hemorrhagic cystitis	1/22 (4%)
Moderate degree of	
dysuria and cystitis	2/22 (9%)
Irritable bladder	2/22[a] (9%)
Diarrhea	3/22 (13%)
Proctitis and rectal	
bleeding (requiring colostomy)	1/22 (4%)

[a] Symptomatic. No volumetric or cystoscopic confirmation of bladder contraction. Both patients died of disease

preoperative radiation therapy (BLOOM et al. 1982; MILLER and JOHNSON 1972; SAGERMAN et al. 1968, 1980; VAN DER WERF-MESSING et al. 1982). BLANDY et al. (1980) reported that following curative irradiation for bladder carcinoma, those patients who achieved a complete response had a 5-year survival rate of 56% as compared to 17% in those patients who did not achieve a complete response. A strong correlation between a complete response and survival has been demonstrated by BATATA et al. (1981), VAN DER WERF-MESSING et al. (1982), and GOODMAN et al. (1982) in patients treated with preoperative or curative irradiation. Numerous attempts have been made to improve survival rates by enhancing local response rates. However, only minimal benefits in local control and survival have resulted from the use of radiosensitizers, hyperbaric oxygen (CADE 1978), high LET radiation, or hyperfractionation.

In 1958, HEIDELBERGER et al. demonstrated the radiosensitizing effect of 5-FU on rodent tumors. Later, in 1961, BAGSHAW used tissue culture to confirm HEIDELBERGER's observation. More importantly, in 1963, WOODRUFF et al. used 5-FU clinically as a radiosensitizer in the treatment of bladder carcinoma. Using preoperative radiation therapy and 5-FU, STEIN and KAUFMAN (1968) demonstrated a greater incidence of tumor regression in surgical specimens.

5-Fluorouracil is a pyrimidine analogue that inhibits de novo synthesis of DNA by binding thymidylate synthetase. It is also taken up as an RNA precursor nucleotide, leading to defective RNA synthesis. The enhanced cell kill by radiation in the presence of 5-FU is not fully understood. VIETTI et al. (1971) suggested that 5-FU may inhibit the repair of sublethal damage produced by radiation. VIETTI et al. (1971) and BYFIELD et al. (1982) subsequently suggested that 5-FU needed to be present during, and up to 48 h after the delivery of radiation for maximum radiosensitization. Obviously, this cannot be achieved by bolus 5-FU due to the short physiological half-life of the drug.

The pharmacodynamics of the drug as well as tumor cell kinetics were used by both CHABNER (1982) and LOCKICH (1984) to explain the benefits of prolonged infusion. Most chemotherapy agents are active in the DNA synthetic phase of the cell cycle. Further, cytotoxic agents tend to have short biological half-lives, and since the synthetic phase of the cell cycle is of short duration as well, bolus administration of these drugs limits their effect to a small fraction of tumor cells.

In a prospective randomized trial, SEIFERT et al. (1975) showed that the radiosensitizing effect of 5-FU is greater when the drug is continuously infused. BYFIELD et al. (1980) suggested that radiosensitization by 5-FU may be only additive when delivered by bolus but synergistic when administered by continuous infusion. Moreover, it is generally agreed that, since peak drug concentrations are avoided with continuous infusion, systemic toxicity is less than with bolus therapy.

Both cisplatin and 5-FU have been used as radiosensitizers in the treatment of bladder carcinoma. SHIPLEY et al. (1984) and SAUR et al. (1988) have used cisplatin with radiation therapy and have enhanced the complete response rates in T_2 and T_3 bladder carcinoma. The use of cisplatin, however, may be limited in older patients or in patients with obstructive uropathy. Mitomycin C has been used extensively in the intravesicular therapy of superficial bladder carcinoma. Five patients in our series received such therapy after the resection of residual tumor. All five patients remained free of disease and with an intact bladder. Mitomycin C is also a hypoxic cell sensitizer and may be more effective when used as a systemic agent in combination with 5-FU against bladder carcinoma, ROTMAN et al. (1990).

Although most of the patients in our series presented with bulky infiltrating disease and one-third of the patients had hydronephrosis, 71% of the patients achieved a complete response within 6 months of starting therapy. The complete response rate was increased to 85% after three patients with residual tumor underwent transurethral resection and intravesical mitomycin C or BCG. Only one patient who had achieved a complete response failed locally. The remaining 21 patients, including those who died of metastases or intercurrent disease, retained tumor-free bladders.

The importance of serial follow-up urine cytologies cannot be overemphasized, as not only recurrent bladder cancers but also second malignancy of the upper urinary tract can be detected by this means. Two of our patients with positive urinary cytology were found to have tumors of the renal pelvis and distal ureter respectively. Both of these patients are alive, without disease at 6 and 6½ years after undergoing salvage procedures.

In this small series it is not possible to evaluate the need for postradiation TURBT (transurethral resection of the bladder) or intravesicular mitomycin C in the achievement of a complete response. Furthermore, because of the addition of chemotherapy to the radiation therapy, it is not possible to compare our dose response data with radiation therapy regimens published by other authors. BLANDY et al. (1980) achieved a complete response for T_{1-2} and T_3 and 49% and 42%, respectively, using 50 Gy in 4 weeks. MILLER and JOHNSON (1972) achieved an overall complete response rate of 43% using a preoperative dose of 50 Gy in 5 weeks. In their preoperative series, BLOOM et al. (1982) and VAN DER WERF-MESSING et al. (1982) delivered 40 Gy in 4 weeks and achieved complete response rates of 31% and 37% respectively. Possibly, this regimen of planned, preoperative radiation therapy does not allow adequate time for tumor regression. Nevertheless, RUSSELL et al. (1988), utilizing CCIC–5-FU and 40 Gy radiation, achieved a complete response rate of 81% when they added cystectomy to the treatment. In our series, the rate of initial complete response rose from 71% to 85% after additional modalities were employed.

As previously mentioned, the 5-year survival for stages A and B_1 was 80%, while for stages B_2, C, and D_1 it was 40%. For superficial stage disease CCIC–5-FU seems to be an effective treatment. For more advanced lesions, the 40% survival rate offers an approximately 15% improvement over historical series employing surgery or radiation therapy alone. The high local complete response obtained for deeply infiltrative tumors has not translated into higher survival rates. This is most probably due to the presence of occult metastases at the start of therapy, as evidenced by the fact that most of these patients have died of metastatic disease within 2 years of treatment. There may be a need in certain cases for prior use of a multidrug chemotherapy regimen such as methotrexate, vinblastine, Adriamycin and cisplatin (M-VAC) or methotrexate, vinblastine, and cisplatin (MCV) followed up by the regimen of concomitant chemotherapy and radiation to provide more effective control of occult metastatic disease (MARKS et al. 1988).

Late complications from CCIC–5-FU therapy were not excessive. One patient required a colostomy for chronic rectal bleeding, one patient had hemorrhagic cystitis, and two others had symptomatic irritable bladder syndrome. RUSSELL et al. (1988) have used CCIC–5-FU in the treatment of bladder cancer and reported no significant bladder complications.

19.6 Conclusion

Effective long-term locoregional control can be obtained in a majority of patients with bladder carcinoma by the use of CCIC–5-FU and radiation therapy. While excellent survival rates are obtained in patients with superficial bladder tumors (A, B_1), survival remains poor in patients with more advanced, infiltrating tumors (B_2, C, D_1). This latter group, while obtaining comparably good locoregional control, are succumbing to distant metastases. Adjuvant M-VAC or MCV chemotherapy hopefully may play a role in reducing distant metastatic disease.

Twenty of 22 patients in our series have retained a functional bladder. On detection of persistent, recurrent, or second tumors in the urothelial tract, a surgical salvage procedure was possible without affecting overall survival.

References

Bagshaw MA (1961) Possible role of potentiators in radiation therapy. AJR 85: 822–833

Batata MA, Chu FCH, Hilaris BS et al. (1981) Factors of prognostic and therapeutic significance in patients with bladder cancer. Int J Radiat Oncol Biol Phys 7: 575–579

Blandy JP, England HR, Evans ST et al. (1980) T3 bladder cancer: the case for salvage cystectomy. Br J Urol 52: 506–510

Bloom HJD, Henry W, Wallace D, Skeet R (1982) Treatment of T3 bladder cancer: a controlled trial of pre-operative radiotherapy and radical cystectomy vs. radical radiotherapy. Br J Urol 54: 136–151

Byfield JE, Barone R, Mendelsohn J et al. (1980) Infusional 5-FU and x-ray therapy for nonresectable esophageal cancer. Cancer 45: 703–708

Byfield JE, Calabro JP, Klisak I, Kulhanian F (1982) Pharmacologic requirements for obtaining sensitization of human tumor cells in vitro to combined 5-FU and x-rays. Int J Radiat Oncol Biol Phys 8: 1923–1933

Cade IS, McEwen JB (1978) Clinical trials of radiotherapy in hyperbaric oxygen at Portsmouth, 1964–1976. Clin Radiol 29: 333–338

Chabner B (1982) Role of drugs in cancer treatment In: Chabner B (ed) Pharmacologic principles of cancer treatment. WB Saunders, Philadelphia, pp 3–14

Coffinet DR, Schneider MJ, Gladstein EJ et al. (1975) Bladder cancer: results of radiation therapy in 384 patients. Radiology 117: 149–153

Cummings BJ, Rieder WD, Hardwood AR et al. (1982) Combination radical radiation therapy and chemotherapy for primary squamous cell carcinoma of the anal canal. Cancer Treat Rep 66: 489–492

Goodman GB, Hislop TG, Elwood JM et al. (1982) Conservation of bladder function in patients with invasive bladder cancer treated by definitive irradiation and selective cystectomy. Int J Radiat Oncol Biol Phys 7: 569–573

Heidelberger C, Greisbach C, Montag BJ et al. (1958) Studies in fluorinated pyrimidin: II. Effects of transplanted tumor. Cancer Res 18: 305–317

John M, Flan M, Wittlinger P, Mowry PA (1987) Inoperable esophageal carcinoma: results of agressive synchronous radiotherapy. Am J Clin Oncol (CCT): 4: 310–316

Lockich JJ (1984) Infusion chemotherapy for cancer. Curr Concepts Oncol 6: 3–8

Marks LB, Kauffman SD, Prout GR Jr, Henry NM, Griffin EF, Shipley WU (1988) Invasive bladder carcinoma: preliminary report of selective bladder conservation by transurethral surgery, up front MCV chemotherapy and pelvic irradiation plus cisplatinum. Int J Radiat Oncol Biol Phys 15: 877–883

Marshall VF (1952) The relation of the preoperative estimate to the pathologic demonstration of the extent of vesical tumors. J Urol 68: 714–723

Miller LS, Johnson DE (1972) Megavoltage irradiation for bladder cancer: Alone, postoperative, and preoperative? In: Proceedings of the National Cancer Conference. JB Lippincott, Philadelphia, pp 771–782

Murthy AK, Taylor WSG, Showell J et al. (1987) Treatment of advanced head and neck cancer with concomitant radiation and chemotherapy. Int J Radiat Oncol Biol Phys 13; 1807–1813

Pearse DD, Reed RR, Hodges CV (1978) Radical cystectomy for bladder cancer. J Urol 119: 216–218

Prout GR Jr (1976) The surgical management of bladder carcinoma. Urol Clin North Am 3: 149–175

Richie JP, Skinner DG, Kaufman JJ (1975) Carcinoma of the bladder: treatment by radical cystectomy. J Surg Res 18: 217–75

Rotman M, Aziz H, Porrazzo, et al. (1990) Treatment of Advanced Transitional Cell Carcinoma of the Bladder with Irradiation and Concomitant 5-FU Infusion. Int J Radiation Oncology Biol Phys Vol 18, pp 1131–1137

RTOG 77-05/81-10 (1981) Phase I and II study, comparing the value of neutron alone, mixed beam and preoperative mixed in bladder carcinoma.

RTOG 81-05 (1981) Phase I/II study on the value of combining misonidazole and radiotherapy in the treatment of bladder cancer.

RTOG 83-08 (1982) Randomized phase II study to evaluate

hyperfractionation radiation for locally advanced carcinoma of the bladder.

Russell KJ, Boileau MA, Ireton RC et al. (1988) Transitional cell carcinoma of the urinary bladder: histologic clearance with combined 5-FU chemotherapy and radiation therapy. Preliminary results of bladder preservation study. Radiology 167: 845–848

Sagerman RH, Veenema RJ, Guttmann R, Dean AL Jr, Uson AC (1968) Pre-operative irradiation of carcinoma of the bladder. Am J Roent Rad Ther Nucl Med 102: 577–580

Sagerman RH, Yo WS, Ryoo MC, King GA, Chung CT, Emanuel IG (1980) Int J Radiat Oncol Biol Phys 6: 607–612

Saur R, Schrott KM, Dunst J, Thiel HJ, Hermanek P, Bornhoff C (1988) Preliminary results of treatment of invasive bladder carcinoma with radiotherapy and cisplatinum. Int J Radiat Oncol Biol Phys 15: 871–875

Scanlon PW, Scott M, Sergura JW (1983) A comparison of short course, low dose, and long course, high dose preoperative radiation for carcinoma of the bladder. Cancer 52: 1153–1159

Seifert P, Baker CH, Reed ML (1975) Comparison of continuous infused 5-FU with bolus injection in treatment of patients with colorectal adenocarcinoma. Cancer 36: 123–128

Shipley WU, Coombs LJ, Einstein AB Jr et al. (1984) Cisplatinum and full dose irradiation for patients with invasive bladder carcinoma: a preliminary report of tolerance and local response. J Urol 132: 899–903

Silowberg E, Lubera JA (1989) Cancer Statistics, 1989. CA 39: 3–20

Stein JJ, Kaufman JJ (1968) Treatment of carcinoma of bladder with special reference to the use of preoperative radiation therapy combined with 5-FU. Am J Roent Rad Ther Nucl Med 102: 519–529

van der Werf-Messing G, Friedell GH, Menon RS, Hop WCJ, Wassif SB (1982) Carcinoma of the urinary bladder T2NXMO treated by pre-operative irradiation followed by cystectomy. Int J Radiat Oncol Biol Phys 8: 1849–1855

Vietti J, Eggerding F, Valeriote F (1971) Combined effect of radiation and 5-FU on survival of transplanted leukemia cells. JNCI 47: 865–870

Woodruff MW, Murphy WT, Hopson JM (1963) Further observation on the use of combination 5-FU and supervoltage irradiation therapy in treatment of advanced carcinoma of bladder. J Urol 90: 747–758

20 Combined 5-Fluorouracil and Irradiation for the Treatment of Invasive Bladder Cancer

Kenneth J. Russell, Celestia S. Higano, Michel A. Boileau, Anthony H. Russell, Caroline Collins, Wui-Jin Koh, Warren H. Chapman, and Thomas W. Griffin

CONTENTS

20.1 Introduction

Extensive clinical experience has demonstrated the efficacy of external beam radiotherapy for selected patients with radioresponsive bladder cancers. Patients who achieve a complete clinical response within 6 months of completion of radical radiotherapy enjoy a 45%–69% survival at 5 years, as opposed to 6%–14% for patients with unresponsive tumors (Bloom et al. 1982; Quilty and Duncan 1986; Hope-Stone et al. 1984). This relationship between tumor radioresponsiveness and prognosis also holds true for patients undergoing combined preoperative radiation followed by planned cystectomy. The 14%–43% of patients whose cystectomy specimens reveal no histological evidence of residual cancer as a result of the radiation enjoy a 64%–80% 5-year survival whereas the 5-year survival for patients without such pathological "downstaging" is 27%–48% (Boileau et al. 1980; DeWeerd et al. 1977; Scanlon et al. 1983; Slack and Prout 1980). Bladder function is retained by the vast majority of patients cured of their bladder cancers by radical radiation, with only 2%–11% experiencing late radiation complications (Quilty and Duncan 1986; Duncan and Quilty 1986; Goodman et al., 1981; Yu et al. 1985).

With this historical background as reference, this clinical trial was designed to address two questions: (a) Can the percentage of patients with complete clinical responses to radiation be increased by the addition of the radiation-potentiating drug 5-fluorouracil (5-FU), and does this increased percentage of downstaged patients translate into a better survival? (b) Can patients who are candidates for cystectomy be treated successfully by chemoradiotherapy alone, provided that there is no histological evidence of residual tumor at the time that planned surgery would normally be performed?

Kenneth J. Russell, MD, Associate Professor, Radiation Oncology, Celestia S. Higano, MD, Assistant Professor, Medical Oncology, Caroline Collins, MD, Assistant Professor, Medical Oncology, Wui-Jin Koh, MD, Assistant Professor, Radiation Oncology, Warren H. Chapman, MD, Professor, Urology, Thomas W. Griffin, MD, Professor and Chairman, Radiation Oncology, University of Washington Medical Center, 1959 N.E. Pacific Street, Seattle, WA 98195, USA

Michel A. Boileau, MD, Bend Urology Associates, 2275 N.E. Doctor's Drive, Bend, OR 97701, USA

Anthony H. Russell, MD, Radiation Oncology Center, 5271 "F" Street, Sacramento, CA 95819, USA

20.2 Materials and Methods

Forty patients have been enrolled on this study since its inception. The majority of the patients have been treated at the University of Washington Medical Center, but patients have been enrolled and treated at seven additional participating regional facilities in Washington and Oregon, as well as two facilities in Kansas and Virginia.

Thirty-four patients completed the prescribed treatment and form the study population. For a variety of reasons, six patients were removed from study prior to completing the protocol (see Sect. 20.3.5) and are excluded from further analysis.

All patients had biopsy-proven transitional cell carcinoma. Patients with both muscle-invading and noninvasive tumors were eligible. All patients with noninvasive tumors had recurrent tumors after prior intravesical chemotherapy, and were thought by their referring urologists to require cystectomy as the best conventional therapy. The age range of the patients was 39–86 years, with a median of 69 years; 27 patients were male and 7 were female.

The pretreatment evaluation included a history and physical examination, routine blood chemistry tests and hematological indices, cystoscopic evaluation, computed tomography of the pelvis (CT), and chest radiographs. The majority of the patients underwent radionuclide bone scanning, and all patients gave written informed consent prior to the initiation of therapy.

At the conclusion of staging, patients were placed into one of two groups: those who were eligible for cystectomy, and those who were not candidates for cystectomy. Patients were considered candidates for cystectomy if their tumors were confined to the bladder or had extravesical spread limited to the vagina or prostate. Patients were enrolled in the nonsurgical group for one of three conditions: surgical inoperability (tumor extension to abdominal wall or rectum, or pelvic lymph node metastases on CT), medical inoperability because of physical frailty, or inoperability due to patient refusal. Of the 34 patients, 18 were deemed to be surgical candidates and 16 were not. As regards the 16 nonsurgical candidates, the criteria for inoperability were surgical inoperability in five cases, medical inoperability in five, and patient refusal in six.

All patients received a preoperative course of 40 Gy pelvic radiation therapy given with two 96-h infusions of 5-FU, over a period of 5 weeks. Pelvic irradiation was administered for an initial 2 weeks, with 5-FU infused on days 1–4 of the radiation therapy at a dose of $1000 \, mg/m^2$ day by continuous intravenous infusion (maximum of 1800 mg/day). This first 2-week cycle of treatment was followed by a week without treatment, with a subsequent second cycle of combined treatment immediately thereafter, again delivering 20 Gy to the pelvis over 2 weeks, with concurrent 5-FU on days 1–4.

Patients ineligible for cystectomy received a third cycle of treatment 1 week after completion of the second cycle. This final cycle differed only from the first two by the shrinking of the radiation treatment portals after the first 4 Gy to include only the bladder for the remaining 16 Gy. There-

fore, the complete treatment consisted of 44 Gy to the pelvic lymph nodes, 60 Gy to the entire bladder, and three concurrent cycles of 5-FU, delivered over 8 weeks.

Patients eligible for cystectomy had a 3-week period of rest after the completion of the first two treatment cycles in order to allow both tumor regression as well as patient recovery from the acute effects of therapy. After this rest period, these patients underwent repeat cystoscopy under anesthesia, with deep-muscle biopsies performed at the original sites. Those patients with histological evidence of residual tumor underwent radical cystectomy 1–2 weeks later. Those without evidence of residual tumor received the third cycle of treatment, as just described, and completed their therapy with an overall treatment time of 11 weeks.

After completion of therapy, all patients received routine follow-up at 3-month intervals. Patients with retained bladders underwent follow-up cystoscopy and directed biopsies, as indicated, at the same intervals. Follow-up (as of March 1989) ranged from 2 to 45 months, with a median of 18 months.

20.3 Results

The distribution of tumor stages for the 34 patients, as well as within the two treatment cohorts, is summarized in Table 20.1.

20.3.1 Surgical Candidates

Of the 18 patients who were surgical candidates, 16 underwent the full urological reevaluation and biopsy after the initial two cycles of treatment, and

Table 20.1. Distribution of Tumor Stages

	Surgical candidates	Nonsurgical candidates	Total
T_1	2	1	3
T_2	3	3	6
T_{3A}	4	3	7
T_{3B}	6	3	9
T_{4A}	3	4	7
T_{4B}	0	2	2
	18	16	34

two underwent cystoscopy without biopsy. The two patients who were not biopsied had no evidence of tumor by visual inspection and were treated as if they had achieved a complete tumor clearance. Of the 16 who were biopsied, 11 (69%) had no tumor in the biopsy specimen and 5 had histological evidence of residual tumor. Of the five patients who underwent planned cystectomy 1–2 weeks later, two had no evidence of tumor in the cystectomy speciment. These two patients had extensive circumferential tumors at initial presentation not readily resectable with a simple biopsy. Assuming that the additional 2 weeks prior to cystectomy allowed for the completion of tumor regression in these two patients, these patients may be considered as complete responders, bringing the percentage of tumor clearance after the initial chemoradiotherapy to 81% (13/16).

Tumor stage, focality, morphology, and pretreatment resectability via transurethral resection (TURBT) have been tabulated for the 16 patients who were evaluated for complete tumor clearance after the initial two cycles of therapy. These data are summarized in Table 20.2.

Of the 18 patients in the surgical cohort, nine remain without evidence of bladder cancer (NED), two have locally recurrent, *noninvasive* bladder cancer at different locations within the bladder managed by TURBT (both patients having had invasive tumors at presentation), one is alive with metastatic disease, two have died of intercurrent illness without bladder cancer, and four are dead of bladder cancer.

In the subgroup of 13 patients who were complete responders following two cycles of treatment, eight are NED (62%), one has recurrent, noninvasive bladder cancer, one has died of intercurrent illness without bladder cancer, and three have died of bladder cancer (one patient died 6 weeks after treatment with widespread liver metastases). The determinental survival for this groups, excluding the death from intercurrent illness, is 75% (9/12 patients), and the survival free of recurrent invasive disease is 69% (9/13 patients).

20.3.2 Nonsurgical Candidates

Of the 16 patients who were not surgical candidates, six remained relapse-free, one is NED after a salvage cystectomy for locally recurrent disease (7/16 patients or 44% overall NED), four are alive with bladder cancer, two have died of intercurrent illness, and three are dead of bladder cancer. The overall survival is 68%, and the determinental survival is 78% (11/14).

20.3.3 Patterns of Failure

The sites of first tumor recurrence have been scored for the 18 surgically eligible patients, the 13 patients in the subgroup of these 18 who were without histological evidence of tumor in the repeat biopsies (a status of P0), and the 16 nonsurgical candidates. These data are summarized in Table 20.3.

20.3.4 Bladder Preservation

Of the 34 patients, 24 (71%) have retained their bladders. Cystectomy was performed in ten patients; six were planned cystectomies and four were salvage cystectomies for local tumor re-

Table 20.2. Factors associated with normal biopsies at 40 Gy (13/16 patients)

Tumor morphology	
Papillary	6/6
Solid	2/4
Unspecified	5/6
Pretreatment TURBT	
Yes	9/12
No	4/4
Tumor multifocality	
Yes	7/9
No	6/7
Tumor stage	
T_1	1/2
T_2	2/2
T_{3A}	3/3
T_{3B}	5/6
T_{4A}	2/3

Table 20.3. Sites of first tumor recurrence

	LF	LF/DM	DM
P0 (13)	2	1	1
S (18)	4	0	2
NS (16)	5	0	3

Abbreviation: LF, local failure; DM, distant metastases; P0, Patients with negative biopsy at 4,000 cGy.; S, surgical candidates; NS, nonsurgical candidates

Table 20.4. Bladder status (34 patients)

10/34 cystectomy (6 primary, 4 salvage)
24/34 retained bladder (71%)
18/24 NED: $T_1 = 1/3$
$T_2 = 5/6$
$T_3 = 5/16$
$T_4 = 7/9$
3/24 noninvasive tumor recurrence
3/24 invasive tumor recurrence
20/24 normal voiding (83%)

currence (one of 11 surgical candidates with a *negative* biopsy after the first two cycles of treatment underwent a planned cystectomy because of physicians' concerns that the large initial tumor had incompletely regressed. Histological evidence of tumor clearance was confirmed by the cystectomy specimen.) The full information with respect to bladder preservation is summarized in Table 20.4. Of the 24 patients with retained bladders, 20 (83%) have normal voiding and four have symptoms of frequency or urgency which developed after the conclusion of the treatment.

20.3.5 Toxicity of Treatment

Of the 40 patients originally enrolled on study, six were unable to complete the treatment. Three of these patients developed angina while receiving the first cycle of 5-FU and were subsequently treated with cisplatin off-study. Two additional patients were off-study, at their request, after the first cycle of treatment, one because of vulvovaginal mucositis and the other for nausea. Finally, one patient developed severe diarrhea during the first cycle of treatment, progressing to sepsis and death.

Of the remaining 34 patients completing the entire treatment, 28 received 100% of the planned 5-FU dosage, with none of the patients receiving less than 80% of the chemotherapy. Specific side-effects of treatment for these 34 patients include one case of excess bleeding following biopsy at 40 Gy, which resulted in a 2-week delay in resuming the last cycle of treatment. Two patients developed dysuria, and most patients developed some degree of diarrhea, limited to the weeks under treatment and generally well controlled with one to three tablets of Lomotil (diphenoxylate hydrochloride with atropine sulfate; Searle Pharmaceuticals) per day.

20.4 Discussion

Tumor radioresponsiveness is a well-established favorable prognostic factor in bladder cancer. More than any individual clinical or pathological feature of an invasive tumor, complete tumor clearance with radiation portends a favorable outcome of treatment relative to its non-responsive counterpart (BLOOM et al. 1982; QUILTY and DUNCAN 1986; HOPE-STONE et al. 1984; BOILEAU et al. 1980; DEWEERD et al. 1977; SCANLON et al. 1983; SLACK and PROUT 1980).

This trial has asked whether the treatment of the bladder cancer patient can be individualized using tumor radioresponsiveness as the criterion by which to decide the need for surgical removal of the bladder. Additionally, the study has sought to determine whether the percentage of patients with radioresponsive tumors can be increased by the use of a radiation potentiator such as 5-FU, and whether increases in the percentage of favorable responses will have consequences in terms of survival as well as bladder preservation. This latter question has been previously addressed in the clinical trial reported on by ROTMAN et al. (1988), who also combined 5-FU and radiation for patients ineligible for cystectomy, with similar results.

Although the short follow-up time for these patients precludes comparison of the current survival data with the 5-year survival data from other series, there is the suggestion that tumor down-staging is enhanced by the addition of 5-FU to the radiation regimen. Historical results obtained from series in which 40–50 Gy of radiotherapy alone was used as a preoperative regimen reveal an expected frequency of complete downstaging on the order of 14%–43% (BLOOM et al. 1982; Boileau et al. 1980; SLACK and PROUT 1980; WHITMORE et al. 1977). The occurrence of complete histological responses in 69%–81% of the patients in the current series is highly suggestive (given the limitations of a small patient numbers) that a biological enhancement is taking place.

To the extent that a deep-muscle biopsy detects residual cancer with the same certainty as pathological examination of the entire cystectomy specimen, these preliminary results may be expected to remain favorable. The requirement in this study of histological confirmation of tumor clearance within 3 weeks of completing relatively low dose radiation would seem to be a more conservative measure of radioresponsiveness than a cystoscopic assessment, without biopsy, at 6 months following completion of high dose radiotherapy. This latter approach has been the accepted endpoint used in prior investigations (Bloom et al. 1982; Quilty and Duncan 1986; Hope-Stone et al. 1984). Nonetheless, recent studies correlating biopsy and cystectomy data to assess combination chemotherapy-induced complete bladder tumor responses suggest that biopsies may underestimate the presence of residual tumor relative to information obtained by examination of the full cystectomy specimen by as much as 34% (Scher et al. 1988). To date, one can conclude from this current series of patients that the incidence of local tumor recurrence in those patients achieving biopsy-proven complete responses has been low.

Much debate has been engendered among investigators as to which clinicopathological features of invasive tumors may predict for radioresponsiveness. Tumor stage, size, grade, focality, morphology, resectability by TURBT, and obstruction of the distal ureters as well as patient age and hemoglobin have all been proposed as pretreatment parameters useful in selecting patients suitable for primary radiotherapy (Bloom et al. 1982; Quilty et al. 1986; Shipley et al. 1985; Batata et al. 1981). Given the small subgroups in the 16 biopsied patients, it is fair only to conclude that there are no obvious trends in radioresponsiveness predictable by these patients' tumor stage, morphology, multifocality, or resectability.

The combined 5-FU and radiation has been well tolerated by most patients, with the one obvious exception. Overall, 80% of patients received full doses of 5-FU. Three patients developed a side-effect of 5-FU infusion, coronary artery vasospasm, clinically manifested as angina, which has been previously well described (Collins and Weiden 1987). Patients who retained their bladders have, to date, experienced little in the way of treatment-related bladder injury.

20.5 Conclusions

The combination of 5-FU with radiotherapy appears to yield a higher percentage of complete tumor responses than historical experiences using radiation alone, and with little additional morbidity from the addition of the chemotherapy. This combined modality approach has permitted bladder preservation in the majority of the patients treated, may prove to be an improvement over radiation alone for patients ineligible for cystectomy, and is an attractive alternative regimen for patients unsuitable for more aggressive chemoradiotherapy approaches.

Acknowledgments. The authors wish to acknowledge the contributions of Drs. Sharon Cole, Lynne Dawson, and Richard Wonderly, who have been very active and supportive participating physicians in this study.

References

Batata MA, Chu FCH, Hilaris BS, Kim YS, Lee MZ, Chung S, Whitmore WF (1981) Factors of prognostic and therapeutic significance in patients with bladder cancer. Int J Radiat Oncol Biol Phys 7: 575

Bloom HJG, Hendry WF, Wallace DM, Skeet RG (1982) Treatment of T3 bladder cancer: controlled trial of preoperative radiotherapy and radical cystectomy versus radical radiotherapy: second report and review. Br J Urol 54:136–151

Boileau MA, Johnson DE, Chan RC et al. (1980) Bladder carcinoma. Results with pre-operative radiation therapy and radical cystectomy. Urology 16: 569–576

Collins C, Weiden PL (1987) Cardiotoxicity of 5-fluorouracil. Cancer Treat Rep 71: 733–736

DeWeerd JH, Colby MY Jr, Myers RP, Cupps RE (1977) Cystectomy after radiotherapeutic ablation of invasive transitional cell cancer. J Urol 118: 260

Duncan W, Quilty PM (1986) The results of a series of 963 patients with transitional cell carcinoma of the urinary bladder primarily treated by radical megavoltage x-ray therapy. Radiother Oncol 7: 299–310

Goodman GB, Hislop TG, Elwood JM, Balfour J (1981) Conservation of bladder function in patients with invasive bladder cancer treated by definitive irradiation and selective cystectomy. Int J Radiat Oncol Biol Phys 7: 569–573

Hope-Stone HF, Oliver RTD, England HR, Blandy JP (1984) T3 bladder cancer: salvage rather than elective cystectomy after radiotherapy. Urology 24: 315–319

Quilty PM, Duncan W (1986) Primary radical radiotherapy for T3 transitional cell cancer of the bladder: an analysis of survival and control. Int J Radiat Oncol Biol Phys 12: 853–860

Quilty PM, Kerr GR, Duncan W (1986) Prognostic indices for bladder cancer: an analysis of patients with transitional cell carcinoma of the bladder primarily treated by radical megavoltage x-ray therapy. Radiother Oncol 7: 311–321

Rotman M, Macchia R, Silverstein M et al. (1988) Treatment of advanced bladder carcinoma with irradiation and concomitant 5-fluorouracil infusion. Cancer 59: 710–714

Scanlon PW, Scott M, Segura JW (1983) A comparison of short-course, low-dose and long-course, high-dose preoperative radiation for carcinoma of the bladder. Cancer 52: 1153–1159

Scher HI, Yogoda A, Herr HW et al. (1988) Neoadjuvant M-VAC (methotrexate, vinblastine, doxorubicin and cisplatin) effect on the primary bladder lesion. J Urol 139: 470–474

Shipley WU, Rose MA, Perrone TL, Mannix CM, Heney NH, Prout GR (1985) Full dose irradiation for patients with invasive bladder carcinoma: clinical and histologic factors prognostic of improved survival. J Urol 134: 679–683

Slack NH, Prout GR Jr (1980) The heterogeneity of invasive bladder carcinoma and different responses to treatment. J Urol 123: 644

Whitmore WF Jr, Batata MA, Ghoneim MA, Grabstald H, Unal A (1977) Radical cystectomy with or without prior irradiation in the treatment of bladder cancer. J Urol 118: 184–187

Yu WS, Sagerman RH, Chung CT, Dalal PS, King GA (1985) Bladder carcinoma. Experience with radical and preoperative radiotherapy in 421 patients. Cancer 56: 1293–1299

21 Protracted (Continuous 5-Fluorouracil) Infusion with Concomitant Radiation Therapy: Indications and Results

Tyvin A. Rich

CONTENTS

5-FU administered by rapid intravenous injection with radiotherapy. Clinical studies using these guidelines ensued in the 1970s and 1980s and a majority of the nonrandomized and randomized trials for patients with adenocarcinomas of the gastrointestinal tract demonstrated a benefit in local control and survival for those receiving chemoradiation (SCHEIN et al. 1982). More recently, interest has grown in using 5-FU given as a continuous infusion employing either short (96–120 h) or protracted (more than 30 days) infusion schedules combined with conventionally fractionated irradiation ("chemoradiation") (RICH et al. 1985b). In this chapter, emphasis will be placed on the use of protracted infusion 5-FU in the Department of Clinical Radiotherapy at M.D. Anderson Cancer Center (MDACC), Houston, Texas.

21.1 Introduction

The favorable therapeutic exploitation by the combination of two cytotoxic agents, namely ionizing radiation and an antimetabolite, in this case the fluorianted pyrimidine, 5-fluorouracil, (5-FU), has been attempted over the past 25 years with variable success. After the discovery of a synergistic effect on cancers in laboratory animals by this combination therapy (HEIDELBERGER et al. 1958), clinical trials in the early 1960s with 5-FU and radiotherapy showed only moderate success, and in some trials there was no superiority over irradiation alone. Nevertheless, investigation continued until the pioneering work at the Mayo Clinic (MOERTEL et al. 1969) which provided the guidelines for the maximum permissible dose of

21.2 Background

Over the last decades, several technical innovations have made the use of continuous infusion clinically practical. The use of Silastic catheters that are inserted into the extremity or placed in the subclavian vein permits long-term vascular access (BOTHE and DALY 1987). Techniques are now standardized that allow safe, convenient, and low cost intravenous administration of a variety of chemotherapeutic agents. A second technical innovation that has permitted outpatient continuous infusion chemotherapy programs to flourish is the development of the low cost ambulatory infusion pump. Electrical mechanical devices are available that permit programmable, intermittent infusion as well as continuous infusion schedules (TUCKER 1987). At MDACC, a balloon pump housed in a plastic cylinder was developed in conjunction with the Travenol Corporation. The pump is small, lightweight, and can be worn under the clothing very easily. The pump is self-contained,

Tyvin A. Rich, MD, Associate Professor, University of Texas System Cancern Center, M.D. Anderson Hospital and Tumor Institute, 6723 Bertner Drive, Houston, TX 77030, USA

and depending on the chemotherapeutic agent can be prepared several days in advance so that the patient can exchange a new pump daily at home. A typical course of continuous infusion chemotherapy combined with radiotherapy for 5–6 weeks will cost approximately $900–$1000 for the infusors.

21.2.1 Background Studies Using Low Dose Continuous 5-Fluorouracil Infusion for Patients with Gastrointestinal Cancers

The mainstay of chemotherapy for patients with advanced adenocarcinoma of the gastrointestinal tract has been 5-FU over the last 25 years. As a single agent, it appears to have produced a consistent objective response rate of 8%–20% when given as bolus injections. In an effort to overcome chemotherapy resistance, drug administration by continuous infusion schedules has been tried with variable success. Relatively short infusion schedules of 8–24 h did not show any significant improvement in responses in patients with advanced colorectal cancers (O'CONNELL 1987). More recently, interest in protracted infusion schedules greater than 24 h have been tried. LOKICH et al. (1981) have reported on a phase I study using continuous venous infusion of 5-FU given for protracted periods through central venous catheters using ambulatory pumps. The initial report showed a dose-limiting toxicity of stomatitis at a daily dose of >300 mg/m^2/day for period of only 8–23 consecutive days. When doses of <300 mg/m^2/day were used, it was possible to administer continuous infusion 5-FU for as long as 60–90 days without significant toxicity. The cumulative doses of 5-FU can be three to four times greater than that achieved by bolus or 5-days infusion schedules. The main toxicity encountered when patients receive low dose continuous 5-FU (>30 days) generally consists of mucocutaneous reactions, most notably stomatitis. Patients may also experience redness and swelling of the distal fingers, palms, and soles associated with paresthesias and a burning sensation referred to as the "hand-foot syndrome." Gastrointestinal toxicity consisting of nausea, vomiting, and diarrhea may also ensue, especially in patients receiving concurrent external beam irradiation to the abdomen or pelvis.

In 1985, we reported on the initial experience using low dose 5-FU infusion and concomitant radiation therapy (RICH et al. 1985b). A total of 41 patients were evaluated at the New England Deaconess Hospital (NEDH), Boston, Mass. The tumor sites were esophagus (9), bile duct (3), pancreas (9), stomach (9), colon (5), rectum (5), and anus (1). Most patients had unresected disease or a high risk of residual disease after resection at the time of referral for irradiation. A 5-FU dose of 250–300 mg/m^2/24 h was infused at rates of 9–12 ml/day.

Cumulative 5-FU doses ranged from 4.6 to 48.2 g (median 14.5 g given over 34 days). An additional infusion of 5-FU or other cytotoxic drugs was used either before or after chemoradiation in 20 patients.

Total radiation doses were planned in most cases to deliver 40–50 Gy for patients receiving adjuvant treatment, and up to 60–70 Gy for those with unresected disease. Irradiation was generally delivered at a rate of 1.8–2 Gy per day although several patients who received palliative radiotherapy (XRT) had fraction sizes of 2.5–3 Gy per day. The median duration of therapy was 5 weeks, which closely coincided with the median duration of 5-FU infusion.

Some toxicity was encountered in all patients. The major categories were gastrointestinal and mucocutaneous reactions with a minority having any hematological toxicity. Acute toxicity was considered mild in 27 patients (66%) and consisted of dysphagia/stomatitis, nausea, and diarrhea. These symptoms were controlled adequately with analgesics, antiemetics, and anticholinergics so that cessation of chemotherapy or radiotherapy was not required. In five patients, additional manifestation of toxicity were conjunctivitis and a macular skin rash. Moderate toxicity was observed in 12 patients (29%) and resulted in treatment interruption of 5-FU and sometimes in interruption of irradiation treatment. This toxicity level was scored in any patient having symptoms not adequately controlled with medications. Stomatitis occurred in nine patients, resulting in temporary interruption of 5-FU, and in five of these the total 5-FU dose given was less then 10 g. Temporary interruption of treatment because of difficulty in controlling nausea and diarrhea occurred in three other patients. Severe toxicity requiring cessation of all therapy occurred in two patients (5%). Both patients had circumstances unrelated to the combined modality therapy which could have also lowered the acute tolerance. Lastly, another toxicity was symptomatic venous thrombosis in three patients (7%), which precluded further chemotherapy. Low hematological toxicity was noted, with the average WBC and platelet count falling by only 20% and 40% of pretreatment values, respectively. An evaluation of the efficacy of treatment showed that 23 patients were alive without evidence of recurrence of disease, or disease progression, with short follow-up (median 8 months). Late radiation toxicity was not encountered above that which was expected with radiation doses used at the sites treated.

This trial demonstrated that the overall toxicity was acceptable when protracted 5-FU was given the concomitant XRT. It was a considerable departure from the standard use of 5-FU given as a bolus intravenous administration for 3 consecutive days, usually at a maximum dosage of 15 mg/kg, at the beginning and end of radiotherapy. A particular attraction in using prolonged infusion schedules is the potential for high total cumulative doses. Also, nondividing tumor cells which are recruited into division during XRT will do so in the presence of this cycle-specific chemotherapeutic agent which has the potential to kill proliferating tumor stem cells.

The possibilities for optimal administration of 5-FU with radiotherapy treatment have recently been addressed by the laboratory studies which emphasized the importance of time–dose relationships for cytotoxicity by 5-FU. BYFIELD et al. (1982) showed that the additive effects of 5-FU plus XRT can be remarkably improved by prolonging drug exposure time beyond the cell cycle time. Other laboratories have confirmed and enhanced cytotoxicity for 5-FU when given for prolonged exposure times without (DREWINKO and YANG 1985) or with irradiation (RICH et al. 1985a). The maximum additive effect of 5-FU plus XRT likely occurs with infusional administration of 5-FU and concomitant XRT.

One of the determinants of the amount of additivity between 5-FU and irradiation is the degree of cytotoxicity achieved with 5-FU infusion. The additive effect appears to require first a concentration × time product that results in cytotoxicity. BYFIELD has concluded that the important clinical implications of this relationship are that (a) radiation enhancement is most likely to occur if the tumor is "responsive" to 5-FU alone and (b) enhancement may be increased depending on the dose (or possibly the time) of 5-FU administered (BYFIELD 1987). There are major differences between the clinical approaches used by BYFIELD and others and our low dose continuous infusion of 5-fluorouracil and radiation. The former tech-

nique generally uses 1000 mg/m^2/24 h over a period of 4–5 days and often in conjunction with other chemotherapy (mitomycin, cisplatin), whereas we have used approximately one-third of the daily dose of 5-FU but have protracted the infusion over a period which is three to three and a half times as long. The pharmacological differences between these different infusion schedules may be considerable. When doses of 25–60 mg/kg/24 h have been used, serum concentrations in man appear to be linearly related to the infused dose rate (BYFIELD 1987). With the 4- to 5-day infusion schedules the mean 5-FU serum concentrations achieved are in the range of 400 ng/ml. This drug concentration is suggested to be the minimum amount for radiation enhancement when short infusion schedules are used. However, lower drug concentrations for longer exposure times may also result in radiation enhancement since the concentration × time product for exposure times up to 240 h in vitro has been shown to result in *both* cytotoxicity and radiation dose modification (BYFIELD et al, 1982). Furthermore, clinical studies using protracted venous infusion alone for patients with advanced colon cancer have shown response rates of >30%, indicating that this administration schedule is at least equal to and is possibly superior to that achieved by bolus intravenous administration of 5-FU. The cytotoxicity found with low dose protracted infusion schedules thus satisfies one of the BYFIELD criteria for radiation enhancement. Comparisons of the cytotoxicity activity in man for short (4- to 5-day) infusions versus either bolus 5-FU or long (>30 days) 5-FU infusion are not available, unfortunately.

Another important aspect of this NEDH pilot trial was the use of conventionally fractionated, external beam irradiation where fraction sizes were 1.8–2 Gy per day. In some trials that have used the short 5-FU infusion schedules, the XRT fractionation has been 2.5 Gy × 4 per week followed by planned treatment interruptions to allow normal tissue recovery. A potential disadvantage of this "cyclic" therapy is the possibility that the tumor may also repopulate during the treatment interruption.

In other clinical trials using low dose continuous infusion 5-FU, the normal tissue toxicity has been reported to be consistent with what we observed in the NEDH trials for stomatitis, hand-foot syndrome, and dermatitis (HANSEN et al. 1987; WADE et al. 1986; BENEDETTO et al. 1986). At the present time, the optimal infusion schedule of 5-FU with irradiation has probably not been determined. Clinical protocols will need to assess the relative effectiveness and toxicity of bolus versus continuous infusion 5-FU with conventional radiation as well as short versus prolonged 5-FU continuous infusion schedules when combined with radiotherapy. There is also the possibility that responses to these different 5-FU infusion schedules may vary for squamous cell carcinomas compared with adenocarcinomas.

21.3 Clinical Studies of Low Dose Continuous 5-Fluorouracil Infusion and Concomitant Irradiation at M.D. Anderson Cancer Center for Gastrointestinal Cancers

Over the past 4 years, a series of gastrointestinal tumor sites have been treated with conventionally fractionated irradiation plus 5-FU given in doses of $300\,mg/m^2/24\,h$ for the entire duration of radiotherapy. Initially these studies were designed to extend the study of toxicity for larger numbers of patients at tumor sites similar to these mentioned in the NEDH pilot study. At MDACC, some clinical protocols have expanded the use of continuous infusion 5-FU via the intraperitoneal route for patients with pancreatic and colorectal adenocarcinomas. In other trials we are investigating the utility of low dose infusion 5-FU plus XRT in a program of postoperative adjuvant therapy for patients with operable rectal cancer.

21.3.1 Esophageal Cancer

Beginning in 1985, a prospective nonrandomized protocol was initiated employing either moderate dose preoperative chemoradiation for marginally resectable patients with squamous cell carcinoma or high dose chemoradiation for those medically unfit or those with tumors unresponsive to induction systemic chemotherapy. The former group received preoperative chemoradiation to a dose of 30 Gy in 15 fractions with 5-FU ($300\,mg/m^2/24\,h$) infused during XRT. Patients with more advanced disease or those who were not surgical candidates were treated to total doses of 60 Gy over 6½ weeks with the same dose of concurrently infused 5-FU. This treatment resulted in a median survival of 24 months for 12 patients. The survival of this

cohort of patients is improved in comparison to patients treated in the previous decade at MDACC. The improved survival probably reflects not only the chemoradiation treatment described above, but also induction systemic therapy used in all patients consisting of infusion 5-FU plus cisplatin. This survival is consistent with that reported by others using shorter, continuous infusion 5-FU schedules and external beam irradiation. Further trials for patients with advanced disease as well as those with "surgical operable" squamous cell carcinoma of the esophagus will need to be performed in the future.

21.3.2 Pancreatic Cancer

For patients with surgically unresectable carcinoma of the pancreas, 5-FU (500 mg/kg) given by bolus intravenous injection for 3 consecutive days at the beginning and end of a course of radiotherapy (to doses of 40 or 60 Gy) has been shown by the Gastrointestinal Tumor Study Group (GITSG) to significantly improve survival over moderate doses (40 Gy) of radiation alone (MOERTEL et al. 1981). Furthermore, 5-FU based adjuvant chemoradiation has been demonstrated to improve local control and survival for patients with resected disease (KALSER and ELLENBERG 1985). These data indicate the utility of combining 5-FU in other ways with external beam irradiation in order to improve local control and survival for patients with pancreatic cancer.

In 1986 at MDACC, we began a prospective, nonrandomized trial employing continuous infusion 5-FU in two different ways for patients with unresected, residual, or recurrent pancreatic cancer or for those with advanced colorectal cancers. First, patients received a single course of intraperitoneal 5-FU infusion starting at 1 g diluted in 1 liter of physiological saline delivered into the peritoneal cavity over 24 h. A treatment course consisted of 5 days of continuous infusion 5-FU. A dose escalation sequence was begun after we determined that 1 g/day was safe. Using incremental doses of 0.25 g per patient, a total dose of 2 g/day for 5 days was found to be the maximum tolerated dose. The most common side-effect was either localized or diffuse abdominal pain, which occurred in 60% and 34% of patients respectively. The systemic side-effects were nausea (34%), diarrhea (12%), and vomiting and mucositis (8%). After a 1- to 2-week treatment break, patients were then started on intravenous 5-FU infusion ($300 \, mg/m^2$/day) with concomitant external beam irradiation directed to the primary or recurrent disease site plus the regional lymph nodes. The median radiation dose was 55 Gy given in 5½ weeks (median 34 days), and the median total 5-FU dose was 16.7 g. The acute toxicities included nausea (74%), diarrhea (65%), vomiting (42%), mucositis (30%), hand-foot syndrome (15%), and leukopenia (24%). These symptoms were usually managed by medications or treatment interruption of 5-FU in 33%. Radiotherapy was also interrupted in 25% of patients. There were 15% of patients hospitalized for a median of 4 days (range 3–27 days). The acute toxicity was not related to site, XRT, or 5-FU dose. Late radiotherapy effects did not appear to be increased. The actuarial local tumor control for the pancreas is 32% and survival 34% at a maximum follow-up of 22 months. One patient in the pancreas group is still radiographically free of disease over 2 years from the beginning of treatment. Although this treatment program was a pilot trial to assess the feasibility of intraperitoneal therapy with chemoradiation, it has allowed us to gain more experience with low dose continuous infusion 5-FU for the treatment of adenocarcinomas arising in the abdomen and pelvis. Most toxicities can be controlled with adequate medication or with brief 5-FU infusion interruption. We have recently begun a new protocol employing chemoradiation for patients with unresectable pancreatic cancer in which the 5-FU infusion is given only 5 days per week with XRT (50.4 Gy) for an overall time of 5½ weeks. This will be followed by laparotomy and resection if feasible, plus electron beam intraoperative radiotherapy. We expect that with planned interruptions of continuous infusion chemotherapy patient tolerance will improve. It is too early for any assessment of this infusion schedule modification to be certain that toxicity is ameliorated.

21.3.3 Biliary Tract Cancer

In contrast to patients with pancreatic cancer, where there is a high transperitoneal and regional lymph node failure pattern, patients with biliary tract cancer of either the extrahepatic biliary ducts or gallbladder usually die of progressive local disease. Our approach in these patients has been to use 5-FU chemoradiation but without intra-peritoneal 5-FU infusion. In our first ten patients, eight of whom had unresectable disease, the treatment program generally consisted of continuous infusion 5-FU continued at $300 \, mg/m^2$/24 h during external beam radiotherapy up to a dose of 45–50.4 Gy. After external beam XRT, the patient was considered for a specialized boost. If a biliary tract catheter could be used, an iridium[192] implant via the transcutaneous route was performed to deliver an additional 25–35 Gy at 1 cm from the lumen of the catheter. In other cases, external beam techniques were used, generally with arc-wedge radiation fields, to deliver an additional 15–20 Gy. The boost treatments were not generally done with 5-FU infusion. Acute toxicity was acceptable and related to both upper gastrointestinal side-effects of nausea and vomiting, as well as mucocutaneous reactions including the hand-foot syndrome and stomatitis. Nine of the first ten patients with biliary cancer were alive at 5–15 months after treatment. In three patients, late radiation-related complications of gastric outlet obstruction or duodenal ulceration became evident, two of which required surgery. At reoperation recurrent tumor was discovered in addition to probable radiation-related changes in the duodenum. These latter changes may be related solely to the XRT, since doses exceeding tolerance of the small intestine were used. In nearly all cases, the entire circumference of the duodenum was in the radiation portal up to a dose of 45–50 Gy. An update of our experience with biliary tract cancer now shows 22 patients have been treated with chemoradiation as described above. An analysis of local control and survival indicates a significant improvement over the results achieved in historical controls treated at MDACC. The improvement in our more recent results of the entire group is a result in part of the more aggressive surgical approaches being used, but appears to be influenced by 5-FU infusion regardless of irradiation technique and total dose. Although this is a nonrandomized study, our data indicate that further trials are warranted to explore the optimal utilization of fluoropyrimidines in conjunction with irradiation for patients with unresectable or marginally resectable biliary tract cancer.

21.3.4 Colorectal Cancer

Continuous infusion 5-FU and external beam radiation has been used for three groups of patients with colorectal disease at MDACC in the last 4 years. The first group were those with localized or recurrent disease above the peritoneal reflection who because of their risk of a transperitoneal failure pattern were candidates for the intraperitoneal 5-FU infusion protocol. The toxicities were described above in the section on pancreatic cancer. The only differences to note between the patients with upper gastrointestinal disease versus those with tumors predominately in the pelvis is the finding of slightly more hematopoietic side-effects with chemoradiation in this group. This toxicity is still rather infrequent when compared with hematopoietic suppression reported with the use of bolus 5-FU infusion with pelvic radiotheraphy. The actuarial local control and survival for the group of 17 colorectal patients is 52% and 45% respectively at 22 months (RICH et al. 1985b). This trial indicates that chemoradiation therapy can also be given feasibly to patients with colon or rectal primaries. The 5-FU intraperitoneal treatment may be marginally effective and needs further investigation, possibly using multiple courses of 5-FU or administration during a perioperative period before adhesions have formed. Assessment of 5-FU in combination with other chemotherapeutic agents (e.g., cisplatin, leucovorin) will also need to be performed in well-designed, prospective trials.

21.3.5 Adjuvant Chemoradiation for Completely Resected Rectal Cancer

Several postoperative randomized trials have recently been reported demonstrating the utility of the combination of systemic 5-FU with methyl-CCNU in conjunction with 5-FU administered durings radiation theraphy as postoperative adjuvant treatment for patients with stage B_2, B_3, and stage C carcinoma of the rectum. Two trials performed at GITSG and Mayo Clinic/North Central Tumor Study Group (NCTSG) indicate the superiority of combined modality therapy compared with a surgical control arm or either adjuvant modality used alone (Gastrointestinal Tumor Study Group 1985; GUNDERSON et al. 1986). In a follow-up trial by NCTSG, the superiority of chemoradiation over irradiation was again confirmed, supporting its use to increase both local control and survival. In 1987 we began with Mayo/NCTSG a cooperative trial investigating the use of systemic adjuvant 5-FU with or without methyl-

CCNU and in conjunction with planned pelvic radiotherapy for all patients. During the radiotherapy, all patients are randomized to receive either (a) continuous infusion 5-FU at a dose of 225 mg/m² for the entire course of radiotherapy to a total dose of 55 Gy over a period of approximately 6 weeks or (b) bolus 5-FU at a dosage of 500 mg/m² during the first 3 and last 3 days of XRT. This trial will hopefully allow assessment of the utility of low dose continuous infusion 5-FU and radiotherapy in the adjuvant setting. There are no data at the present time to indicate which method is superior.

21.3.6 5-Fluorouracil Infusion and Radiotherapy for Advanced Rectal Cancer

At MDACC over the past 4 years we have treated patients with residual or recurrent rectal cancer with continuous 5-FU infusion and external beam radiotherapy. Among 121 patients who served as historical controls, there were no statistically significant differences between those patients who were treated for residual disease and those who had unresectable, gross disease at the initiation of treatment with only postoperative radiotherapy. A preliminary analysis shows an improvement in both local control and survival for the 5-FU chemoradiation group when compared with previously treated patients who received only radiotherapy in the prior decade. This is a nonrandomized study and the comparison must be viewed with caution. Nevertheless, patients are now appearing to enjoy a symptom-free and possibly disease-free interval of up to 2 years following 5-FU infusion and pelvic radiotherapy. The acute complications have been somewhat less than those seen in the trial with intraperitoneal therapy and chemoradiation, largely because of irradiation therapy technique. Patients with rectal cancer are all treated at MDACC on an open-table top device which is designed to maximize the small bowel shift away from the posterior pelvis. This permits the overlapping toxicities of 5-FU infusion and pelvic radiotherapy to be minimized and allows us to take patients to doses in excess of 55 Gy.

21.3.7 Anal Canal Cancer

In 1985 at MDACC, we began a prospective, nonrandomized protocol employing continuous infusion 5-FU (300 mg/m^2) plus external beam radiotherapy to 45 Gy for patients with squamous cell or basaloid carcinoma of the anal canal. The majority of patients received treatment via parallel-opposed 18- to 25-MeV photon fields to the pelvis, perineum, and medial inguinal regions at 1.8 Gy per fraction over 5 weeks. An examination under anesthesia (EUA) was performed 4–6 weeks after radiotherapy in order to assess tumor response in the first nine patients. All were found to have no evidence of disease, including five who had negative biopsies. Nevertheless, seven were given a single plane iridium^{192} implant and one an external beam arc rotation boost. We have subsequently discontinued EUA for patients who have a complete clinical response. All patients are followed with routine anoscopy every 8–12 weeks thereafter. An abdominal perineal resection is performed in those with persistent or recurrent disease. Eighteen of the first 24 patients evaluable achieved a complete response. In two patients there was recurrence the primary site at 7 and 8 months. The local control rate with chemoradiation alone for the entire group is 67% (16/24). The colostomy-free local control rate is 78% (14/18) for T_1, T_2, and T_3 and 33% (2/6) for T_4 patients. The median follow-up is 14 months (range 1–30 months).

Eight patients who had persistent recurrent disease after chemoradiation underwent APR. In one specimen, there is no evidence of tumor. Two patients have subsequently failed in the pelvis after Abdomino-perineal resection (APR) yielding an overall local control rate including surgical salvage of 92% (22/24). Local control was significantly better for patients with tumors less that one-third of the circumferential extent versus patients who presented with massive tumors causing incontinence ($P = 0.03$). We could find no statistical differences between T stages according to the American Joint Committee Tumor Staging. Those patients receiving an implant had a higher tumor control than those who were treated to only 45–50 Gy. There was no difference in local control depending on the total chemotherapy dose.

21.4 Summary

In summary, we have demonstrated the feasibility of using low dose continuous infusion with conventionally fractionated irradiation for the patient with gastrointestinal diseases. Delivery of a 5-FU dose of 300 mg/m^2/day is achievable with irradiation when directed to the upper abdomen or pelvis. Those patients with adenocarcinoma arising in the pancreas, biliary tract, or colorectal area appear to be responsive. Compared with historical control groups treated at this institution without chemoradiotherapy but by x-ray therapy alone, there appears to be an improvement in both local control and survival for those with colorectal primaries.

Our present scheme for patients with colorectal disease is directed toward using 5-FU in conjunction with radiation for only 5 days per week with planned weekend interruptions. We believe this may ameliorate some of the gastrointestinal toxicity and allow us to continue achieving the therapeutic benefit of combined therapy. This is being assessed in new prospective trials.

Future possibilities using continuous infusion 5-FU chemotherapy include building further onto our experience with intraperitoneal prophylaxis for patients with tumors who are at high risk for transperitoneal failure. We have demonstrated the feasibility and potential therapeutic efficacy of one cycle; however, the best timing for the delivery of intraperitoneal chemotherapy as well as combination with other chemotherapeutic agents needs further investigation. Low dose whole abdominal XRT could also possibly be used although we have not tried this scheme.

Finally, conventional irradiation treatment schedules for gastrointestinal primaries in conjunction with not only 5-FU infusion but also other potentiators (leucovorin) or other chemotherapeutic agents (mitomycin C or cisplatin) offer several exciting possibilities for selective enhancement of 5-FU cytotoxicity and possibly augmented radiation enhancement.

References

Benedetto P, Bogos M, Morillo G, Sfakiauakis G (1986) Chronic continuous infusion of 5-fluorouracil in previously untreated patients with measurable metastatic colorectal cancer. In: (Abstract) Proceedings of the Am Soc Clin Oncol. p 92

Bothe A, Daly J (1987) Technical aspects of vascular access for infusional chemotherapy. In: Lokich J (ed) Cancer chemotherapy by infusion. Precept, Chicago, pp 59–73

Byfield JE (1987) The clinical use of 5-fluorouracil and other halopyrimidines as radiosensitizers in man. In: Lokich J (ed) Cancer chemotherapy by infusion. Precept, Chicago, pp 479–501

Byfield JE, Calabro-Jones P, Klisak I (1982) Pharmacologic requirements for obtaining sensitization of human tumor cells in vitro to combined 5-fluorouracil or ftorafur and x-rays. Int J Radiat Oncol Biol Phys 8: 1923–1933

Drewinko B, Yang L-Y (1985) Cellular basis for the inefficacy of 5-FU in human colon carcinoma. Cancer Treat Rep 69:1391–1398

Gastrointestinal Tumor Study Group (1985) Prolongation of the disease-free interval in surgically treated rectal carcinoma. N Engl J Med 312: 1465–1472

Gunderson LL, Collins R, Earle JD et al. (1986) Adjuvant treatment of rectal cancer: randomized prospective study of irradiation ± chemotherapy: a NCCTG, Mayo Clinic study. Int J Radiat Oncol Biol Phys 12: 169

Hansen R, Quebbeman E, Ausman R, Ritch P, Anderson W, Schulte W, Frick J (1987) Continuous 5-fluorouracil infusion in colorectal cancer. In (Abstact) Proceedings of the Am Soc Clin Oncol. p 80

Heidelberger C, Griesbach L, Montag BJ (1958) Studies on fluorinated pyrimidines. II. Effects on transplanted tumors. Cancer Res 18: 305–317

Kalser MH, Ellenberg SS (1985) Pancreatic cancer: adjuvant combined radiation and chemotherapy following curative resection. Arch Surg 120: 899

Lokich JJ, Bothe A, Fine N (1981) Phase I study of protracted venous infusion of 5-fluorouracil. Cancer 48: 2565–2568

Moertel CG, Childs DS, Retemeier RJ (1969) Combined 5-fluorouracil and supervoltage radiation therapy of locally unresectable gastrointestinal cancer. Lancet II: 865–867

Moertel CG, Frytak S, Hahn RG et al. (1981) Therapy of locally unresectable pancreatic carcinoma: a randomized comparison of high dose (6000 rads) radiation alone, moderate dose radiation (4000 rads + 5-fluorouracil), and high dose radiation + 5-fluorouracil. Cancer 48: 1705–1710

O'Connell MJ (1987) Antipyrimidines: 5-fluorouracil and 5-fluoro-2'-deoxyuridine. In: Lokich J (ed) Cancer chemotherapy by infusion. Precept, Chicago, pp 117–122

Rich TA, Kavanagh B, Williams M, Bock S, Murray D, Meyn R, Brock WA (1985a) Effects of continuous post-irradiation low dose 5-fluorouracil on log and plateau-phase CHO cells. In: (Abstract) Proceedings on chemical modifiers. Clearwater, FL

Rich TA, Lokich JJ, Chaffey JT (1985b) A pilot study of protracted venous infusion of 5-fluorouracil and concomitant radiation therapy. J Clin Oncol 3: 402–406

Schein PS, Gore ME, Buckman RA (1982) Radiation therapy and 5-fluorouracil. Drugs Exptl Clin Res 8: 587–592

Tucker EM (1987) Drug administration for infusion chemotherapy. In: Lokich J (ed) Cancer chemotherapy by infusion. Precept, Chicago, pp 41–58

Wade JL, Herbst S, Greenberg A (1986) Prolonged venous infusion of 5-fluorouracil for metastatic colon cancer. In (Abstract) Proceedings of the Am Soc Clin Oncol. p 88

Section IV
Radiopotentiation by Cisplatin in Continuous Infusion

22 Radiopotentiation in a Murine Tumor (MTG-B) by Continuous Infusion Platinum

Evan B. Douple, Marcia L. Wills, and Ellen L. Jones

CONTENTS

22.1 Introduction

For more than a decade, studies have shown that the chemotherapeutic drug cisplatin can interact with ionizing radiation, resulting in what is often described as a potentiation of radiation-induced cell kill (for review see DEWIT 1987, and DOUPLE 1986, 1988). At least two distinguishable effects have been identified in cell culture experiments which might account for the supra-additive therapeutic effects reported in animal tumors when the two agents are combined. The first, radiosensitization of hypoxic cells, requires that the cisplatin be present at the time of irradiation. The second, post-irradiation potentiation, enhances cell kill when the cisplatin is added shortly after irradiation, and might include an inhibition of sublethal and potentially lethal damage repair processes. These effects are not limited to the combination of only cisplatin with radiation, since other platinum complexes have also produced these effects (NIAS 1985; DOUPLE 1988), including the second genera-tion platinum complex carboplatin, also known as paraplatin (DOUPLE 1985; DOUPLE et al. 1985, 1987; O'HARA et al. 1986). The precise mechanisms responsible for the interactions remain elusive, but because of the potential for therapeutic gain represented by the two effects, numerous clinical trials with varying protocols have been instituted in an effort to exploit the interactions between the two modalities (DOUPLE 1985, 1988).

Since most cell culture and animal tumor studies have combined a limited number of administrations of bolus platinum with a limited number of irradiations, it is not known whether platinum levels associated with more prolonged administration schedules will approach concentrations of approximately $10 \mu M$ which might be necessary to produce the interactions with radiation mentioned above (DOUPLE et al. 1988; FU et al. 1988). Furthermore, it is not known whether the platinum levels attained will interact with clinically relevant radiation fractions. However, pioneering studies by FU and her co-workers (FU et al. 1984, 1985, 1986) have demonstrated supra-additive tumor cell killing in two murine tumors (SCC VII/SF and RIF-1) when cisplatin was infused continuously over 48 h through intraperitoneal Alzet osmotic minipumps (0.22 mg/kg/h) concomitant with continuous low dose rate whole-body irradiation. In these studies the tumor cells were explanted immediately after irradiation and cell survival was measured by clonogenic assay in vitro.

The current studies were designed to investigate the effects of continuous infusion platinum in combination with radiation therapy on tumors in situ, using a murine mammary adenocarcinoma (MTG-B) and a tumor doubling volume endpoint. Two different localized tumor irradiation protocols were used, either five daily fractions of x-irradiation (RT) or low dose rate ^{125}I brachytherapy (BT). In addition, the effects of cisplatin were compared with those effects obtained using the second generation platinum complex paraplatin for both irradiation protocols.

Evan B. Douple, PhD, Marcia L. Wills, Ellen L. Jones, PhD, Radiobiology Laboratories, Dartmouth-Hitchcock Medical Center, Hanover, NH 03756, USA

22.2 Methods and Materials

22.2.1 Tumor System

MTG-B is a murine mammary adenocarcinoma maintained via serial passage in 5- to 7-week-old female C3H/HeJ mice (Jackson Laboratories, Bar Harbor, ME). Tumor cell suspensions were injected subcutaneously in the flanks of host mice as described elsewhere (JONES et al. 1989). Tumor therapy was initiated on the day tumors first reached 9.5 mm diameter.

22.2.2 Platinum Therapy

Cisplatin or paraplatin (carboplatin) was obtained courtesy of Johnson-Matthey, Inc. (West Chester, PA), dissolved fresh in normal saline, and loaded in a volume of 200 µl into Alzet 2001 osmotic minipumps (Alza Corporation, Palo Alto, CA) to deliver doses of 10 mg/kg body weight (cisplatin) or 30, 60, or 80 mg/kg (paraplatin). The pumps were implanted intraperitoneally and remained in the mice, delivering the drug at a rate of 1 µl/h.

22.2.3 Radiation Therapy

Tumors were irradiated locally, beginning 24 h after pump implantation, using either a Maxitron-300 x-ray machine (General Electric Corporation, Milwaukee, WI) or ^{125}I seeds (Model 6711, 3M Corporation, St. Paul, MN). The RT was delivered as five consecutive daily fractions (2 or 4 Gy/day) using a 2-cm cone, 3 mm Al filtration, 20 mA and 140 kVp, and a skin dose rate of 5.17 Gy/min. Mice were anesthetized with 60 mg/kg sodium pentobarbital (Butler Company, Columbus, OH) prior to irradiation. The BT dose of approximately 7.75 Gy was delivered over 48 h (0.16 Gy/h) using a cap containing three ^{125}I seeds. The BT irradiation system is described in detail elsewhere (JONES et al. 1989).

22.2.4 Tumor Regrowth Analysis

Tumor diameters were measured daily in two orthogonal directions using a template, and tumor volumes were computed using the average diameter for each mouse. A monotonic, semilogarithmic fit to the volumetric regrowth data was used to estimate the time needed to double the treatment volume (GD_{DV}). Approximately eight to ten mice were evaluated in each treatment group. The fraction of tumors which had not reached the GD_{DV} at various times was also computed and the effects of the treatments were analyzed by comparing median GD_{DV}. Additional details regarding the statistical analysis methods are described by JONES et al. (1989).

22.2.5 Platinum Level Measurements

Groups containing three mice with implanted pumps were sacrificed by cervical luxation on days 1 through 5, and tumors were removed and stored frozen at −20°C. The tumors were halved into samples of approximately 100–200 mg. The samples were weighed and digested in 0.5 ml 1 M hyamine (methylbenzethonium hydroxide, Sigma Chemical Company, St. Louis, MO) at 60°C for 12 h. After digestion, the solution was neutralized with 0.5 ml 1 M HCl and diluted 1:1 with distilled water. This digestion is a modification of SIDDIK et al. (1986). Total platinum concentrations were measured as peak area absorbance at 266.1 mm using a Perkin-Elmer Model 2380 AAS with a deuterium arc lamp background correction and an HGA 400 graphite furnace. The ppm of platinum in each sample was determined from a standard curve generated by spiking appropriate control tumor digests with known weights of cisplatin, and total µg of platinum per gram of tissue was computed.

22.3 Results

22.3.1 Cisplatin Combined with Radiation Therapy

Cisplatin (10 mg/kg) by continuous infusion produced significant therapeutic effects on the MTG-B as summarized in experiment A in Table 22.1. The mean GD_{DV} was 28.2 days and the median GD_{DV} was 29.1 days. The cisplatin was also more toxic than expected, since 3 of 30 mice died following the 10 mg/kg, a dose that was not lethal when injected as a bolus in 0.2 ml i.p. The combination of the cisplatin with five daily RT doses of 2 Gy/day beginning 1 day after pump implantation did not increase the mean or median GD_{DV}. However, the combination of five daily RT fractions of 4 Gy/day produced a mean GD_{DV} and median

Table 22.1. Mean and median growth delays to double the treatment volumes (GD_{DV}) for MTG-B treated with radiation and continuous infusion cisplatin or paraplatin

Treatment (dose)	Mean $GD_{DV} \pm$ SD (days)	Median GD_{DV} (days)	Cures/survivors
Experiment A			
Sham control	2.9 ± 1.16	3.1	0/8
RT (10 Gy)	4.4 ± 1.02	5.2	0/8
RT (20 Gy)	9.0 ± 3.23	7.6	0/7
Cisplatin (10 mg/kg)	28.2 ± 3.08	29.1	0/8
Cisplatin + RT (10 Gy)	28.4 ± 3.14	28.8	0/8
Cisplatin + RT (20 Gy)	35.6 ± 4.60	41.3	3/10
Experiment B			
Sham control	2.4 ± 0.73	2.6	0/7
RT (10 Gy)	3.1 ± 1.10	3.6	0/7
RT (20 Gy)	7.8 ± 1.22	6.0	0/7
Paraplatin (30 mg/kg)	24.3 ± 3.68	24.3	0/5
Paraplatin + RT (10 Gy)	23.6 ± 2.11	23.4	0/6
Paraplatin + RT (20 Gy)	27.9 ± 3.18	27.9	0/7
Experiment C			
Sham control	4.6 ± 1.92	4.3	0/8
BT (7.75 Gy)	5.8 ± 0.95	6.0	0/10
Cisplatin (10 mg/kg)	31.2 ± 5.73	30.1	1/8
Paraplatin (60 mg/kg)	32.4 ± 6.85	33.1	0/6
Cisplatin + BT	30.7 ± 4.95	31.8	1/9
Paraplatin + BT	39.3 ± 15.49	37.2	1/9

GD_{DV} of 35.6 and 41.3 days, respectively, compared with values of 34.3 and 33.6 days predicted on the basis of additive effects of the two agents acting independently [GD_{DV} RT (4 Gy × 5) + GD_{DV} cisplatin − GD_{DV} sham control]. The results of this combined treatment suggest a potentiation by the combined therapy since three of ten tumors were cured (no palpable tumor at least 60 days post-treatment), and these three best responses were not included in the mean GD_{DV} computations. The tumor growth curves for this experiment are illustrated in Fig. 22.1. The asterisk and the dashed line denote the predicted mean GD_{DV} and regrowth curve, respectively, if the effect of the cisplatin and RT were strictly additive.

22.3.2 Paraplatin Combined with Radiation Therapy or Brachytherapy

Paraplatin also proved to be more effective and more toxic when administered by continuous infusion compared with i.p. injections. A dose of 80 mg/kg, nonlethal if injected as a bolus in 0.2 ml, produced 100% lethality in this experiment. Doses of 60 mg/kg and 30 mg/kg produced 5/17 and 9/27 deaths, respectively. All tumors in mice which survived the 60 mg/kg paraplatin plus daily fractions of 4 Gy × 5 RT (3/3) were cured. However, when the dose of paraplatin was reduced to 30 mg/ kg, no cures were obtained with the combined therapy, and the mean and median GD_{DV} values were not greater than predicted by additive effects, as summarized in experiment B in Table 22.1. However, when a 60 mg/kg dose of paraplatin was combined with a low dose (7.75 Gy) of BT,

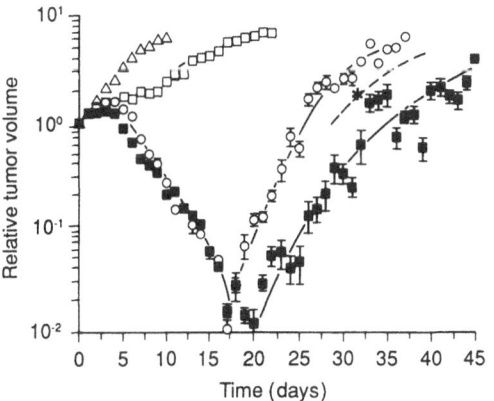

Fig. 22.1. Mean relative tumor volumes for MTG-B as a function of time posttreatment (data from experiment A). *Key:* sham control (*open triangles*); 2; Gy RT in 4 Gy daily fractions × 5 (*open squares*); 10 mg/kg cisplatin (*open circles*); cisplatin plus RT (*solid squares*). *and *dashed curve* denote predicted additive effect for cisplatin plus RT. *Error bars* are standard errors of the means

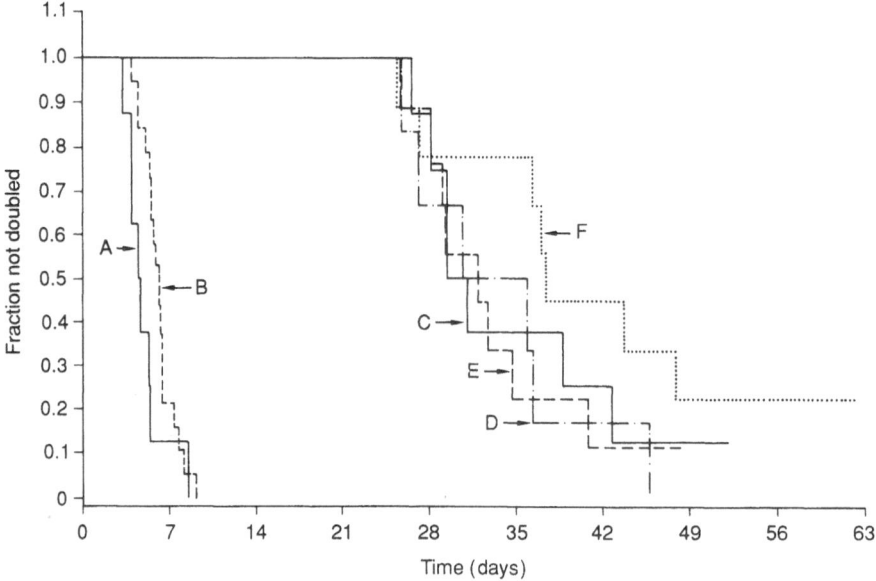

Fig. 22.2. Fraction of mice having not doubled treatment volumes for MTG-B (data from experiment C). *Key*: sham control (A); 7.75 Gy BT in 48 h (B); sham plus 10 mg/kg cisplatin (C); sham plus 60 mg/kg paraplatin (D); cisplatin plus BT (E); paraplatin plus BT (F)

cure was obtained in one of nine tumors and a median GD_{DV} of 39.3 days was obtained, which was greater than the value predicted by paraplatin alone (32.4 days) plus BT alone (5.8 days) minus the sham control (4.6 days), or 33.6 days (see experiment C in Table 22.1). As illustrated in Fig. 22.2, paraplatin plus BT appears to be more effective than cisplatin plus BT for doses of cisplatin (10 mg/kg) and paraplatin (60 mg/kg) which are approximately equally effective when administered without BT.

22.3.3 Concentrations of Total Platinum

The concentrations of total platinum measured in the tumors at various times after initiation of continuous infusion of cisplatin (10 mg/kg in 0.2 ml saline) are illustrated in Fig. 22.3. The days 1 through 5 correspond to the times when daily fractionated RT was delivered in experiments A and B, and the BT was delivered continuously on days 1 through 3. The concentration of total platinum is represented as total μg Pt/g wet tumor, and these values continue to increase with infusion time. A concentration of 1 μg Pt/g tumor obtained after 4 days corresponds to a concentration of

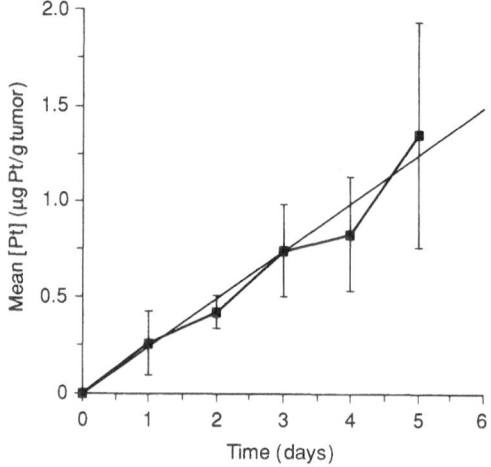

Fig. 22.3. Mean total platinum per gram of wet MTG-B tissue measured as a function of time following pump implantation. *Error bars* denote standard deviations

approximately 5 μM if 1 g of tumor tissue is considered equivalent to 1 ml of water.

22.4 Discussion

At least two types of interactions leading to enhanced cell kill have been characterized for cisplatin or paraplatin in combination with radiation in cultured cell studies, radiosensitization of hypoxic cells and a postirradiation potentiation which appears to be an inhibition of recovery from potentially lethal damage. While it is not clear that these are mechanisms responsible for the potentiation that has been reported in animal tumor systems, studies have shown greater therapeutic potentiation when the platinum is administered before RT compared with immediately after RT, presumably since the drug will be present for both interactions when it is injected a short time before RT. Continuous infusion of platinum chemotherapy offers the potential for delivering significant levels of drug before, during, and after the RT. However, for the design of clinical studies, it is important to know (a) the levels of platinum required to produce the interactions, (b) whether the effects are demonstrable at clinically relevant doses of radiation and drug, and (c) whether there is a difference in the interaction with radiation produced by the second generation platinum drug, paraplatin, compared with cisplatin.

In this mouse MTG-B system, the delivery of cisplatin or paraplatin by infusion is therapeutically more effective, producing larger GD_{DV} values than when the drugs are delivered by a bolus i.p. injection. This effect may result from a larger area under the curve of concentration over time, or it may reflect an effect on cell kinetics or altered chemosensitivity when the drug is present for a longer time. Attendant with the improved therapeutic efficacy was an increase in toxicity at doses which did not produce lethality following single i.p. administrations. Some cures were obtained with the combination of cisplatin or paraplatin with noncurative radiation doses. While these results suggest there might be therapeutic potentiation, the tumor cures and enhanced GD_{DV} from the combined treatments, illustrated in Table 22.1 and Fig. 22.1, required the larger of the two fractionated RT doses, 20 Gy, and were not evident using the platinum with 10 Gy. Whether an increase in the platinum dose would produce an interaction at lower RT doses is not clear. Recent results reported by KORBELIK et al. (1989) suggest that cisplatin produces a significant radiosensitization of hypoxic cell kill in the low dose (<3 Gy) region of the survival curve in cultured cells.

Lowering the dose of paraplatin to 30 mg/kg did not produce greater than additive therapeutic efficacy, suggesting that potentiation requires a certain level of platinum drug. The enhancement by the combination of paraplatin with BT is especially interesting since the total radiation dose was very low (7.75 Gy). FU et al. (1984, 1985, 1986) re-

ported a potentiated tumor cell kill when cisplatin was combined with continuous irradiation at BT dose rates. These earlier studies used a different murine tumor, the pumps were implanted only 48 h, the dose of cisplatin was 12 mg/kg, the irradiation was delivered whole body, and the tumor cells were excised following irradiation and survival was determined by colony forming unit analysis in vitro.

The BT plus paraplatin appears to be more effective than the BT plus cisplatin at doses of drug which have approximately the same toxicity and therapeutic efficacy. Whether this is due to the presence of the larger total platinum metal present in the tumor following the paraplatin compared with cisplatin (DOUPLE et al. 1988) is not known. The levels of cisplatin measured after 4 days (5 µM) approach the level of 10 µM required in cell culture studies to produce radiosensitization of hypoxic cells (DOUPLE 1988), exceed the levels which produce potentiation postirradiation (CARDE and LAVAL 1981; O'HARA et al. 1986), and approach the peak levels measured in MTG-B (DOUPLE et al. 1988) as well as in human xenografts in nude mice (BOVEN et al. 1985) after i.p. bolus injections.

The increasing concentration of total platinum in the tumors with time of infusion suggests that the peak concentration is not reached at 5 days. Therefore, the interaction between RT or BT and platinum chemotherapy might be potentiated if the irradiation were delivered later during the infusion. It should be noted that the platinum levels were measured in unirradiated tumors and there is some evidence to suggest that radiation therapy may alter the pharmacokinetics of certain platinum complexes after bolus i.p. injections (DOUPLE et al. 1988). However, this effect was not observed following whole-body low dose irradiation and continuous infusion of cisplatin in a different tumor system (FU et al. 1988).

In conclusion, these results support a rationale for combining continuous infusion cisplatin or paraplatin chemotherapy concomitantly with either fractionated RT or BT. Therapeutic potentiation, which has been previously reported following bolus administration of platinum complexes and irradiation, may also result under the infusion conditions at relatively low radiation doses. However, the radiation dose and the tumor platinum concentration may be very important in determining the degree of interaction between the two modalities.

Acknowledgments. This work was supported in part by Grant CA40500 from the U.S. National Institutes of Health, National Cancer Institute. The authors gratefully acknowledge the biostatistical assistance provided by Bradley J. Dain and Daniel H. Freeman.

References

Boven E, van der Vijgh WJF, Nauta MM, Schluper HMM, Pinedo HM (1985) Comparative activity distribution studies of five platinum analogues in nude mice bearing human ovarian carcinoma xenografts. Cancer Res 45: 86–90

Carde P, Laval F (1981) Effects of *cis*-dichlorodiammineplatinum(II) and x-rays on mammalian cell survival. Int J Radiat Oncol Biol Phys 7: 929–933

Dewit L (1987) Combined treatment of radiation and *cis*-diamminedichloroplatinum(II): a review of experimental and clinical data. Int J Radiat Oncol Biol Phys 13: 403–426

Douple EB (1985) The use of platinum chemotherapy to potentiate radiotherapy: preclinical results encourage clinical trials. Platinum Metals Rev 29:118–125

Douple EB (1986) Cis-diamminedichloroplatinum(II): effects of a representative metal coordination complex on mammalian cells. In: Dethlefsen LA (ed) Cell cycle effects of drug. Pergamon, Oxford, pp 215–250

Douple EB (1988) Keynote address: platinum-radiation interactions. NCI Monogr 6: 315–319

Douple EB, Richmond RC, O'Hara JA, Coughlin CT (1985) Carboplatin as a potentiator of radiation therapy. Cancer Treat Rev 12[Suppl A]: 111–124

Douple EB, O'Hara JA, Jones EL (1987) Paraplatin enhancement of radiation therapy in a murine tumor (MTG-B). In: Lapis K, Eckhardts (eds) Anticancer drug research, lectures and symposia of the 14th International Cancer Congress, 1986, vol 9. Akademiai Kiado, Budapest, pp 71–80

Douple EB, Totten MD, Spencer F (1988) Platinum levels in murine tumor following intraperitoneal administration of cisplatin or paraplatin. NCI Monogr 6: 129–132

Fu KK, Rayner PA, Lam KN (1984) Modification of the effects of continuous low dose rate irradiation by concurrent chemotherapy infusion. Int J Radiat Oncol Biol Phys 10: 1473–1478

Fu KK, Lam KN, Rayner PA (1985) The influence of time sequence of cisplatin, administration and continuous low dose rate irradiation (CLDRI) and their combined effects on a murine squamous cell carcinoma. Int J Radiat Oncol Biol Phys 11: 2119–2124

Fu KK, Lam KN, Rayner PA (1986) Effects of continuous low dose rate irradiation and concurrent infusion of mitomycin, cisplatin and 5-fluorouracil on three murine tumors. Endocurietherapy/Hyperthermia Oncol 2: 157–162

Fu KK, DeGregorio MW, Phillips JW (1988) Plasma and tumor concentrations of cisplatin following intraperitoneal infusion or bolus injection with or without continuous low-dose-rate irradiation. NCI Monogr 6: 123–127

Jones EL, Lyons BE, Douple EB, Filimonov A, Dain BJ (1989) Response of a brachytherapy model using ^{125}I in a murine tumor system. Radiat Res 118: 112–130

Korbelik M, Palcic B, Skov KA (1989) Cisplatin enhancement of response to low radiation doses in hypoxia. Abstracts of papers for the 37th Annual Meeting of the Radiation Research Society and the 9th Annual Meeting of the North American Hyperthermia Group

Nias AHW (1985) Radiation and platinum drug interaction. Int J Radiat Biol 48: 297–314

O'Hara JA, Douple EB, Richmond RC (1986) Enhancement of radiation-induced cell kill by platinum complexes (carboplatin and iproplatin) in V79 cells. Int J Radiat Oncol Biol Phys 12: 1419–1422

Siddik ZH, Boxall FE, Harrap KR (1986) Tissue solubilization in hyamine hydroxide for the flameless atomic absorption spectrophotometric determination of platinum. In: McBrien DCH (ed) Biochemical mechanisms of platinum antitumor drugs. Oxford University Press, Oxford, pp 355–360

23 Locally Advanced Paranasal Sinus and Nasopharyngeal Cancers – Effects of Hyperfractionated Radiation and Concomitant Continuous Infusion Cisplatin

KWANG CHOI, MARVIN ROTMAN, HASSAN AZIZ, RICHARD S. STARK, C. JULIAN ROSENTHAL, and JOSE R. MARTI

CONTENTS

23.1 Introduction

Management of advanced cancers involving the paranasal and nasopharyngeal complex is complicated by the locally invasive nature of this tumor. The spread of this disease is along mucosal linings and often extends directly into the orbit, or involves the base of skull with cranial nerve dysfunction. The role of surgery is limited because of the structures involved in these strategic locations. Conventional radiotherapy, as pointed out by LEDERMAN (1970), has difficulty in sterilizing malignant cells in compact facial and base of skull bones due to physical and radiobiological limitations. In addition, there is the therapeutic dilemma

KWANG CHOI, MD, Associate Professor, Radiation Oncology, MARVIN ROTMAN, MD, Professor and Chairman, Radiation Oncology, HASSAN AZIZ, MD, Associate Professor, Radiation Oncology, C. JULIAN ROSENTHAL, MD, Professor of Medicine and Oncology, SUNY Health Science Center at Brooklyn, 450 Clarkson Avenue, Brooklyn, NY 11203, USA

RICHARD S. STARK, MD, Director Medical Oncology, Interfaith Medical Center, 555 Prospect Place, Brooklyn, NY, 11238, USA

JOSE R. MARTI MD, Associate Professor of Surgery – SUNY, Chairman of Surgery, The Brooklyn Hospital, 121 Dekalb Ave., Brooklyn, NY 11201, USA

of producing optic nerve, chiasmal, and brain damage. A successful treatment regimen must improve the local control of this disease with a higher therapeutic ratio.

Recently, hyperfractionation regimens have been used to treat locally advanced tumors. The most important phenomenon occurring between dose fractions is the repair of sublethal damage. This phenomenon occurs most consistently with late responding tissues compared to early responding tissues. Therefore, late responding tissues are spared more by hyperfractionation. This allows the total dose of radiation to be increased by 10%–20% for the same normal tissue reaction, thus achieving an improved therapeutic ratio (THAMES et al. 1982)

Cisplatin is an active agent in squamous cell carcinoma. In addition, it may enhance the effect of radiation on tumor and normal tissues in vitro and in vivo (AL-SARRAF et al. 1984; DOUPLE and RICHMOND 1979; DRISTSCHILO et al. 1979; HASELOW et al. 1983), especially when given by intravenous infusion (SIDGESTAD 1979). In an attempt to improve the therapeutic ratio, a strategy using split courses of hyperfractionated radiation and concomitant infusion of cisplatin was tried at the State University of New York.

23.2 Material and Methods

Thirteen patients with locally advanced or recurrent cancer of the nasopharynx and paranasal sinuses were treated with split courses of hyperfractionated radiation and concomitant infusion of cisplatin. Table 23.1 lists the characteristics of the 13 patients. Four of them had nasopharynx, six maxillary antrum, 2 ethmoid sinus, and one lacrimal gland cancers. Eleven of the 13 patients had squamous cell carcinoma, and two had adenoid cystic carcinoma. Eight had primary T_4 lesions, and five had locally advanced recurrent

Table 23.1. Patient characteristics ($n = 14$ patients)

Primary site	
Nasopharynx	4
Maxillary antrum	6
Ethmoid sinus	2
Lacrimal Gland	1
Pathology	
Squamous cell carcinoma	11
Adenoid Cystic carcinoma	2
Stage	
T_4 primary	8
Massive recurrent disease	5

Table 23.2. Treatment regimen

2 wk Tx (10 Tx days) 24–25 Gy Cisplatin	1 or 2 wk rest	2 wk Tx (10 Tx days) 48–50 Gy Cisplatin	1 or 2 wk rest	1–2 wk Tx (7–10 Tx days) 67.2–67.5 Gy Cisplatin

Each Course
Radiation – hyperfractionated (b.i.d.)
24–25 Gy
   Daily: 1.2 Gy, 4- to 6-h interval, 1.2 Gy
   Daily: 1.25 Gy, 4- to 6-h interval, 1.25 Gy
Cisplatin – continuous infusion
   5–7 mg/m²/day

disease after initial surgery or radiation treatment. Eleven patients received a curative dose of radiation treatment and two of the patients with recurrent disease received only palliative treatment due to previoius curative radiation treatment. The treatment program consisted of three courses of 2 weeks of concomitant continuous cisplatin infusion and twice-a-day irradiation with 1 or 2 weeks' rest between courses (Table 23.2). The daily radiation dose was 2.4–2.5 Gy given at 1.2–1.25 Gy/fraction spaced by a 4- to 6-h interval. The curative regimen consisted of three courses of radiation to a total tumor dose ranging from 60–69 Gy with a modal dose of 67.5 Gy. Nasopharyngeal cancers were treated with parallel opposing ports, including nasopharynx, base of skull, cranial extensions of the disease, and upper neck. The lower neck was treated using a single anterior field. Two patients were treated exclusively using parallel opposing ports and shrinking field technique because of oropharyngeal extension. One patient was switched to three field technique (one anterior and two wedged lateral) after 52 Gy. Patients with bilateral massive neck metastases were treated with parallel opposing ports including nasopharynx up to 57.8 Gy, and the neck was

treated using anterior, posterior parallel opposing ports up to a total dose of 66.3 Gy. The techniques used for paranasal sinuses were conventional two wedged anterior and lateral oblique ports or three field technique using one anterior and two wedged lateral ports. All patients received their treatments either on a 4-MeV linear accelerator or cobalt 60 machine.

Cisplatin was given as a continuous infusion using a Hickman catheter or peripheral i.v. line at a dose of 5–7 mg/m²/day. The average total dose of cisplatin was 200 mg/m². The survival figure was calculated from the onset of treatment using the KAPLAN-MAIER product limit method.

23.3 Treatment Results

23.3.1 Tumor Response

One of the therapeutic goals for such advanced disfiguring disease is the local clearance of the tumor. The tumor response is quite impressive, as shown in Table 23.3 and Figs. 23.1a and 23.2. Of the 11 patients treated with curative intent, all but one achieved complete locoregional response. One patient showed almost a complete response of the primary tumor but died in 6 months with a neck recurrence. Of the 10 patients with a complete response, six were confirmed by follow-up CT scans, two by biopsy, and two by clinical examination (one patient for massive neck disease, one through open hard palate). One of the patients who received less than 50 Gy as palliation achieved 90% regression of the tumor and died in 8 months. The other patient achieved a complete remission but died of pneumonia and cachexia several weeks after completion. With this regimen, a complete response was usually obtained dur-

Table 23.3. Tumor response

Curative treatment group (n = 11)
10 CR: 5 NED (26–63 mo)
           2 alive with local recurrence (31.36 mo)
           2 died of bone mets.; locally controlled (7.22 mo)
           1 died of local recurrence (12 mo)
1 PR (90%): Died in 6 mo

Palliative treatment group (n = 2)
1 CR: Died in 2 mo of pneumonia
1 PR (90%): died in 8 mo of disease

Abbreviations: CR, complete response; PR, partial response; NED, no evidence of disease

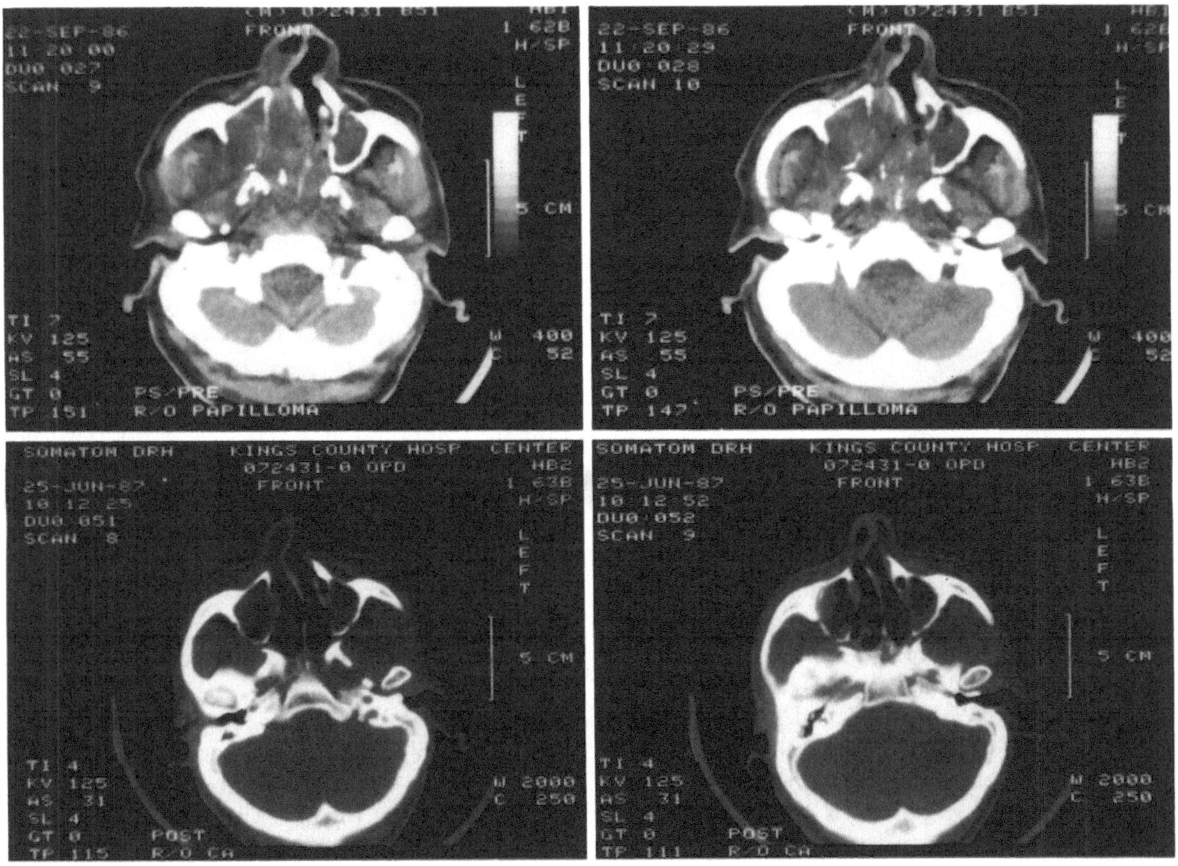

Fig. 23.2. *Upper row*: 49-year-old male presented with a $T_4N_0M_0$ nasopharyngeal paranasal sinus cancer. CT scan (9/22/86) showed a tumor filling the entire nasal, paranasal, and nasopharyngeal spaces, destroying cribriform plates, bilateral maxillary walls, and pterygoid plates. Tumor extended into both orbits. *Lower row:* CT scan (6/25/89) showed complete remission of tumor leaving only some mucosal swelling

ing the second course (4–6 weeks) or the second rest period (6–8 weeks). Of the 11 patients who achieved a complete response, three developed local recurrence: two had in-field recurrences at 12 and 25 months and the third patient developed outside field recurrence in the opposite orbit at 30 months.

23.3.2 Dose–Tumor Volume Relationship

Two patients were excluded from this analysis because one died 2 months after completing palliative treatment and the other died in 7 months with the local tumor controlled. There were 14 measurable lesions in 11 patients. The average diameter of the three dimensions of each lesion varied from 2 to 10 cm. The status of tumor control was plotted against the total dose delivered and the average

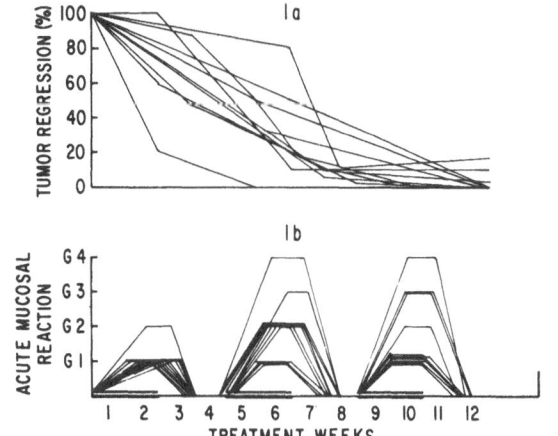

Fig. 23.1. Tumor regression (**a**) and acute mucosal reaction (**b**)

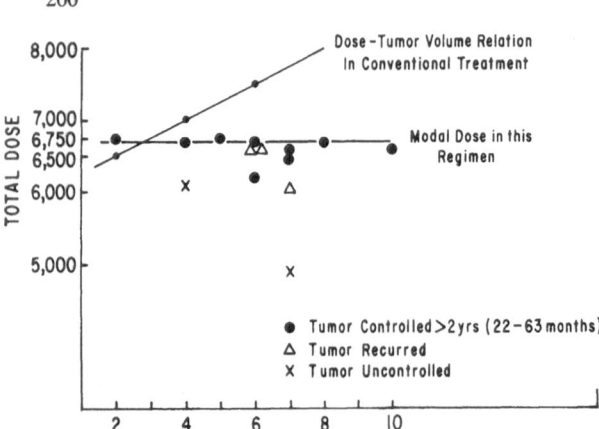

Fig. 23.3. Dose–tumor volume and control relationship

diameter of tumor, as shown in Fig. 23.3. Nine lesions were controlled with a median follow-up of 38 months (22–63 months) and five had failed. There were two failures out of 10 which received more than 65 Gy. Of nine lesions ranging from 4 to 10 cm in diameter, only two failed, with a radiation dose of 65–72 Gy (modal dose of 67.5 Gy). In conventional once-a-day radiation treatment the radiation dose required for a lesion larger than 6 cm in diameter to be controlled with 90% confidence is 75–80 Gy (FLETCHER 1980). With the addition of cisplatin infusion in our regimen, the radiation dose was approximately 15%–18% less than the conventional treatment dose. This is in contrast to other hyperfractionation regimens, which usually require a dose escalation. A dose-modifying factor of 1.15–1.18 was calculated with the addition of cisplatin. Of particular interest is the fact that as tumor size increases, the separation between the tumor dose required in conventional

treatment and modal dose in this regimen gets wider. In other words, the therapeutic ratio increases as the tumor size increases.

23.3.3 Survival

Figure 23.4 shows the survival of 11 patients treated with curative intent. Seven patients (64%) were alive at the time of analysis (26–63 months); five of the seven had no evidence of disease, and two were alive with recurrence of the primary. Two patients died of bone metastases with the primary controlled at 7 and 22 months. Two patients died due to recurrence of the primary at 6 and 12 months. As expected, two patients treated palliatively survived a short interval (2 and 8 months).

23.3.4 Complications – Acute Reactions

Acute skin reactions consisted of mild erythema which became dry hyperpigmented skin. The degree of acute mucosal reactions was within an acceptable range. Figure 23.1b illustrates the pattern of mucosal changes during the overall courses of treatment. Erythemal reactions gradually increased during the 2nd week of the first course and then subsided during the rest of the first course. Intense erythema or petechial mucositis developed towards the end of the second course and resolved by the end of the second rest period. These same reactions occurred during the third course and were sometimes less because of smaller ports and less treatment days. Confluent mucositis developed in two patients. Three patients developed

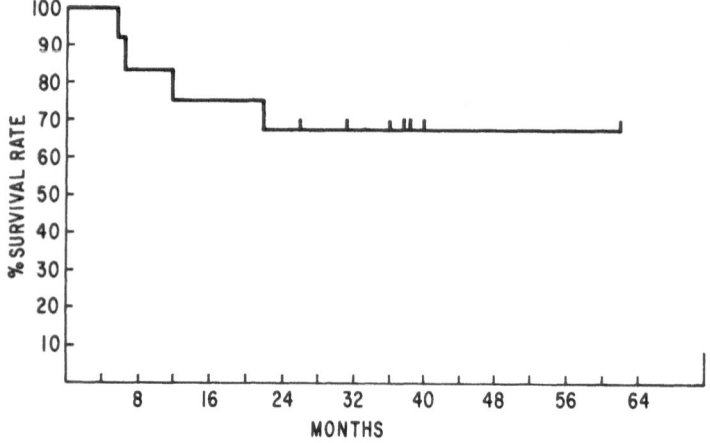

Fig. 23.4. Absolute survival of 11 curative patients

oral candidiasis which responded to antifungal medication.

Hematological reactions were within acceptable ranges. In only three patients was the WBC count less than 3000 (1800, 2200, 2500), and there was no significant thrombocytopenia (nadir platelet count was 76 000).

23.3.5 Late Complications

Late effects on the soft tissues or muscles were not different from those of conventional once-a-day treatment. Care was taken not to exceed a dose of 40 Gy to the cervical spinal cord.

The eyes or optic nerve had to be included in the treatment ports in nine patients (Table 23.4). In four patients, the optic nerve received 20–55 Gy due to the proximity to the tumor and none of them developed optic nerve damage (36–40 months). In five patients, eyes and optic nerve tract received the same total tumor dose (60–69 Gy) because tumor involved either the orbit or frontal base of skull. It is difficult to determine the late effect because three of these six patients died within 2 years after treatment. One of the five developed corneal ulceration which resulted in white corneal cloudiness. No cataracts developed in the three patients treated with a lens block. In this series, one case of late complications occurred. The patient developed blindness from total corneal cloudiness of the ipsilateral eye, and at the same time a recurrence developed in the

Table 23.4. Dose to eye or optic nerve

Patient	Whole eye	Optic nerve	Follow-up in months	Result
1		2000	36A	No eye symptoms
2		5000	38A	
3		5000	38A	
4		5500	40A	
5		6000	22D	
6	3000 (lens block)	6480	26A	
7	6645 (lens block)	6645	12D	
8	6960 (lens block)	6960	7D	
9[a]	6000	6000	31A	Ipsilateral blindness, corneal cloudiness

A, alive; D, dead
[a] Patient had previously two frontal craniotomies for recurrence after maxillectomy and 50 Gy

contralateral orbit. This patient had previously undergone two surgical craniotomies for a large recurrent mass occurring above the cribriform plate after maxillectomy and postoperative 50 Gy. The development of late complication thus occurred in patient who were predisposed by either surgical procedures or extensive tumor involvement. In addition, such occurrences are not unusual in conventional radiation therapy, as reported by Parsons et al. (1988b); 16 of 48 patients who received 60–70 Gy for nasal cavity and ethmoid and sphenoid sinus cancers developed blindness. In order to achieve meaningful treatment results in such advanced cases, the acceptable criteria evaluating morbidity should be lowered to accept some inevitable side-effects.

23.4 Discussion

The overall 5-year survival rate of patients with the nasopharyngeal cancers ranges from 28% to 56% when they are treated with radiotherapy alone (Chu et al. 1984; Schabinger et al. 1985; Wang et al. 1988). When the base of skull is involved, the 5-year survival rate decreases to 0%–27% (Chu et al. 1984; Marcial et al. 1985). With paranasal sinus cancers the combination of extensive surgery and high dose irradiation gives an overall survival of 35%–50% and a local control rate of approximately 30%–43% in T_4 lesions (Bush et al. 1982; Cheng and Wang 1977).

The combination of chemotherapeutic agents with radiation has been an area of great expectations in the management of advanced head and neck cancers. Recently, with the advent of neo-adjuvant therapy, chemotherapeutic agents have been administered prior to radiation or surgery, achieving sometimes dramatic responses. The benefits from this treatment, however, are yet to be clearly defined, as the results of the randomized trials are still controversial (Kun et al. 1986; Taylor 1987; Taylor et al. 1985).

Another encouraging way to combine chemotherapy and radiation is with their concomitant use, thus taking advantage of the potential radiation-sensitizing properties of the chemotherapeutic agents. Marcial and colleagues from RTOG 81–17 (1985) reported the treatment results of 124 patients who presented with advanced head and neck cancers using concomitant cisplatin (100 mg i.v.) every 3 weeks for three daily doses during a definitive course of radiation of 70 Gy in 7 weeks. A complete remission was achieved in 71% (88 of 124 patients) with a 3-year survival of 43%. MURPHY et al. (1987), treated 44 patients using a more effective combination consisting of 5-FU (800 mg/m^2 × 5 days) and i.v. cisplatin (60 mg/m^2) on days 1 and 5 with 2 Gy/day. The weekly treatment cycle was repeated every 2 weeks for seven cycles. Regional control was obtained in 87% with surgical salvage (minimal follow-up 24 months) and actuarial 2-year survival was 66%. Therefore, concomitant combination of radiation and radiation-potentiating chemotherapeutic agents shows promise in local control.

The combination of chemotherapeutic agents and radiation, however, increased normal tissue toxicity and may therefore result in no therapeutic gain. PETERS et al. (1988) reported on the M.D. Anderson Hospital experience of treating 33 patients with nasopharyngeal cancers with radiation therapy and adjunctive chemotherapy of combined bleomycin, cytoxan, methotrexate, and 5-fluorouracil (BCMF), or cisplatin, methotrexate, and bleomycin (PMB). The treatment outcome in these patients was compared with that of a stage-matched group of 71 patients treated during the same period with radiation alone. The actuarial risk of developing severe late reaction (soft tissue and muscle fibrosis) by 2 years was 68% in a combined modality group vs 8% in the radiation therapy only group ($p = 0.001$). Therefore, the ultimate value of combined modality therapy has to be assessed based on acute and late toxicity against any potential benefit in survival. The acute mucosal reactions from combined treatments can be minimized by splitting the treatment courses. It should be remembered, however, that such split-course schedules will not reduce the late effects because they are related to dose per fraction and total dose, not overall treament time.

Lately, hyperfractionated irradiation has been investigated extensively with the promise that two smaller fractions separated by 4–6 h per day favor the repair of cellular damage in late responding normal tissue. PARSONS et al. (1988a) were able to increase tumor dose by as much as 10%–15% (total dose of 74.4–79.2 Gy) over that conventionally used for once-a-day treatment and produced results of local control that are higher by 10%–15%.

In this hyperfractionated scheme, instead of increasing the total tumor dose, concurrent low dose cisplatin infusion was used to have a sensitiz-ing effect, hoping for a greater effect on tumor cells. With this regimen, only two out of nine lesions ranging from 4 to 10 cm in diameter failed with a radiation dose of 65–69 Gy (modal dose of 67.5 Gy). The late effects were not increased over those of conventional treatment, thus increasing the therapeutic ratio. Figure 23.5 shows schematically a possible explanation of the increasing therapeutic ratio of this regimen. With minimal or perhaps no increase of late tissue effect a marked increase in local control was achieved with an estimated dose-modifying factor range from 1.15 to 1.18. The therapeutic ratio becomes larger as tumor size increases.

23.5 Summary

With the use of concomitant infusion cisplatin and radiation, a radiosensitizing effect is achieved without the toxicities of the drug which usually accompany its bolus use. Hyperfractionated radiation further provides a means of avoiding late effects, without compromising local control of the tumor. Instead of escalating the total dose by hyperfractionation, we lowered the total dose by 15%–18% as compared with conventional irradiation due to the effective radiosensitization offered by the infusion cisplatin. The net effect of radiosensitization and split-course hyperfractionated radiation is to increase the therapeutic ratio. Ten of 11 patients who were treated curatively had achieved complete local response, with late complications in only one patient. The number of

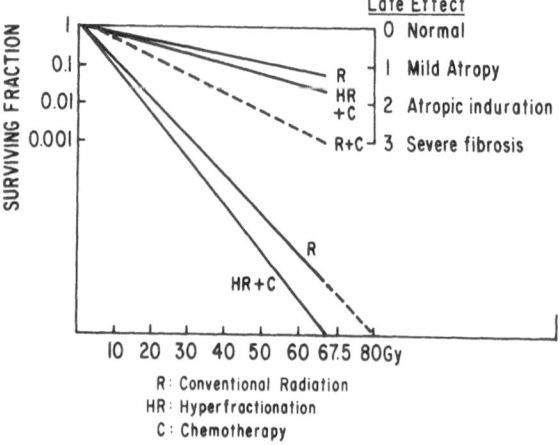

Fig. 23.5. Schematic illustration of therapeutic benefit

patients in this series is small, and results cannot be regarded as conclusive. It will take a randomized trial to prove the advantages of this regimen of treatment, i.e., an increased therapeutic ratio, with better tumor control with acceptable toxicity.

References

Al-Sarraf M, Kinzie J, Marcial V, et al. (1984) Combination of cis-platinum and radiotherapy in patients with advanced head and neck cancer. Radiation Therapy Oncology Group Progress Report. Proc Am Soc Clin Oncol 3: 180

Bush SE, Bagshaw MA (1982) Carcinoma of the paranasal sinuses. Cancer 50: 154–158

Cheng VST, Wang CC (1977) Carcinoma of the paranasal sinuses. Cancer 40: 3038–3041

Chu AM, Flynn MB, Achinoe, Mendoza EF, Scott RM, Jose B (1984) Irradiation of nasopharyngeal carcinoma: correlations with treatment factors and stage. Int J Radiat Oncol Biol Phys 10: 2241–2249

Douple EB, Richmond RC (1979) A review of platinum complex biochemistry suggests a rationale for combined platinum–radiotherapy. Int J Radiat Oncol Biol Phys 5: 1335–1339

Dristschilo A, Pieo AJ, Kelman AD (1979) The effect of cis-platinum on the repair of radiation damage in plateau phase Chinese hamster (V-79) cells. Int J Radiat Oncol Biol Phys 5: 1345–1349

Fletcher G (1980) Textbook of radiotherapy, 3rd edn. Lea and Febiger, Philadelphia, PA, pp 195–196

Haselow RE, Adams GS, Oken MM, Goudsmit A, Leenez HJ, Marsh JC (1983) Cisplatinum with radiation therapy for locally advanced unrestectable head and neck cancer. Proc Am Soc Clin Oncol 2: 160

Kun LE, Toohill RJ, Holoye PY, et al. (1986) A randomized study of adjuvant chemotherapy for cancer of the upper aerodigestive tract. Int J Radiat Oncol Biol Phys 12: 173–178

Lederman M (1970) Tumours of the upper jaw. J Laryngol 84: 369–401

Marcial VA, Paiak TF, Al-Saraf M, Kinzie J, Velez G (1985) Concurrent radiotherapy and cisplatinum chemotherapy in inoperable mucosal squamous cell carcinoma of the head and neck: a RTOG Report. Int J Radiat Oncol Biol Phys 11: 89

Murpthy AK, Taylor SG, Showel J, et al. (1987) Treatment of advanced head and neck cancer with concomitant radiation and chemotherapy. Int J Radiat Oncol Biol Phys 13: 1807–1813

Parsons JT, Merdenhall WM, Marcus AA, Cassisi NJ, Million RR (1988a) Hyperfractionation for head and neck cancer. Int J Radiat Oncol Biol Phys 14: 649–658

Parsons JT Merderhall WM, Cassisi NJ, Issacs JH, Million RR. (1988b) Malignant tumors of the nasal cavity and ethmoid and sphenoid sinuses. Int J Radiat Oncol Biol Phys 14: 11–22

Peters LJ, Harrison ML, Dimery IW, et al. (1988) Acute and late toxicity associated with sequential bleomycin containing chemotherapy regimens and radiation therapy in the treatment of carcinoma of the nasopharynx. Int J Radiat Oncol Biol Phys 14: 623–633

Schabinger PR, Reddy S, Herdrickson FR, Phillips RL, Saxena V (1985) Carcinoma of the nasopharynx: survival and patterns of recurrence. Int J Radiat Oncol Biol Phys 11: 2081–2084

Sidgestad CD (1979) Cell cycle phase preferential killing of fibrosarcoma tumor cells by cis-di-chlorodi-chlorodiamminineplatinum or adriamycin. Proc Am Assoc Cancer Res 20: 178

Taylor SG (1985) A randomized trial of adjuvant chemotherapy in head and neck cancer. J Clin Oncol 3: 672–679

Taylor SG (1987) Integration of chemotherapy into the combined modality therapy of head and neck squamous cancer. Int J Radiat Oncol Biol Phys 13:779–783

Thames HD, Withers RH, Peters LJ, Fletcher GH (1982) Changes in early and late radiation responses with altered dose fractionation: implications for dose-survival relationships. Int J Radiat Oncol Biol Phys 8:219–226

Wang DC, Cai WM, Hu YH, Gu XZ (1988) Long-term survival of 1035 cases of nasopharyngeal carcinoma. Cancer 61:2338–2341

24 Cisplatin plus Radiotherapy in Bladder Cancer

Rolf Sauer and Jürgen Dunst

CONTENTS

24.1 Clinical Aspects of Bladder Cancer and Rationale for Conservative Treatment Approaches

Bladder cancers currently account for approximately 3% of all malignancies. The incidence of new cases per year is estimated to be about 10 000 in the Federal Republic of Germany and about 40 000 in the United States (KLIMBERG and WAJSMAN 1986; RICHIE et al. 1985; ROTMAN and AZIZ 1987). About 70%–80% of newly diagnosed bladder cancers are so-called superficial tumors (T_a, T_{is}, T_1). Standard treatment for these tumors is conservative surgery in the form of transurethral resection (TUR) and/or intravesical chemother-

apy. Radiation therapy is only indicated in a limited number of patients whose tumors cannot be controlled conservatively, e.g., unresectable T_1 tumors. Patients with superficial tumors have a good prognosis as regards survival, although 70% of patients will develop recurrences or new bladder tumors with a 30% incidence of progression to higher T stage or poorer differentiation of the tumor. About 15% of patients with superficial tumors will ultimately progress to deeply infiltrating cancers.

Deeply infiltrating tumors with invasion of the muscle or beyond the bladder wall account for 30% of all bladder tumors. Muscle invasion worsens prognosis in two ways as compared with superficial tumors: *Firstly*, conservative surgery alone is normally unable to definitively control the local tumor. TUR alone may be an effective treatment in a small number of tumors with muscle invasion, provided that careful follow-up and re-examination are performed. Most muscle-invading cancers, however, cannot be treated curatively by conservative surgery alone and in most institutions, radical cystectomy has become the standard treatment for these patients. *Secondly*, the incidence of occult micrometastatic spread increases with T stage, and more than 50% of patients with muscle-invading tumors will subsequently develop metastatic disease.

The discrepancy between local control and cure rate makes muscle-invading bladder cancer a "systemic disease." Improvement of treatment seems possible in two ways: *Firstly*, control of micrometastatic disease is necessary in order to improve survival. Adjuvant chemotherapy has been initiated with this in mind and is being studied in clinical trials (DANIELS et al. 1986; HAVSTEEN et al. 1987; LOGOTHETIS et al. 1986; SOLOWAY 1987; STERNBERG et al. 1985; YAGODA et al. 1976). Preliminary results show a prolongation of the disease-free interval in high-risk bladder cancer patients. Whether there might be an increase in survival remains questionable. A considerable number of

Prof. Dr. med. ROLF SAUER, Dr. med. JÜRGEN DUNST, Department of Radiation Therapy, University of Erlangen, Universitätsstraße 27, W-8520 Erlangen, FRG

patients with bladder cancers are not suitable for aggressive multiagent chemotherapy because of age and poor general condition. *Secondly*, function- or organ-preserving treatment seems possible even in advanced bladder tumors. Large series, especially series with preoperative irradiation and cystectomy, have shown a discrepancy between excellent local control rates of more than 90% and unchanged survival figures of 50% or less. On the other hand, local failure after bladder-sparing treatment can be treated curatively (Svanson et al. 1981). Both facts are strong arguments for a conservation treatment approach (comparable to breast cancer or larynx cancer).

Currently, cystectomy is the most widely used therapy for muscle-invading bladder cancers if the patient is suitable for radical surgery. Nevertheless, large series with irradiation alone and the randomized trial from the Royal Marsden Hospital have shown that definitive irradiation is an alternative to cystectomy (BATATA et al. 1981; BLOOM et al. 1982; GOFFINET et al. 1975; GOODMAN et al. 1981; QUILTY and DUNCAN 1986; YU et al. 1985). Survival rates after 5 years were slightly lower than after radical cystectomy, but half of the patients achieved cure *with* maintained bladder function. In contrast to radical cystectomy, the number of local failures was high in irradiated patients. This has focused the radiotherapists' interest on improving local control. A correlation between local control and survival has been shown, suggesting a survival improvement with increasing the local control rate (SHIPLEY et al. 1985, 1987b).

Bladder cancer is a chemosensitive malignancy, and several antineoplastic drugs have proven clinical efficacy. Cisplatin is the most effective single agent in advanced bladder cancer (RICHIE et al. 1985) and it seems reasonable to combine this drug with irradiation. Thus several institutions, including our own, have used primary radiotherapy in bladder cancer in combinaton with concurrent (simultaneous) cisplatin. In this chapter, we present a critical analysis of our own results after 3 years and give an overview of the current data from other institutions.

24.2 Irradiation plus Cisplatin in Bladder Cancer: Results at the University of Erlangen After Three Years

24.2.1 Protocol

At the University of Erlangen, primary cystectomy was abandoned in 1982 in favor of a bladder-sparing treatment concept including TUR plus radiotherapy and also salvage cystectomy for irradiation failures. Patients were irradiated up to a total dose of 41.4 Gy to the pelvis and 50.4 Gy to the bladder (calculated on the 90% isodose surrounding the target volume) with 1.8 Gy per fraction. An interim analysis in 1985 showed poor local control in patients who had an incomplete TUR prior to radiotherapy.

On the basis of the data from the University of Innsbruck (JAKSE et al. 1986) as well as from the National Bladder Cancer Group (SHIPLEY et al. 1987a), we started to add cisplatin to the radiotherapy (radiochemotherapy = RCT) in October 1985. Until the end of 1986, cisplatin was restricted to patients with poor risk for local control. Since 1987, cisplatin has been used in all patients without contraindications to this chemotherapeutic agent. During recent years, however, more and more patients with advanced tumors have been referred to our department from other hospitals. This has led to an increasing number of patients who receive radiation therapy alone without cisplatin because of contraindications to chemotherapy.

From 1982 through 1988, 160 patients were treated at the Department of Radiotherapy at Erlangen University for locoregional bladder cancer (excluding patients with metastases or recurrences after cystectomy). Sixty-four patients received irradiation alone from January 1982 through September 1985. Between the introduction of cisplatin chemotherapy in October 1985 and December 1988, 96 patients were treated, 29 of them with irradiation alone. This analysis deals with the 67 patients treated during this period with irradiation and simultaneous cisplatin chemotherapy. There were 52 males and 15 females with a mean age of 63 years (range: 42–77 years). Sixty-four patients had transitional cell carcinoma and three had squamous cell carcinoma of the bladder. The date of this analysis is 1 January 1989, and the median follow-up is 18 months.

Staging included TUR of primary tumor, a bladder mapping with resection of all suspicious lesions and at least six random biopsies from definite areas, urine cytology, computed tomography (CT) scans of pelvis and abdomen (not routinely performed prior to 1985), chest x-ray, bone scan, and laboratory workup. Definition of T stage was based on histological examination of TUR specimens except in two patients with histologically proven muscle-invading cancers, in whom the diagnosis of a T_4 cancer was made on the basis of the CT findings. In eight patients with proven muscle invasion and treatment prior to 1987, no differentiation between T_2 and T_3 was made and these patients are included in the T_3 group. Positive regional (pelvic) lymph nodes were found in eight patients.

Radiotherapy usually started 3–6 weeks after TUR. After simulator treatment planning with contrast filling of bladder and rectum, patients were treated in supine position with a 10-MV photon beam. The daily dose was 1.8 Gy (on the 90% isodose surrounding the target volume) on 5 days per week. The pelvis was treated with a box technique and individual shielding up to 41.4 Gy and the whole bladder was boosted with a rotation technique with five additional fractions up to 50.4 Gy.

Cisplatin chemotherapy was administered in the first and fifth irradiation week on five consecutive treatment days as short infusion prior to irradiation. The daily dose was 25 mg/m^2 with a total dose of 250 mg/m^2 in two courses. Contraindications to cisplatin were a serum creatinine level > 1.6 mg/dl or a creatinine clearance <50 ml/min.

Response was examined 6 weeks after radiochemotherapy by control cystoscopy with deep biopsies, bladder mapping, and urine cytology. Complete response means the absence of visible tumor, negative biopsies from the primary tumor region, negative random biopsies, and a negative cytology. *Follow-up examinations* included cystoscopies with resection of suspicious areas every 3 months as well as chest x-ray and pelvic and abdominal CT scans every 6 months.

Salvage cystectomy was performed in the case of persistent or recurrent invasive bladder tumor without evidence of distant disease, provided that patients were medically fit for radical surgery. Figure 24.1 gives an overview of our treatment schedule.

Table 24.1. Radiotherapy (50.4 Gy) plus simultaneous cisplatin chemotherapy in bladder cancer: complete remission rates according to T stage. Erlangen University, October 1985 through December 1988

Stage	% complete remissions
T_1	8/11 (73%)
T_2	14/16 (88%)
$T_{2-3/3}$	27/36 (75%)
T_4	1/4 (25%)
Total	50/67 (75%)

24.2.2 Results

24.2.2.1 Local Control According to T Stage

Local control according to initial T stage is shown in Table 24.1. Overall complete response after TUR and radiotherapy plus cisplatin was 75% (50/67) at control cystoscopy. Complete remission was achieved in 8/11 (73%) T_1, 14/16 (88%) T_2, 27/36 (75%) $T_{2-3/3}$, and 1/4 (25%) T_4 tumors. Six additional patients had noninvasive tumors at control cystoscopy. Therefore, 56/67 patients (84%) were free of invasive tumor after completed treatment.

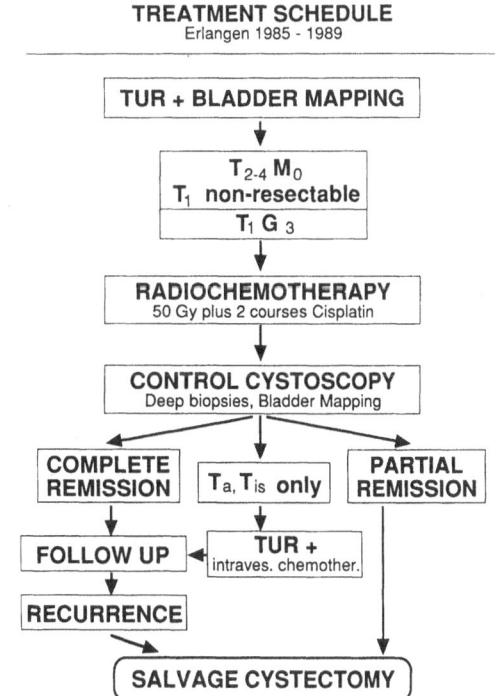

Fig. 24.1. Bladder-preserving treatment schedule for muscle-invading bladder cancer and poor prognostic T_1 cancers at the University of Erlangen

24.2.2.2 Local Control According to the Extent of TUR

Twelve patients had a complete TUR with negative biopsies from the margins of resection (R_0) prior to radiochemotherapy. Eight of them (67%) had a complete response and four had noninvasive tumors at reevaluation after treatment. Twenty-four patients received radiochemotherapy after macroscopically complete TUR but with tumor-positive biopsies from the margins of resection (R_1). Twenty (83%) of them were complete responders and two had noninvasive cancers. Thirty patients were treated because of macroscopic residual bladder tumor after TUR, and 21 of them (70%) had a complete response. A total of 11 patients out of 67 had only a partial response with residual invasive tumor after radiochemotherapy, either microscopically or macroscopically. Partial response was related to the extent of TUR: 0% vs 9% vs 30% partial response in R_0 vs R_1 vs R_2 resections, respectively. The results are summarized in Table 24.2.

24.2.2.3 Maintenance of Local Control

After a median follow-up of 18 months, ten bladder recurrences have occurred. Two of them were noninvasive second tumors (T_a, T_{is}). At least one of the remaining eight invasive recurrences was thought to be a second bladder tumor: this was a T_1 recurrence outside the primary tumor region and in the salvage cystectomy specimen; the former tumor region was histologically negative. Nine of

Table 24.2. Radiotherapy (50.4 Gy) plus simultaneous cisplatin chemotherapy in bladder cancer: complete remission rates according to the extent of preceding transurethral surgery (R_0, complete resection; R_1, microscopically incomplete resection; R_2, macroscopically incomplete resection)[a]. Patients without complete remission, but with exclusively noninvasive tumors (T_a, T_{is}) are listed separately. Erlangen University, October 1985 through December 1985

Extent of TUR	Histopathological status at control cystoscopy 6 weeks after radiotherapy plus simultaneous cisplatin	
	% complete remissions	% T_a/T_{is}
R_0	8/12 (67%)	4/12 (33%)
R_1	20/24 (83%)	2/24 (8%)
R_2	21/30 (70%)	0/30 (0%)

[a] One patient is excluded because of unknown extent of surgery.

Table 24.3. Intravesical recurrences after radiochemotherapy (50.4 Gy plus simultaneous cisplatin) in invasive bladder cancer. Patients with preserved bladders include complete responders and patients without complete response but with conservative salvage treatment. Erlangen University, October 1985 through December 1988. Median follow-up, 18 months

Recurrences	In complete responders	In preserved bladders
Total recurrences	9/50 (18%)	10/60 (16%)
Invasive recurrences	7/50 (14%)	8/60 (13%)

the patients with recurrences were complete responders after initial treatment. One recurrence was observed in a patient who had a T_a tumor at reevaluation after treatment for a T_4 cancer. He was treated with TUR and intravesical chemotherapy, but developed a T_4 recurrence 6 months later.

The local relapse rate is 18% (9/50) after initial complete response: there were invasive recurrences in 14% and noninvasive recurrences in 4% (Table 24.3). If all patients with preserved bladders are analyzed, including those without complete response but with preserved bladders after conservative salvage treatment, the local relapse rate is 16% (10/60).

24.2.2.4 Cystectomy Rate

Eleven cystectomies have been performed. Six were part of initial treatment because of residual invasive tumor after radiochemotherapy. Four patients underwent cystectomy because of subsequent recurrence after initial bladder preservation. One patient required cystectomy because of a bladder shrinkage; the bladder shrinkage was present prior to radiochemotherapy and was likely caused by multiple TURs and was not thought to be related to radiochemotherapy.

24.2.2.5 Toxicity

We have not noted an increase in severe or late toxicity. However, mild to moderate acute toxicity is higher with additional cisplatin treatment. Mild to moderate nausea and vomiting occurred in most of our patients, even with antiemetic treatment. Hematological toxicity grade I–II (WHO score) was noted in 61% and grade III toxicity in 27% with no case of grade IV reactions. Transient elevation of the serum creatinine level was measured in 35% of our patients. One patient (2%) developed severe dysuria requiring hospital treatment. One patient had a pulmonary embolism after 40 Gy and one course of cisplatin, and further therapy was omitted.

24.2.2.6 Survival

The 3-year survival (Kaplan-Meier method) according to T stage is 73% for T_1, 68% for T_{2-3}, and 25% for T_4 tumors, with an overall survival of 66%. Patients with complete TUR (R_0) had a 3-year survival of 100% as compared with 54% for patients with incomplete TUR (R_{1-2}). The data are shown in Table 24.4.

24.2.2.7 Radiotherapy plus Cisplatin Versus Radiotherapy Alone

We have compared the results in patients with additional cisplatin and the results in those patients who were treated prior to October 1985 with irradiation alone (Table 24.5). Surgical and pathological staging, surgical treatment, and irradiation technique and dosage were the same in both series (January 1982 through September 1985 versus October 1985 through December 1988). Nevertheless, the comparison must be interpreted carefully because it is a historical control and selection criteria might have contributed to better results in one group.

Overall, cisplatin has increased the complete response rate after incomplete TUR, i.e., in patients with macroscopic tumor after TUR or positive margins of resection (R_{1-2}). Prior to October 1985, the complete remission rate was 45% (24/53) in this group. Since the introduction of cisplatin chemotherapy, local complete response rate has increased significantly to 76% (41/54) for patients with R_{1-2} resections receiving cisplatin. This has led to a decrease in the rate of initial cystectomies from 20% to 9% for the whole group (13/64 vs 6/67). However, the increase in local control is significant only for the cisplatin group and is only slight if all patients with treatment after October 1985, i.e., after the initiation of additional cisplatin, are compared with those patients who received treatment prior to October 1985 (55% vs 45%). Cisplatin had no influence on local control in patients with complete TUR prior to radio (chemo) therapy (complete remission rate 7/9 vs 8/12).

Concerning survival, cisplatin has not been able to improve the 3-year survival figures. Prior to the initiation of cisplatin, irradiation alone yielded a 3-year survival of 66% for the whole group, and the survival is now 66% for the cisplatin group (Table 24.5).

24.2.3 Conclusions from Our Results

We conclude from our data that cisplatin will likely increase the complete remission rate after incomplete TUR. The acute treatment morbidity is higher with simultaneous cisplatin (hyperemesis, hematological toxicity), but there has been no increase in severe complications or late toxicity. Therefore, cisplatin means a local benefit for the patient. However, we have failed to demonstrate an increased survival. Cisplatin in our series has not been able to control micrometastatic disease. Our data are in contrast to the theory that increasing local control in irradiated patients would be associated with an increased survival.

Table 24.4. Radiotherapy (50.4 Gy) plus simultaneous cisplatin chemotherapy in bladder cancer. Survival after 3 years (Kaplan-Meier method). Erlangen University, October 1985 through December 1988; analysis, 1 January 1989. R_0, complete transurethral surgery prior to radiochemotherapy; R_{1-2}, microscopically or macroscopically incomplete transurethral surgery prior to radiochemotherapy

Stage	3-year survival
Overall	66%
T_1	73%
T_{2-3}	68%
T_4	25%
T_{1-3} R_0	100%
T_{1-4} R_{1-2}	54%

Table 24.5. Radiochemotherapy (50.4 Gy plus cisplatin, October 1985 through December 1988) versus radiotherapy alone (50.40 Gy, January 1982 through September 85) in bladder cancer. Results of the University of Erlangen. CR, complete remission; R_{1-2}, microscopically or macroscopically incomplete TUR prior to radio (chemo) therapy

	XRT alone	XRT plus cisplatin
CR in T_{1-4} R_{1-2}	45% (24/53)	76% (41/54)
Initial bladder preservation	80%	91%
Severe complications	0%	0%
3-year survival	66% !	66% !

24.3 Radiotherapy plus Cisplatin in Bladder Cancer: Review of Current Data

24.3.1 Cisplatin Alone in Advanced Bladder Cancer

Cisplatin is the most effective single-agent drug in advanced bladder cancer. In metastatic disease, clinically complete remissions are achieved in 20%–30% of all patients and in 50% or more when cisplatin is used in combination with other drugs. The same seems to hold true for the advanced tumor in the bladder (Table 24.6). Cisplatin alone or in combination with other drugs can produce 15%–50% clinically complete remissions. However, the percentage of histologically confirmed complete remissions does not exceed 20%–30%. If one excludes the possibility of sensitizing (overadditive) effects in the combination of cisplatin and irradiation, an optimal increase in local control would appear to be limited to a percentage of about 20%–30% (additive effect).

24.3.2 Local Control

Major prognostic factors for local tumor control are the *amount of residual tumor at the start of radiation therapy* and the *radiation dose* (SHIPLEY et al. 1985, 1987b). Definitive local control rates are high in those patients who have undergone a complete TUR prior to irradiation. Local control

rates after 5 years are in the range of more than 70%.

On the other hand, local control is relatively poor in patients with macroscopic residual disease prior to radiotherapy. Tumor control increases with radiation dose. Data from preoperative regimens suggest that radiation doses of 40–50 Gy will eradicate not more than 35% of all bladder tumors (Table 24.7). In these series, about 25%–35% of patients had no residual tumor in the cystectomy specimen after preoperative radiation. In the series with full-dose irradiation, macroscopic residual tumor has been controlled in about 50%–60% (Table 24.7). The best results have been obtained by EDSMYR and co-workers (1985), who have reported a 62% local control rate of T_{2-4} tumors at 6 months after hyperfractionated radiotherapy.

From these figures, a relationship between radiation dose and local control can be obtained. It can be suggested that doses of 60–70 Gy will yield a complete remission rate of about 40%–60%. Higher local control rates are unlikely in the case of macroscopic residual tumor after TUR.

Several institutions have used radiotherapy in combination with concomitant cisplatin chemotherapy in order to improve local control. At the University of Innsbruck (JAKSE et al. 1986), irradiation to a total dose of 60 Gy (split after 40 Gy) has been combined with cisplatin bolus injections at 3-week intervals. At the same institution, a second regimen has been used with weekly adriamycin, cisplatin at 3-week intervals, and a hyperfractionated irradiation scheme with six fractions

Table 24.6. Cisplatin-based chemotherapy alone in advanced bladder cancer: complete remissions

Reference	Drugs	Complete remissions	Toxic deaths
RAGHAVAN et al.1985	Cisplatin	8/47 pCR	
MAATMAN et al. 1986	CISCA i.v./i.a.	5/16 cCR, 3/13 pCR	0%
	Cisplatin i.a.	1/8 cCR, 0/3 pCR	(16% plexopathy)
LOGOTHETIS et al. 1985	CISCA i.v./i.a.	19/38 total	0%
DENIS and HENDRICKS 1986	Cisplatin/MTX × 4	6/16 total	2/25 (8%)
		6/10 previously untreated	
		0/6 previously treated	
JACOBS et al. 1984	Cisplatin i.a. + HT	2/6 pCR	0%
MEYERS et al. 1985	MCV	6/12 pCR without RT	
		5/5 pCR with RT	
STERNBERG et al. 1985	MVAC	12/24 cCR,	
		60% of cCR were pCR	
		4/5 cCR in the bladder	

Abbreviations: CISCA, cisplatin +cyclophosphamide + adriamycin; MTX, methotrexate; MCV, methotrexate + cisplatin + vinblastine; MVAC, methotrexate + vinblastine + adriamycin + cisplatin; HT, hyperthermia; cCR, clinical complete remission; pCR, pathologically confirmed complete remission; RT, radiotherapy

Table 24.7. Local control of macroscopic bladder cancer by irradiation alone

I. Preoperative irradiation plus planned cystectomy

Reference	Dose (Gy)	%pT$_0$ at cystectomy
van der Werf-Messing 1979	40	30
Bloom et al. 1982	40	31
Shipley et al. 1982	40	24
Prout et al. 1973	45	32
Miller 1977	50	29
Chan and Johnson 1978	50	35

II. Full-dose irradiation series

Reference	Daily dose (Gy)	Total dose (Gy)	No. of cases	Complete remissions (%)
Morrison 1975	2.12	42.5	38	38
	2.50	50	40	55
Quilty and Duncan 1986	2.25	50–52.5	99	33
	2.25	55–57.5	124	52
Edsmyr et al. 1985	2	64	40	33
	3 × 1	84	36	62
Bloom et al. 1982	2	60	81	40

Table 24.8. Local complete response rates in macroscopic tumor: full-dose irradiation plus cisplatin

Institution/reference	Treatment	Complete response rates		
		T$_{2-3}$	T$_4$	Total
National Bladder Cancer Group (Shipley et al. 1987a)	64.8 Gy + cisplatin	40/47 (85%)	5/10 (50%)	44/57 (77%)
University of Innsbruck (Jakse et al. 1986)	60 Gy + cisplatin	12/16 (75%)		12/16 (75%)
	57.6 Gy Hyp + Cis/Adr	14/18 (78%)		14/18 (78%)
GU Tumor Group Vancouver (Coppin and Brown 1986)	Full-dose/40 Gy + Cis			22/29 (76%)
University of Erlangen (this report)	50.4 Gy + cisplatin	18/25 (72%)	1/3 (33%)	19/28 (68%)
Overall		84/106 (79%)	6/13 (46%)	111/148 (75%)

Abbreviations: Cis, cisplatin; Adr, adriamycin; Hyp, hyperfractionated irradiation

of 1.6 Gy twice daily on 3 days per week up to a total dose of 57.6 Gy. The National Bladder Cancer Group (Shipley et al. 1987a) has combined full-dose irradiation (64.8 Gy without split) with cisplatin bolus injections every 3 weeks. A comparable treatment scheme has been used in Vancouver (Coppin and Brown 1986). In Erlangen, we have administered 25 mg/m^2 cisplatin on 5 days in the 1st and 5th weeks of a conventionally fractionated irradiation scheme (total dose of 50.4 Gy). These regimens differ somewhat in terms of total radiation dose and cisplatin administration (Fig. 24.2). However, all four regimens are a combination of an effective radiotherapeutic regimen with an effective chemotherapeutic regimen. The results concerning local control are quite similar (Table 24.8). The complete remission rate for patients with macroscopic residual tumor lies in the range of 70%–80%. As compared with the literature, there seems to be an increase of about 20% or more when using cisplatin in addition to radiotherapy. These figures correspond well with our

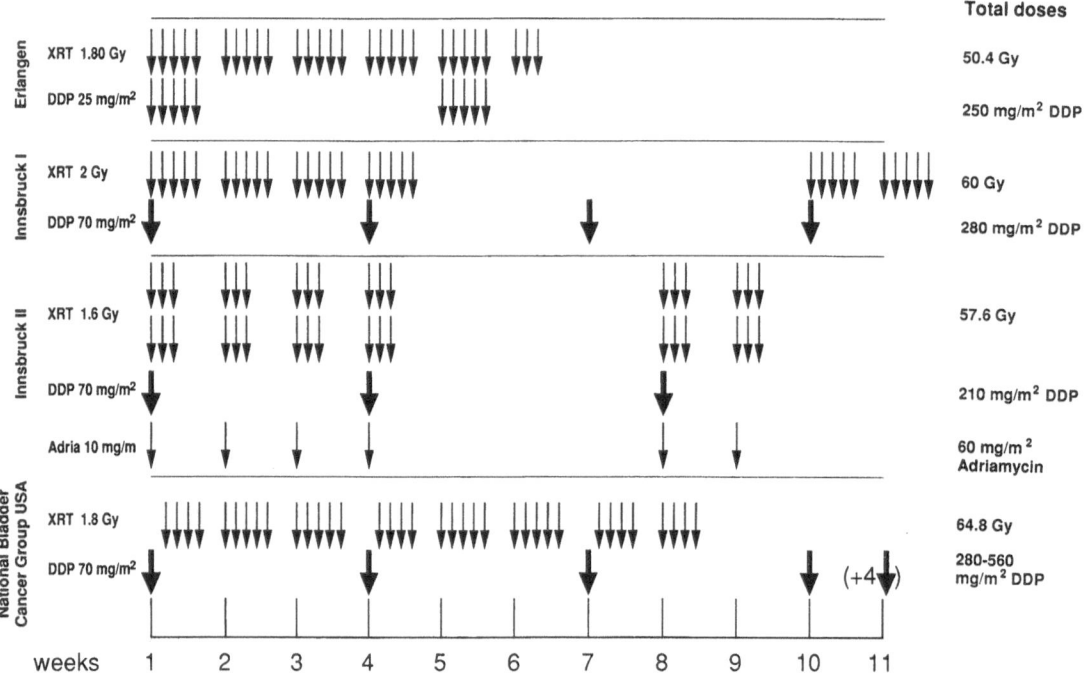

Fig. 24.2. Comparison of different treatment regimens including radiotherapy and simultaneous chemotherapy in muscle-invading bladder cancer. The regimen of the University of Erlangen, the two regimens from Innsbruck, and the regimen used by the National Bladder Cancer Group are shown. Each *arrow* means one radiation fraction or one single dose of drug. On the *left*, single doses are shown, on the *right*, the total doses after whole treatment. *XRT*, radiotherapy; *DDP*, cisplatin; *Adria*, adriamycin

own results (SAUER et al. 1988). The combination of irradiation and cisplatin seems to be superior to a combination of irradiation with other active drugs such as 5-fluorouracil or adriamycin (CROSS et al. 1976; RICHARDS et al. 1983; ROTMAN et al.1987).

The *question of the optimal radiation dose* in combination with cisplatin cannot be answered clearly from the currently available data. After 40 Gy plus cisplatin, 44% of the patients in Innsbruck (JAKSE et al. 1986) and 65% of the patients in the RTOG protocol 85–12 (TESTER et al. 1989) achieved a complete remission. In Erlangen, 70% complete remissions were observed after 50 Gy plus cisplatin. Higher radiation doses seem to produce an increase in local control of 5%–10%, but are possibly associated with a higher complication rate (JAKSE et al. 1986).

24.3.3 Maintenance of Local Control

In most series with definitive full-dose irradiation, about 50% of all patients with initial complete response have failed subsequently in the bladder (GOFFINET et al. 1975; GOODMAN et al. 1981; MORRISON 1975; QUILTY and DUNCAN 1986; SHIPLEY et al. 1987b; TIMMER et al. 1985; YU et al. 1985). The long-term rate of local tumor control lies in the range of 25%–50% for all patients.

The influence of cisplatin on long-term control is difficult to estimate because of the limited follow-up in patients with cisplatin treatment. However, in patients with proven muscle invasion, most recurrences occur during the first 2–3 years (SHIPLEY et al. 1987b; TIMMER et al. 1985). In patients with additional cisplatin treatment, the incidence of local recurrences seems to be equal to or lower than that after irradiation alone. So far, the initial increase in local control achieved by cisplatin has been maintained in the reported series (JAKSE et al. 1986; SHIPLEY et al. 1987; this report).

24.3.4 Toxicity

Up to now, no toxic deaths or notable increase in severe toxicity have been reported after radiotherapy plus cisplatin. This is remarkable as even patients with advanced age have been treated who were not suitable for radical surgery (JAKSE et al. 1986; SHIPLEY et al. 1987a). However, additional cisplatin treatment will surely increase acute hematological and gastrointestinal toxicity.

24.3.5 Survival

The data from Innsbruck (JAKSE et al. 1986) as well as from the National Bladder Cancer Group (SHIPLEY et al. 1987a) and from the GU Tumor Group in Vancouver (COPPIN and BROWN 1986) show excellent survival figures after 3 years (Table 24.9). Survival rates were improved as compared with historical controls. This is encouraging if one considers the fact that the National Bladder Cancer Group has treated only patients not suitable for radical surgery and therefore carrying a worse prognosis. However, our data from Erlangen show no increase in survival. The 3-year survival in our series was 66% for patients receiving irradiation plus cisplatin and 66% for a historical group treated with radiotherapy alone. A possible explanation for the lack of a survival benefit even with increased local control is the use of salvage cystectomy whenever possible. Local persistent tumor was rare in our patients and death related to an exclusively local tumor progression has not been observed.

On the other hand, our data demonstrate that simultaneous cisplatin in a total dosage of 250 mg/m² is not able to prevent systemic metastases. A better survival with a more aggressive chemotherapeutic approach cannot be excluded from our data.

24.3.6 Upfront Chemotherapy Prior to Irradiation plus Cisplatin

At the Massachusetts General Hospital (MGH) (KAUFMAN et al. 1989; MARKS et al. 1988) as well as at the University of Florida (TESTER et al. 1989), so-called upfront multiagent chemotherapy prior to irradiation plus cisplatin has been used (Table 24.10). Patients received two courses of combination chemotherapy including methotrexate, cisplatin, and vinblastine (MCV) as initial treatment. Although 48% of the patients in the MGH series showed a complete response after upfront chemotherapy, the local complete response after additional irradiation (40 Gy) plus cisplatin was only 67%. At the University of Florida, two courses of MCV chemotherapy were followed by an irradiation scheme identical to that of the National

Table 24.9. Survival rates after full-dose irradiation ± cisplatin

Institution/reference	RT alone	RT plus cisplatin	Comment
University of Innsbruck (JAKSE et al. 1986)	T_{2-3}: 23%	T_{3-4}: 62%	4-year survival, historical control
National Bladder Cancer Group (SHIPLEY et al. 1987a)	–	T_2: 62% T_{3-4}: 24%	4-year survival, no control
GU Tumor Group Vancouver (COPPIN and BROWN 1986)	T_{3-4}: 49%	T_{3-4}: 82%	3-year survival, historical control
University of Erlangen (this report)	T_{1-4}: 66%	T_{1-4}: 66%	3-year survival, historical control

Table 24.10. Local complete response rates in patients with macroscopic tumor: upfront multiagent chemotherapy followed by full-dose irradiation plus cisplatin

Institution	Stage	Treatment regimen[a]	Complete response
Massachusetts General Hospital	T_{2-4}	2x MCV 40 Gy + cisplatin	22/46 (48%) after 2x MCV 26/39 (67%) after additional 40 Gy + cisplatin
University of Florida	T_{2-4}	24.8 Gy + cisplatin 2x MCV ± A 64.8 Gy + Cis	34/51 (66%) after total treatment

[a] 2x MCV, two courses of methotrexate + cisplatin + vinblastine (A, adriamycin); Cis, cisplatin

Bladder Cancer Group. However, complete response after the end of the total treatment was only 66%. The data suggest that more aggressive chemotherapeutic approaches will not increase the local control rate. The effect on survival remains unclear at the moment because of limited follow-up.

24.3.7 Irradiation plus Intra-arterial Cisplatin

EAPAN and co-workers have recently published their results with irradiation combined with preceding and concurrent intra-arterial cisplatin (EAPAN et al. 1989). The drug ($60-120 \, mg/m^2$) was administered via both iliac arteries over 2 h. Three courses were performed at 3-week intervals prior to and concurrent with irradiation. Radiotherapy consisted of a standard fractionation regimen up to a total dose of 60 Gy in 6 weeks. 25 patients with T_{3-4} bladder cancers were treated; 22 had macroscopic residual tumor. The complete remission rate was 96% with an estimated 2-year survival of 90%. These are the best results concerning local control and survival. However, the authors have reported a 4% incidence of toxic deaths and a 46% rate of neurological complications in their patients. Further evaluation of this treatment concept is necessary.

24.4 Therapeutic Recommendations

It is well-known from the literature that bladder-sparing treatment by TUR and irradiation is an effective treamtent in muscle-invading bladder cancer. Cystectomy can be restricted to irradiation failures. However, it is nearly impossible to give recommendations concerning the role of cisplatin in bladder-preserving treatment programs. Randomized trials are necessary to evaluate the local and systemic efficacy of cisplatin when used in combination with full-dose irradiation. Recently, ABRATT and co-workers have reported that the addition of misonidazole in bladder cancer treatment improved local control when compared with a historical group, but they failed to demonstrate a significant effect in a randomized trial (ABRATT et al. 1987). The study shows clearly that comparisons with historical controls should be interpreted carefully in bladder cancer treatment. Therefore, cisplation should be tested mainly in randomized

trials, and widespread uncritical use of cisplatin seems unjustifiable. Nevertheless, the questions of whether cisplatin can be used outside clinical trials and, if so, what is the optimal regimen remain to be answered:

1. *Can we treat patients with cisplatin outside clinical trials?* All currently available studies have shown an excellent local control without enhanced severe complications when cisplatin was added to irradiation in patients with incomplete TUR prior to radiotherapy. This group of patients seems to profit concerning local control and bladder preservation. We therefore believe that it is ethically justified to treat this subgroup of bladder cancer patients with additional cisplatin even outside clinical trials, provided that there are no contraindications to this drug.

2. *Is there an optimal regimen for irradiation plus simultaneous cisplatin?* The current results have been obtained with a combination of simultaneous cisplatin and full-dose irradiation. Radiation doses varied from 50 to 65 Gy. The local control rate is possibly higher with doses over 60 Gy. Careful treatment planning is necessary, especially in patients with macroscopic residual tumor, in order to exclude a geographical miss (EMAMI and PILEPICH 1983). Concerning simultaneous cisplatin, a regimen with proven efficacy as single-agent chemotherapy in bladder cancer should be used. We believe that one should use a less toxic cisplatin regimen if one treats a patient outside a clinical trial. Aggressive multiagent chemotherapy should be avoided because a benefit concerning local control and survival has not yet been shown and because of a treatment-related mortality of about 5% in several trials.

24.5 Summary

In summary, a combination of full-dose irradiation and simultaneous cisplatin chemotherapy is possible and well tolerated. Several institutions, including the University of Innsbruck, the National Bladder Cancer Group, and the University of Erlangen, have used different regimens in advanced bladder cancer. In patients with macroscopic residual tumor, histological complete remission rates of 70% and more have been achieved. At Erlangen University, additional cis-

platin has significantly increased the complete remission rate after macroscopically or microscopically incomplete transurethral surgery as compared
with a historical group: 45% complete remissions
after 50.4 Gy versus 76% complete remissions
after 50.4 Gy plus cisplatin. The maintenance of
local control seems to be as good or better with
cisplatin as compared with irradiation alone. An
increase in severe or late toxicity has not been
reported although mild to moderate acute toxicity
is higher with additional cisplatin (hyperemesis,
hematological toxicity). It can be concluded from
these nonrandomized (phase II) trials that cisplatin is well tolerated and will likely increase the
local control rate by about 20% in patients with
incomplete TUR. The effect of cisplatin on survival remains unclear at the moment. Preliminary
results from several studies (National Bladder
Cancer Group, University of Innsbruck, GU
Tumor Group in Vancouver) suggest an increased
survival with cisplatin as compared with historical
groups. At the University of Erlangen, however,
increased local control with additional cisplatin
was not associated with an increased survival: the
3-year survival was 66% after irradiation plus cisplatin versus 66% in a historical group treated with
radiotherapy alone.

At the moment, randomized trials are necessary
for further evaluation of the efficacy of cisplatin.
Outside clinical trials, the use of cisplatin seems
ethically justified in patients with incomplete TUR.
Cisplatin should be given in a dosage with proven
efficacy but low toxicity. More aggressive chemotherapeutic approaches should be restricted to
randomized clinical trials.

References

Abratt RP, Barnes DR, Pontin AL, Sarembock LA,
Williams AM (1987) Radical radiation and oral and
intra-vesical misonidazole for bladder cancer. Int J
Radiat Oncol Biol Phys 13: 1053–1055

Batata MA, Chu FCH, Hilaris BS, Kim YS, Lee MZ,
Chung S, Whitmore WF (1981) Factors of prognostic and
therapeutic significance in patients with bladder cancer.
Int J Radiat Oncol Biol Phys 7: 575–579

Bloom HJG, Hendry WF, Wallace DM, Skeet RG (1982)
Treatment of T3 bladder cancer: controlled trial of preoperative radiotherapy and radical cystectomy versus
radical radiotherapy. Br J Urol 54: 136–151

Chan RC, Johnson DE (1978) Integrated therapy for invasive bladder carcinoma: experience with 108 patients.
Urology 12: 549–552

Coppin C, Brown E (1986) Concurrent cisplatin with radiation for locally advanced bladder cancer: a pilot study

suggesting improved survival. Proc Am Soc Clin Oncol
5: 99

Cross RJ, Glashan RW, Humphrey CS, Robinson MRG,
Smith PH, Williams RE (1976) Treatment of advanced
bladder cancer with adriamycin and 5-fluorouracil. Br J
Urol 48: 609–615

Daniels JR, Skinner DG, Lieskovsky G, Turcillo P, Daniels
AM, Krailo M (1986) Adjuvant chemotherapy following
radical cystectomy for carcinoma of the bladder: a randomized trial. Proc Am Soc Clin Oncol 4: 105

Denis L, Hendricks G (1986) Preoperative chemotherapy
in T3/T4–Nx–M0 bladder cancer. J Urol 135: 222A

Eapan L, Stewart D, Danjoux C et al. (1989) Intraarterial
cisplatin and concurrent radiation for locally advanced
bladder cancer. J Clin Oncol 7: 230–235

Edsmyr F, Andersson L, Esposti PL, Littbrand B, Nilsson
B (1985) Irradiation therapy with multiple small fractions
per day in urinary bladder cancer. Radiother Oncol 4:
197–203

Emami B, Pilepich MV (1983) Anatomic considerations in
radiotherapeutic management of bladder cancer. Am J
Clin Oncol 6: 593–597

Goffinet DR, Schneider MJ, Glatstein EJ, Ludwig H, Ray
GR, Dunnick NR, Bagshaw MA (1975) Bladder cancer:
results of radiation therapy in 348 patients. Radiology
117: 149–153

Goodman GB, Hislop G, Elwood JM, Balfour J (1981)
Conservation of bladder function in patients with invasive bladder cancer treated by definitive irradiation
and selective cystectomy. Int J Radiat Oncol Biol Phys 7:
569–573

Havsteen H, von der Maase H, Stroyer I, Rasmussen F
(1987) Cisplatin as a first-line treatment in T_2 and T_3
bladder carcinoma. Cancer Treat Rep 71: 1285–1287

Jacobs SC, McCellan SL, Maher C, Lawson RK (1984)
Pre-cystectomy intra-arterial cis-diamminedichloroplatinum II with local bladder hyperthermia for bladder
cancer. J Urol 131: 473–476

Jakse G, Rauschmeier H, Fritsch E, Frommhold H,
Marberger H (1986) Die integrierte Radiotherapie und
Chemotherapie des lokal fortgeschrittenen Harnblasen-
karzinoms. Aktuel Urol 17: 68–73

Kaufman DS, Prout GR, Shipley WU et al. (1989) Upfront
MCV chemotherapy plus cisplatin and radiotherapy: its
efficacy in successful bladder preservation in 50 patients
with invasive cancer. Proc Am Soc Clin Oncol 8: 129

Klimberg IW, Wajsman Z (1986) Treatment for muscle
invasive carcinoma of the bladder. J Urol 136: 1169–
1175

Logothetis CJ, Samuels LM, Ogden S, Dexeus FH, Svanson
D, Johnson DE, von Eschenbach A (1985) Cyclophosphamide, doxorubicin and cisplatin chemotherapy for
patients with locally advanced urothelial tumors with or
without nodal metastases. J Urol 134: 460–464

Logothetis C, Samuels M, Ogden S, Dexeus F, Johnson D,
Svanson D, von Eschenbach A (1986) Adjuvant chemotherapy for invasive bladder carcinoma: a preliminary
report. Proc Am Soc Clin Oncol 4: 108

Maatman TJ, Montie JE, Bukowski RM, Risius B, Gei-
singer M (1986) Intra-arterial chemotherapy as an adjuvant to surgery in transitional cell carcinoma of the
bladder J Urol 135: 256–260

Marks LB, Kaufman SD, Prout GR, Heney NM, Griffin
PP, Shipley WU (1988) Invasive bladder carcinoma:
preliminary report of selective bladder conservation by
transurethral surgery, upfront MCV (methotrexate, cis-

platin, and vinblastine) chemotherapy and pelvic irradiation plus cisplatin. Int J Radiat Oncol Biol Phys 15: 877–883

Meyers FJ, Palmer JM, Freiha FS et al. (1985) The fate of the bladder in patients with metastatic bladder cancer treated with cisplatin, methotrexate and vinblastine: a Northern California Oncology Group Study. J Urol 134: 1118–1120

Miller LS (1977) Bladder cancer: superiority of preoperative irradiation and cystectomy in clinical stages B_2 and C. Cancer 39: 973–980

Morrison R (1975) The results of treatment of cancer of the bladder – a clinical contribution to radiobiology. Clin Radiol 26: 67–75

Oliver RTD, Hope-Stone HF, Blandy JP (1989) Radiotherapy and radical surgery in management of invasive bladder cancer. In: Oliver RTD, Blandy JP, Hope-Stone HF (eds) Urological and genital cancer. Blackwall Scientific, Oxford, p 105

Prout GR, Slack NH, Bross IDJ (1973) Preoperative irradiation and cystectomy for bladder carcinoma IV: results in a selected population. In: Seventh National Cancer Conference Proceedings. J.B. Lippincott, Philadelphia, p 783

Quilty PM, Duncan W (1986) Primary radical radiotherapy for T3 transitional cell cancer of the bladder: an analysis of survival and control. Int J Radiat Oncol Biol Phys 12: 853–860

Raghavan D, Pearson B, Duval P et al. (1985) Initial intravenous cis-platinum therapy: improved managment for invasive high risk bladder cancer? J Urol 133: 399–402

Richards B, Bastable JRG, Freedman L et al. (1983) Adjuvant chemotherapy with doxorubicin (Adriamycin) and 5-fluorouracil in T3, Nx, M0 bladder cancer treated with radiotherapy. Br J Urol 55: 386–391

Richie JP, Shipley WU, Yagoda A (1985) Cancer of the bladder. In: deVita VT, Hellman S, Rosenberg SA (eds) Cancer. Principles and practice of oncology, 2nd edn. J.B. Lippincott, Philadelphia, p 915

Rotman M, Aziz H (1987) Bladder carcinoma. In: Perez CA, Brady LW (eds) Principles and practice of radiation oncology. J.B. Lippincott, Philadelphia, p 847

Rotman M, Macchia R, Silverstein M et al. (1987) Treatment of advanced bladder carcinoma with irradiation and concomitant 5-fluorouracil infusion. Cancer 59: 710–714

Sauer R, Schrott KM, Dunst J, Thiel HJ, Hermanek P, Bornhof C (1988) Preliminary results of treatment of invasive bladder carcinoma with radiotherapy and cisplatin. Int J Radiat Oncol Biol Phys 15: 871–875

Shipley WU, Cummings KB, Coombs LJ, Hawkins IR, Einstein AB, Penick G (1982) 4000 rad preoperative irradiation followed by prompt radical cystectomy for invasive bladder carcinoma: a prospective study of patient tolerance and pathologic downstaging. J Urol 127: 48–51

Shipley WU, Rose MA, Perrone TL, Mannix CM, Heney NM, Prout GR (1985) Full-dose irradiation for patients with invasive bladder carcinoma: clinical and histological factors prognostic of improved survival. J Urol 134: 679–683

Shipley WU, Prout GR, Einstein AB et al. (1987a) Treatment of invasive bladder cancer by cisplatin and radiation in patients unsuited for surgery. JAMA 258: 931–935

Shipley WU, Prout GR, Kaufman SD, Perrone TL (1987b) Invasive bladder carcinoma. The importance of initial transurethral surgery and other significant prognostic factors for improved survival with full-dose irradiation. Cancer 60: 514–520

Soloway MS (1987) Is there a role for induction therapy for locally advanced bladder cancer? Urology 29: 577–583

Sternberg CN, Yagoda A, Scher HI et al. (1985) Preliminary results of M-VAC (methotrexate, vinblastine, doxorubicin and cisplatin) for transitional cell carcinoma of the urothelium. J Urol 133: 403–407

Svanson DA, Eschenbach AC, Johnson DE (1981) Salvage cystectomy for bladder carcinoma. Cancer 47: 2275–2279

Tester W, Porter A, Asbell S et al. (1989) Combined modality program with possible organ preservation for invasive bladder carcinoma. Proc Am Soc Clin Oncol 8: 141

Timmer PR, Hartleff HA, Hooijkaas JAP (1985) Bladder cancer: patterns of recurrence in 142 patients. Int J Radiat Oncol Biol Phys 11: 899–905

van der Werf-Messing B (1979) Preoperative irradiation followed by cystectomy to treat carcinoma of the urinary bladder category T3 Nx, 0–4 M0. Int J Radiat Oncol Biol Phys 5: 395–401

Yagoda A, Watson RC, Gonzalez-Vitale JC, Whitmore WF (1976) cis-Dichlorodiammineplatinum(II) in advanced bladder cancer. Cancer Treat Rep 60: 917–923

Yu WS, Sagerman RH, Chung CT, Dalal PS, King GA (1985) Bladder carcinoma. Experience with radical and preoperative radiotherapy in 421 patients. Cancer 56: 1293–1299

25 Small-Cell Carcinoma of the Lung

Andrew T. Turrisi, III

CONTENTS

25.1 Platinum in Lung Cancer

cis-Diamminedichloroplatinum (cisplatin) has a broad range of activity. Since its development in the early 1970s, it has become the crucial drug for the management of testicular and ovarian cancers, and the drug yielding the most impressive responses in bladder, esophagus, and head and neck cancers. It has been combined with other drugs, thereby providing the best available results in the treatment of lung cancer. DDP has been used both as a single agent and in a variety of combinations for lung cancer. Its activity against small-cell carcinoma of the lung is actually quite marginal, but most, if not all, phase II studies were conducted on heavily pretreated patients (MORSTYN et al. 1984). The cisplatin analog, carboplatin, has a single-agent response rate of 65%–79% (SMITH et al. 1985; JACOBS et al. 1987). Although extrapolation to cisplatin is speculative, it is reasonable to postulate that cisplatin will have an excellent single-agent response rate when used in previously untreated patients.

25.2 Small-Cell Carcinoma of the Lung: Current Concepts

Small-cell carcinoma of the lung (SCLC) has unique characteristics. Unlike other solid tumors, it has a large growth fraction (MUGGIA et al. 1974). Distinct from other lung cancers, it is very responsive to chemotherapy and radiotherapy. In the late 1960s and early 1970s, SCLC was projected to be the next disease that would be cured by chemotherapy. Although most agree that SCLC is a systemic disease at the time of presentation, local failure at the site of tumor bulk after chemotherapy alone remains a problem for the majority of patients. For limited disease, this has led to attempts at integration of thoracic radiotherapy (TRT). TRT was found to improve local control and survival in three recent large studies (PEREZ et al. 1984; BUNN et al. 1987; PERRY et al. 1987). However, the optimal chemotherapy remains unsolved. The chemotherapeutic strategy of alternating non-cross-resistant regimens has been somewhat disappointing (AISNER 1983) but there have been some conflicting recent positive studies (Havemann et al. 1987; ETTINGER et al. 1986). Etoposide by itself yields excellent responses against SCLC (MORSTYN et al. 1984). However, a 24-h infusion was inferior to a multiday dose, when total dose was kept constant (SLEVIN et al. 1986). The optimal etoposide dose and schedule, including longer than 24 h continuous infusion, have not been established (EINHORN 1986), but many doses and schedules of cisplatin-etoposide (PE) are active, and a variety are in clinical use. PE has provided a source of new hope. It has caused responses in patients having progressed from other cyclophosphamide-based regimens (LOPEZ et al. 1985; OCHS et al. 1983; PORTER et al. 1985; EVANS et al. 1985a; BATIST et al. 1986). Furthermore, PE has excellent response rates when used as a front-line regimen (EVANS et al. 1985b; SIEROCKI et al. 1979). In extensive disease, two studies, from the *(SEG)

Andrew T. Turrisi, III, MD, Associate Professor, Department of Radiation Oncology, University of Michigan, UH-B2C490, Box 0010, 1500 E. Medical Center Drive, Ann Arbor, MI 48109, USA

and from Japan, conflict. The SEG study shows no difference between CAV (cyclophosphamide, Adriamycin, and vincristine) vs PE vs alternation between the two regimens (JOHNSON 1989, personal communication). The study from Japan, using a similar design, indicates the alternating arm to be superior (FUKUOKA et al. 1988 – updated at oral presentation, Interlaken 1988).

25.3 Rationale for Continuous Infusion Platinum

The rationale for continuous infusion (CI) is based on a number of factors. Although cisplatin can cause cytotoxicity in all phases of the cell cycle, cisplatin exerts its maximal cell kill in G_1 (SIDGESTAD et al. 1979). Therefore, cells in cycle increase their exposure to cisplatin if it is continuously infused. Pharmacologically, cisplatin is quickly bound to serum proteins, but the free form is the only active species (DECONTI et al. 1973). CI allows for saturation of these binding sites but facilitates longer exposure, albeit at lower peak levels. It appears that the continuous exposure results in less toxicity, but this is based on non-randomized, single-arm studies of 5 day CI in selected patients of various primary tumor site. (SALEM et al. 1984; POSNER et al. 1985; TISMAN et al. 1984). Five day-infusions have been used employing doses of $20-40 \, mg/m^2$/day (Table 25.1). For each tumor site, phase II data are hard to discern, but the lung data shown in Table 25.1 are for tumors of non-small-cell histology.

25.4 Platinum as a Radiation Sensitizer

The role of cisplatin as a radiation sensitizer has been reviewed by DEWITT (1987). It appears that cisplatin potentiates radiation by (a) abrogating the shoulder, (b) steepening the exponential portion of the single cell survival curve (sensitization), (c) altering split-dose and potentially lethal repair, and (d) influencing both hypoxic and euoxic cellular response (DEWITT 1987; CARDE and LAVAL 1981). Also cisplatin may deplete endogenous thiols. The independent cell kill of each modality may also cause synergism by improving oxygenation and increasing access of chemotherapeutics.

Table 25.1. Continuous Infusion of Cisplatin: dose escalation for 5-day schedule and phase II lung data.

Authors	Dose $(mg/m^2$/day)	No. of patients	Resp Lung	Toxicity
SALEM et al. 1984	20	96	1/10	Minimal
POSNER et al. 1985	25	22	1/6	Minimal
TISMAN et al. 1984	20–40	14	6/7	Minimal

Resp Lung: Response lung cancer.

25.5 Issues of Continuous Infusion

Continuous infusion has not been often tried in SCLC. Two fundamental issues stand out. First, it is important to define whether CI DDP alone or CI DDP plus etoposide produces better response rates in either (a) limited disease or (b) extensive disease. Second, since TRT may improve both local control and survival, it will be important to evaluate, both for normal tissues and for SCLC, CI vs other infusion schedules (i.e. daily pulse, weekly, Q 3 weekly), as a potentiator of radiation response, Clearly, if normal tissue toxicity is increased, no therapeutic gain will be achieved. Using rodents, LELIEVELD and colleagues (1985) have shown cisplatin to produce net gains against tumors vs normal tissues. As of yet there are no data regarding CI DDP and this issue of therapeutic ratio. Suggesting an advantage for CI in tumor control, DREWINKO et al. (1973) have demonstrated that concentration × time (area under curve) provides better cytotoxicity in an in vitro human lymphoma model than the cytotoxicity of pulsed doses. SALEM, Posner, and TISMAN have used CI cisplatin for 5 days, which caused a response in some non SCLC patients (SALEM et al. 1984; POSNER et al. 1985; TISMAN et al. 1984). As regards to CI of other drugs in lung cancer, TAYLOR et al. (1988) have used continuous 5-day infusions of 5-FU plus bolus DDP and radiation therapy prior to surgery and ROWLAND et al. (1988) have described the use of CI etoposide in previously treated SCLC.

It is not clear that interference with the above radiation response endpoints is dose related or schedule dependent, in regard to cisplatin. Furthermore, it is not clear whether there is a threshold dose for either DDP efficacy or radiotherapy potentiation, below which no interaction is detected. The optimal sequence of platinum and irradiation has not yet been established. The pharmacodynamics suggest rapid plasma clearance (T 1/2 30 min), but there are few data on tissue concentrations, and what the necessary tissue levels might be and when these levels may be achieved in relation to time after infusion, or relationships to plasma levels. Furthermore, it will be helpful to know the duration of the effects on normal tissue and tumor in order to optimize timing with irradiation. Data regarding these issues, both for normal tissues and for tumors, may point toward better methods than the empiricism which directs that platinum be infused "just before" radiotherapy. Also, they may tell us that the doses we can now achieve are either too high, too low, or just right to produce radiation modification. An advantage of CI therapy is prolonged delivery of free DDP at levels low enough to circumvent toxicity but possibly sufficient to increase tumor cytotoxicity. It is yet to be established whether these low levels effectively modify radiation responses or cause direct cytotoxicity to tumors to any meaningful degree.

In attempt to correlate tumor platinol concentrations with serum levels, Mattox reported a study that infused $50-100 \, mg/m^2$ in 10 minutes. Plasma disappearance and tumor platinum concentration, measured at 2, 6 and 24 hours post infusion, were obtained in 5 patients. Six hours post infusion marked the peak time of tissue concentrations, which exceeded the plasma concentrations at this point. In other experiments, Mattox also explanted tumor specimens making single-cell, tissue cultures. DDP concentrations of $0.02-100$ micro grams/ml were added to these tumor specimens suspended in soft agar. Although a majority showed response, which seemed dose related, this was not universal. In many, the platinol was only slightly inhibiting of growth potential, if at all.

This study demonstrates how difficult it is to define proper timing of peak levels in tissue, and minimum level necessary to inhibit human head and neck cancer. It may provide some impetus to do continuous infusions if tumor concentrates platinol, at least to a level that might potentiate radiation's effect.

Two recent studies detail DDP CI pharmaco-

kinetic data in children (DOMINICI et al. 1989) and adults with solid tumors (REECF et al. 1989). The study in children used high dose DDP ($40 \, mg/m^2/$ day) and multiple courses. The subsequent courses were associated with increased mean plasma DDP concentrations and decreased urinary excretion of DDP. The higher concentrations of DDP did not create an increased response, but did increase the frequency of emesis. It is not clear whether the same observations would be found in previously untreated patients or at lower daily doses. It may be of some importance of radiation–modifying effects or responses prove to be related to plasma levels or area-under-curve parameters. Also, it is not clear that the apparent cumulative effect of increased DDP retention creates toxicity. In previous studies, longer infusions have been associated with less nephrotoxicity and ototoxicity. REECE et al. compared a 2-h infusion with a 24-h infusion and found the longer infusion to be better tolerated and to be associated with higher mean plasma levels. Urinary clearance of DDP was less with the prolonged infusion. Again, how these findings influence clinical endpoints is yet to be determined.

25.6 The CEPi Regimen

FRYTAK et al. (1987) at the Mayo Clinic have used CI cisplatin plus etoposide both alone and together with split-course, twice-daily TRT. They call this regimen CEPi. Table 25.2 demonstrates the doses and schedules of chemotherapy. CEPi was infused for three courses in three patients, two courses in eight patients, and one course in one patient. Patients had either progressed or plateaued on standard chemotherapy. Nausea and vomiting were common place but considered acceptable. One case of neuropathy was reported. Because of substantive prior chemotherapy it was difficult to chavacterize myelotoxicity and to know whether the observations would forecast for previously untreated patients. Using these drugs by themselves without TRT, 9 of 12 (75%) previously

Table 25.2. Mayo Clinic CEPi regimen

Cyclophosphamide	$500 \, mg/m^2$	Day 1
Etoposide	$60 \, mg/m^2$	Days 1–3
Platinum	$20 \, mg/m^2$	CI, days 1–5

treated patients responded. In a subsequent trial, CEPi was used for three cycles followed by sequential, split-course 48 Gy given in two courses of 24 Gy, separated by 2 1/2 weeks. In each course twice-daily irradiation doses of 1.5 Gy were given for 8 days. During radiotherapy, patients continued to receive cyclophosphamide and etoposide, but *not* the CI DDP. Fourteen patients entered the study, but only 11 are evaluable. Toxicity to esophagus was found in four but caused hospitalization of only one. Median leukocyte nadir was 1800/mm^3, and median platelet count was 127 000/mm^3. All patients responded; 4/11 (36%) had a complete response (FRYTAK et al., submitted for publication).

25.7 The Challenge of Future Trials

The results of many ways of integrating chemotherapy with radiotherapy have been reported for limited SCLC (TURRISI 1988). CI platinum needs further study both alone, preferably in previously untreated extensive disease patients, and subsequently in a variety of schedules, with sequential, alternating, and concurrent chemotherapy. Whether large peak doses or larger total doses spread continuously over time (areas under the curve) are preferable awaits further elucidation by well-designed clinical trials. The issues that must be addressed are:

1. Does infusional DDP cause more or less toxicity?
2. Do DDP infusions provide good response rates?
3. Do infusions of DDP provide radiation modification, and are the infusions superior or inferior to bolus doses?
4. What is the optimal duration of infusion (either as a chemotherapeutic or as a radiation modifier), and what is the maximum tolerated dose per day?
5. What is the optimal timing of platinum with radiotherapy?
6. Can DDP infusions be integrated with other drugs without reducing effectiveness, increasing toxicity, or spoiling radiation modification?
7. Are these infusions cost-effective?

These are interesting leads to pursue in aiming to establish exactly how infusions alter the therapeutic ratio.

References

Aisner J (1983) Alternating chemotherapy for the treatment of small cell carcinoma of the lung. Proceedings of the International Congress of Chemotherapy 205: 15–23

Batist G, Carney DN, Cowan KH, Veach SR, Gilliom M, Bunn PA, Ihde DC (1986) Etoposide (VP-16) and cisplatin in previously treated small-cell lung cancer: clinical trial and in vitro correlates. J Clin Oncol 4: 982–986

Bonomi P, Rowland KM, Taylor IV SG et al. (1988) Phase II trial of therapy with etoposide, 5-fluorouracil by continuous infusion, cisplatin, and simultaneous split-course radiation in stage III non-small cell bronchogenic carcinoma. NCI Monogr 6: 331–334

Bunn Jr PA, Lichter AS, Makuch RW et al. (1987) Chemotherapy alone or chemotherapy with chest radiation therapy in limited stage small cell lung cancer. Ann Intern Med 106: 655–662

Carde P, Laval F (1981) Effect of cis-dichlorodiammine platinum II and xrays on mammalian cell survival. Int J Radiat Oncol Biol Phys 7: 929–933

DeConti RC, Toftness BR, Lange RC, Creasey WA (1973) Clinical and pharmacological studies with cis-diamminedichloroplatinum (II). Cancer Res 33: 1310–1315

Dewitt L (1987) Combined treatment of radiation and cis-diamminedichloroplatinum (II): a review of experimental and clinical data. Int J Radiat Oncol Biol Phys 13: 403–426

Dominici C, Petrucci F, Caroli S, Alimonti A, Clerico A, Castello MA (1989) A pharmacokinetic study of high-dose continuous infusion cisplatin in children with solid tumors. J Clin Oncol 7: 100–107

Drewinko B, Brown BW, Gottlieb JA (1973) The effect of cis-diamminedichloroplatinum (II) on cultured human lymphoma cells and its therapeutic implications. Cancer Res 33: 3091–3095

Einhorn LH (1986) Initial therapy with cisplatin plus VP-16 in small-cell lung cancer. Semin Oncol 13: 5–9

Ettinger DS, Mehta CR, Abeloff MD, Ruckdeschel JC, Aisner S (1986) A randomized comparison of conventional chemotherapy with immediate alternation of non-cross resistant chemotherapy in extensive disease (ED) small cell lung cancer (SCLC). Proc ASCO 5: 170

Evans WK, Osoba D, Feld R, Shepherd FA, Bazos MJ, DeBoer G (1985a) Etoposide (VP-16) and cisplatin: an effective treatment for relapse in small-cell lung cancer. J Clin Oncol 3: 65–71

Evans WK, Shepherd FA, Feld R, Osoba D, Dang P, DeBoer G (1985b) VP-16 and cisplatin as first-line therapy for small-cell lung cancer. J Clin Oncol 3: 1471–1477

Frytak S, Eagan RT, Richardson RL, Creagan ET, Jett JL, Coles DT, Lee RE (1987) Cyclophosphamide, etoposide, and infusion cisplatin in refractory small cell lung cancer. Am J Clin Oncol (CCT) 10: 33–35

Frytak S, Shaw EG, Eagan RT, Creagan ET, Richardson RL, Jett JR (submitted for publication) Hyperfractionated thoracic radiotherapy (HTRT) and infusion cisplatin based chemotherapy (CT) for small cell lung cancer (SCLC) – a preliminary report. Proc ASCO

Fukuoka M, Furuse K, Saijo N, Nishiwaki Y, Ikegami H, Suemasw K (1988) A randomized study in the treatment of small cell lung cancer (SCLC): cyclophosphamide (C), adriamycin (A), and vincristine vs cyclophosphamide, adriamycin, vincristine alternating with cisplatin etoposide. Lung Cancer 4 [Suppl]: A101

Havemann K, Wolf M, Holle R et al. (1987) Alternating versus sequential chemotherapy in small cell lung cancer: a randomized German multicenter trial. Cancer 59: 1072–1082

Jacobs RH, Bitran JD, Deutsch M, Hoffman PC, Sinkule J, Purl S, Golomb HM (1987) Phase II study of carboplatin in previously untreated patients with metastatic small cell lung carcinoma. Cancer Treat Rep 71: 311–312

Lelieveld P, Scoles MA, Brown JM, Kallman RF (1985) The effect of treatment in fractionated schedules with the combination of x-irradiation and six cytotoxic drugs on the RIF-1 tumor and normal mouse skin. Int J Radiat Oncol Biol Phys 11: 111–121

Lopez JA, Mann J, Grapski RT, Nassif E, Vannicola P, Krikorian JG, Finkel H (1985) Etoposide and cisplatin salvage chemotherapy for small cell lung cancer. Cancer Treat Rep 69: 369–371

Mattox DE, Sternson LA, Von Hoff DD, Kuhn JG, Repta AJ (1983) Tumor concentration of platinum in patients with head and neck cancer. Otolaryngol Head Neck Surg 91: 271–275

Morstyn G, Ihde DC, Lichter AS, Bunn PA, Carney DN, Glatstein E, Minna JD (1984) Small cell lung cancer 1973–1983: early progress and recent obstacles. Int J Radiat Oncol Biol Phys 10: 515–539

Muggia FM, Krezoski SK, Hansen H (1974) Cell kinetic studies in patients with small cell carcinoma of the lung. Cancer 34: 1683

Ochs JJ, Tester WJ, Cohen MH, Lichter AS, Ihde DC (1983) "Salvage" radiation therapy for intrathoracic small cell carcinoma of the lung progressing on combination chemotherapy. Cancer Treat Rep 67: 1123–1126

Perez CA, Einhorn L, Oldham RK et al. (1984) Randomized trial of radiotherapy to the thorax in limited small-cell carcinoma of the lung treated with multiagent chemotherapy and elective brain irradiation: a preliminary report. J Clin Oncol 2: 1200–1208

Perry MC, Eaton WL, Propert KJ et al. (1987) Chemotherapy with or without radiation therapy in limited small-cell carcinoma of the lung. N Engl J Med 316: 912–918

Porter III LL, Johnson DH, Hainsworth JD, Hande KR,

Greco FA (1985) Cisplatin and etoposide combination chemotherapy for refractory small cell carcinoma of the lung. Cancer Treat Rep 69: 479–481

Posner MR, Belliveau JF, Ferrari L et al. (1985) Clinical and pharmacokinetic study of 5-day continous infusion cis-platinum. Proc ASCO 4:38

Reece PA, Stafford I, Abbott RL et al. (1989) Two-versus 24-hour infusion of cisplatin: pharmacokinetic considerations. J Clin Oncol 7: 270–275

Rowland Jr KM, Bonomi P, Taylor IV SG, Maffey S, Reddy S, Lee MS (1988) Continuous infusion of etoposide, bolus administration of cisplatin, and simultaneous radiation therapy in previously treated patients with small cell bronchogenic carcinoma. NCI Monogr 6: 323–325

Salem P, Khalyl M, Jabboury K, Hashimi L (1984) Cisdiamminedichloroplatinum (II) by 5-day continuous infusion. Cancer 53: 837–840

Sidgestad CP, Grdina DJ, Peters LJ, Stutesman J (1979) Cell cycle phase preferential killing of fibrosarcoma tumor by cis-diamminedichloroplatinum or adriamycin. Proc AACR 20: 178

Sierocki JS, Hilaris BS, Hopfan S (1979) Cis-diamminedichloroplatinum (II) and VP-16-213: an active induction regimen for small cell lung carcinoma. Cancer Treat Rep 63: 1593–1597

Slevin ML, Clark PI, Osborne RJ et al. (1986) A randomized trial to evaluate the effect of schedule on the activity of etoposide in small cell lung cancer. Proc ASCO 5: 175

Smith IE, Harland SJ, Robinson BA et al. (1985) Carboplatin: a very active new cisplatin analog in the treatment of small cell lung cancer. Cancer Treat Rep 69: 43–46

Taylor IV SG, Murthy AK, Bonomi P, Reddy S, Lee MS, Faber LP, Mathisen DJ (1988) Concomitant therapy with infusion of cisplatin and 5-fluorouracil plus radiation in stage III non-small cell lung cancer. NCI Monogr 6: 327–329

Tisman G, Flener V, Hsu MYK et al. (1984) Outpatient high dose cis-platinum continuous infusion chemotherapy. Proc ASCO 3:27.

Turrisi AT (1988) The role of radiotherapy for limited small cell lung cancer. Oncology 2(7): 19–25

26 Non-Small-Cell Carcinoma of the Lung

Hassan Aziz, C. Julian Rosenthal, Louis Potters, Mohan Nuthakki, and Marvin Rotman

CONTENTS

26.1 Introduction

It is estimated that in the United States during 1989, 155 000 cases of carcinoma of the lung will occur and that close to 142 000 of these patients will die within 1 year from their disease (Silverberg and Lubera 1989). At present in the United States, the incidence and death rate from this disease for females has surpassed that for breast cancer in the 55–74 year age group (Silverberg and Lubera 1989) and is directly related to cigarette smoking. There is clearly an overwhelming need for the implementation of programs directed at the prevention of this disease. Meanwhile, in the face of current statistics, it is a priority among multi-specialty cancer physicians to improve and discover new treatment modalities for this most intractable form of the disease.

Surgical resection of a non-small-cell carcinoma of the lung (NSCLC) can provide a 28%–38% 5-year survival (Holmes 1988). Unfortunately, only 20% of all patients will have localized tumors that may be resectable at the time of diagnosis

Hassan Aziz, MD, Associate Professor, Radiation Oncology, C. Julian Rosenthal, MD, Professor of Medicine and Oncology, Louis Potters, Department of Radiation Oncology, Mohan Nuthakki, Department of Medical Oncology, Marvin Rotman, MD, Professor and Chairman, Department of Radiation Oncology, SUNY Health Science Center at Brooklyn, 450 Clarkson Avenue, Brooklyn, NY, 11203, USA

(Holmes 1988). Despite the high propensity to distant metastasis, improved control of intra-thoracic disease, according to several studies, can be directly correlated with improved survivals (Perez et al. 1982, 1986, 1987).

In head and neck (Showell et al. 1983) and esophageal carcinomas (Leichman et al. 1984) there has been an encouraging enhancement of locoregional control using concomitant infusion of 5-FU, cisplatin bolus and radiation. Bearing this in mind and using the data generated by a phase I study previously conducted at our center (Rosenthal et al. 1986), we started a phase II study of the use of concomitant infusion of cisplatin and radiation for the treatment of advanced inoperable NSCLC. We report here on two small series of patients. The first consists of eight patients who received a cisplatin dose of $5–7\,mg/m^2/24\,h$ (low dose) concomitant with radiation therapy, while the second consists of 12 patients who received $20\,mg/m^2/24\,h$ (intermediate dose) of cisplatin concomitant with radiation therapy.

26.2 Methods and Materials

For this phase II study employing continuous concomitant infusion of cisplatin with radiation, two different dose schedules of cisplatin were used.

In the low dose group, eight patients in the age of group of 50–65 years, with inoperable squamous cell carcinoma of the lung were included (six males and two females). In this series seven patients had squamous cell and one patient had giant cell carcinoma substantiated by a transbronchial biopsy. All patients underwent a staging workup that included a CT scan of the chest and abdomen, a bone scan, and a routine blood chemistry screening that included liver function tests. Mediastinoscopy was also performed if required. Using the TNM staging system, three patients had stage $T_3N_1M_0$, two patients had stage $T_3N_2M_0$, two patients had stage $T_3N_2M_1$, and one patient had stage $T_2N_2M_0$ disease (Table 26.1). In this study, cisplatin was given at a constant slow rate of 5 mg/m^2/24 h in 14-day cycles with concomitant radiation delivered to the lung lesion with 2-cm margin, to the mediastinum, and to the supraclavicular regions if indicated by the location of tumor. Radiation treatment was given once daily 5 days a week in 2-week cycles. The total radiation dose, including the boost dose, ranged from 42 Gy to 60 Gy at 1.6–1.8 Gy/fraction. The concomitant cycles of radiation and cisplatin were repeated after a 1- and 2-week break, which the phase I study had shown was necessary for hematological recovery (ROSENTHAL et al. 1986). Cisplatin was usually administered through a central indwelling port inserted in the subclavian vein and connected to a battery-activated pump (Cormed Medino, N.Y.) or through a Hickmann catheter inserted in the subclavian vein.

In the intermediate dose cisplatin series, 12 patients were registered. All patients had inoperable NSCLC. There were six males and six females, and their ages ranged from 35 to 60 years. Four patients were staged as $T_2N_1M_0$, three as $T_2N_2M_0$,

and three as $T_3N_2M_0$. One patient had $T_4N_XM_0$, and one patient had $T_2N_1M_1$ disease. Histologically, six patients had cell adeno-carcinoma, three patients had squamous cell carcinoma, and three had large cell carcinoma. These patients received an infusion of cisplatin at 20 mg/m^2/24 h for 5 days in the 1st and the 4th week of radiation (Fig. 26.1) through a peripheral i.v. line or through a central indwelling port. Radiation was given at 1.6–1.8 Gy/fractions for 5 days/week without any break. A total radiation dose of 40–55 Gy was delivered, including the boost dose.

For the determination of response, chest x-rays and CT scans were repeated at 3–4 weeks after the completion of treatment, and thereafter every 2 months. Survival was calculated in months from the data of first treatment. Acute and late toxicities were recorded as percentages of the total number of patients.

26.3 Results

26.3.1 Tumor Response and Survival

In the low dose (5 mg/m^2/24 h) group of eight patients, two (25%) achieved a complete and three (37.5%) a partial response. Two (25%) patients had stable disease, while in one patient disease progressed during treatment. The survival time of the entire group ranged between 16 and 78 weeks. One of two patients who achieved a complete response survived more than 76 weeks. All three patients achieving partial responses have died. Two such patients survived 60 and 72 weeks, respectively. The median survival of the entire group of patients was 40 weeks.

Among patients who received the intermediate dose cisplatin infusion (at a rate of 20 mg/m^2/24 h),

Table 26.1. Patient characteristics

	Low dose group		Intermediate dose group	
No. pts.	8		12	
Age (years)	50–65		35–60	
M:F	3:1		1:1	
Stages	$T_2N_2M_0$	1	$T_2N_1M_0$	4
(TNM system)	$T_3N_1M_0$	3	$T_2N_2M_0$	3
	$T_3N_2M_0$	2	$T_3N_2M_0$	3
	$T_3N_2M_1$	2	$T_2N_1M_1$	1
			$T_4N_XM_0$	1
Pathology	Squamous Cell	7	Adenocarcinoma	6
	Giant Cell	1	Squamous Cell	3
			Large Cell	3

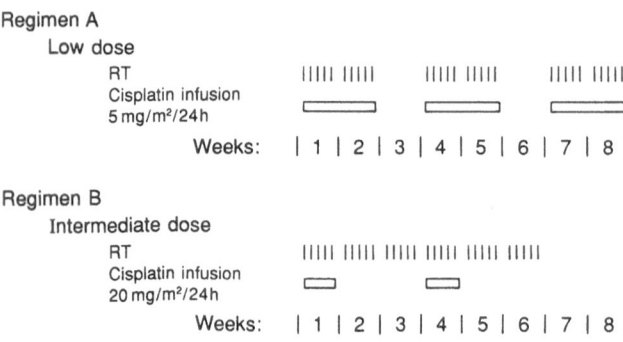

Fig. 26.1. Schematic representation of the two regimens employed in the study (radiotherapy delivered in 1.6–1.8 Gy daily fractions)

there were a greater number of responders (Tables 26.2, 26.3) than in the low dose group. Of the 12 patients, five (41.5%) achieved a complete response and five (41.5%) a partial response. Three of the five who achieved a complete response are still in complete remission with a follow-up period of 56–60 weeks. Three of the five who achieved a partial response are alive at 44–50 weeks. The mean duration of partial response was 30 weeks. Patients who progressed after achieving either partial or complete response did so in- or outside the irradiated port.

Analyzing the response rate by histological type, the results of both groups together showed that patients with adenocarcinoma and large cell carcinoma achieved a high rate of complete response (44%) as compared with patients with squamous cell carcinoma, who attained only a 30% complete response (Table 26.4). The rate of partial response in adenocarcinoma and large cell type was 33%, as compared with 40% in squamous cell carcinoma. Median survival, however, was better in squamous cell type at 48 weeks, as compared with 37 weeks for adenocarcinoma and large cell type. These figures indicate that more deaths due to metastases occurred in adenocarcinoma and large cell type tumors.

Table 26.2. Tumor response and survival in the low and intermediate dose groups

	Low dose group	Intermediate dose group
Complete response	2/8 (25%)	5/12 (41.5%)
Partial response	3/8 (37.5%)	5/12 (41.5%)
Stable disease or progression	3/8 (37.5%)	2/12 (17%)
Median survival (weeks)	40	52

Table 26.3. Survival according to complete or partial response to concomitant cisplatin infusion and radiation

	Complete response	Partial response
Low dose group (median follow-up 1.5 yrs)	2/8 pts Alive, 76 wks Dead, 16 wks	3/8 pts Dead, 72 wks Dead, 60 wks Dead, 16 wks
Intermediate dose group (median follow-up 1 yr)	5/12 Alive, 60 wks Alive, 60 wks Alive, 56 wks Dead, 26 wks Dead, 26 wks	5/12 Alive, 50 wks Alive, 44 wks Alive, 44 wks Dead, 42 wks Dead, 26 wks

Table 26.4. Response and survival according to cell type in the low and intermediate dose groups combined

	Squamous cell	Adenocarcinoma and large cell	Giant cell
Complete response	3/10 (30%)	4/9 (44%)	–
Partial response	4/10 (40%)	3/9 (33%)	1/1
Total response	7/10 (70%)	7/9 (78%)	–
Median survival (weeks)	48	37	Alive at 76 weeks

Table 26.5. Toxicity in the low and intermediate dose groups

Toxic effect	Low dose group ($n = 8$ pts)	Intermediate dose group ($n = 12$ pts)
Vomiting	0	5 (41.5%)
Mucositis	4 (50%)	3 (25%)
Esophagitis	2 (25%)	6 (50%)
Pneumonitis	2 (25%)	0
Neutropenia (<2500, $>2000\,\mu l$)	0	3 (25%)
Renal toxicity (creat. $>1.5\,mg/dl$)	0	3 (25%)

26.3.2 Toxicity

Cisplatin given by continuous infusion for 2 weeks with split courses of radiation at a dose of $5\,mg/m^2/24\,h$ was well tolerated. The most common toxicity at this dose was mild bone marrow suppression. In two of the eight (25%) patients, the total WBC count had fallen below $2000/\mu l$. At this dose level none of the patients experienced nausea or vomiting or abnormally high blood creatinine levels. However, in two (25%) patients (Table 26.5) the concomitant administration of radiation and cisplatin infusion was associated with the development of pneumonitis, and in two patients (25%) with the development of moderate esophagitis.

Intermediate dose cisplatin therapy ($20\,mg/m^2/24\,h$) given only in the 1st and the 4th weeks of radiation was also associated with limited toxicity. Bone marrow suppression and pneumonitis were not encountered but esophagitis and slight renal dysfunction were more frequently seen – grade II esophagitis in 6/12 (50%) patients, serum creatinine $> 1.5 < 2.2$ in three (25%) patients. Nausea and vomiting were also frequently reported but were easy to control and did not lead to interruptions in treatment.

26.4 Discussion

Distant metastases are the main cause of death in patients with bronchogenic carcinoma. There is, however, a small group of patients who die from locoregional disease only. Several studies (KATZ 1983; The Lung Cancer Study Group 1986) have shown that, among the NSCLCs, squamous cell carcinoma may have the greatest propensity for remaining confined to the thorax. Approximately 50% of patients with this diagnosis die from locoregional disease with infection, hemorrhage, and respiratory failure. In patients with adenocarcinoma and large cell carcinoma, death may be due to the effects of locoregional disease in only 30% and 37% of cases, respectively (PEREZ et al. 1982). It has been shown (PEREZ et al. 1986) that enhanced control of locoregional disease improves the survival rate for all patients with NSCLC. One can postulate, then, that the increase in locoregional control may lead to a decrease in mortality because of the control of intrathoracic disease and the reduced rate of distant metastases.

Several authors have shown a dose–response relationship with radiation (KATZ 1983). PEREZ et al. (1980) in the RTOG 73-01 study demonstrated the relationship between radiation dose and response: with an improved complete response rate, there was an improved survival rate. As the radiation dose in that study increased from 40 Gy given as a split course to 60 Gy given as a continuous course, the complete response rate improved from 8% to approximately 24%. This improvement in complete response translated to an overall improvement in survival, with a median 36 weeks'

survival in the patients treated with 40 Gy (split course) versus 47 weeks in patients treated with continuous 60 Gy. (Table 26.6) KATZ and ALBERTS (1983) have also shown similar dose–response relationship. The rate of sterilization of NSCLCs with 40, 50, and 60 Gy is 17%, 22%, and 30%, respectively (RTOG 73-01 study). In our study it was shown that the complete response rate is directly related to the volume of the primary lesion. In patients with T_1 disease a complete response rate of 53% was noted, as compared with 14% in patients with T_3 disease. This relationship to tumor volume has been shown in several other studies (PEREZ et al. 1980, 1982). Despite the trends noted with dose response to radiotherapy, the complete response rate and sterilization of this disease remains poor.

A number of approaches that were thought to hold out the hope of improving locoregional control have met with poor results. Hypoxic cell sensitizers such an misonidazole (SIMPSON et al. 1982) and escalating doses of radiation with hyperfractionation (SEALY et al. 1982) have been tried with no apparent benefit in controlling the disease. In addition, neutron therapy and the use of hyperbaric oxygen trials have also shown no improvement (CADE and McEWEN 1978). The use of chemotherapeutic drugs as sensitizers has therefore been strongly pursued for the treatment of advanced NSCLC.

WODINSKY et al. (1974), working on some experimental tumors, first showed and enhancement of the cytotoxic effect with the use of combined cisplatin and radiation. Later, DOUPLE and RICHMOND (1978) found that *E. coli* bacteria and V79 Chinese hamster cells, when irradiated in the presence of cisplatin, sustained increased cellular damage due to the inhibition of DNA repair. This same mechanism also enhanced the response of hypoxic cells to radiation. KYRIAZIS et al. (1983)

Table 26.6. Response and survival in patients with NSCLC according to radiation dose administered

	Complete response		Partial response		Survival (weeks)	
	RTOG 73-01 (Perez, 1980)	SIMPSON et al. 1985 73-02	RTOG 73-01 (Perez, 1980)	SIMPSON et al. 1985 73-02	RTOG 73-01 (Perez, 1980)	SIMPSON et al. 1985 73-02
30 Gy continuous		17%		24%		25.6
40 Gy split course	8%	12%	41%	27%	36.8	24.8
40 Gy continuous	21%	15%	28%	29%	45.5	27.6
50 Gy continuous	20%		33%		41.0	
60 Gy continuous	24%		32%		47.2	

have shown an enhanced radiation reaction with the use of cisplatin on human bladder carcinoma cells implanted in nude mice. Experimental data suggest that the delivery of cisplatin should preferably be given by continuous infusion in order to achieve more effective radiosensitization. It may be that a phase cycle nonspecific drug, such as cisplatin, has preferential action on the G_1 phase of the cell cycle.

REIMER et al. (1981) used cisplatin $20-50 \, mg/m^2$ weekly along with radiation in 13 patients with advanced nonbronchogenic tumors, with a response rate of approximately 91%. Fifty-four percent of these patients developed a complete response. The complication rate, however, was quite high. Twelve of the 13 patients experienced vomiting, four had enhanced radiation toxicity, and four developed hematological toxicity. SCHAAKE-KONING et al. (1983) treated 20 patients with advanced NSCLC with a split course of radiation therapy consisting of 30 Gy in ten fractions given twice with 2 weeks' rest between the courses of radiation and infusion of cisplatin. Cisplatin was given at $35 \, mg/m^2$ once weekly as an i.v. bolus during the radiation treatments. A total of 17/20 patients (85%) had responses, with 10/20 (50%) having complete responses. In this series of patients, however, vomiting was a dose-limiting toxic effect. Later, COUGHLIN et al. (1986) used both bolus and concomitant infusion cisplatin in 13 patients with advanced locoregional squamous carcinoma of the lung. Toxicity rate was improved and a 1-year survival rate of 46% was shown.

Encouraged by the radiosensitization offered by 5-FU and cisplatin in the treatment of advanced head and neck carcinomas (SHOWELL et al. 1983) and advanced esophageal and bladder carcinomas (LEICHMAN et al. 1984), we treated two groups of patients with concomitant cisplatin and radiation therapy. This was done after a phase I study was completed obtaining the MTD of cisplatin and radiation therapy for two different schedules of concomitant administration of the two therapeutic modalities. One group received $5 \, mg/m^2/24 \, h$ (low dose group) and the other received $20 \, mg/m^2/24 \, h$ (intermediate dose group) concomitantly with radiation.

In our series, the use of prolonged low dose cisplatin infusion during split-course irradiation showed a lower rate of local response and survival when compared with the use of the intermediate dose of $20 \, mg/m^2/24 \, h$ during the 1st and 4th weeks of irradiation. The total response rate with the use of prolonged continuous infusion was 62.5%, with 25% achieving a complete response and 37.5% a partial response. The range of survival in this series was 16–76 weeks, excluding two patients who had metastatic disease at the start of treatment. Of the five patients who achieved at least a partial response, three (60%) survived more than 1 year. This survival rate compares favorably with the radiation alone series (PEREZ et al. 1986). The results in the patients receiving an intermediate dose of cisplatin infusion during the 1st and 4th weeks of irradiation appeared to be superior to those of the low dose group, as well as to the radiation therapy alone series (PEREZ et al. 1986). In this group, the rate of both complete and partial responses was 41.5%, and the total response rate was 83%. In addition, 6/12 (50%) are alive from 44 to 60 weeks, as compared with only one of eight surviving at 76 weeks in the low dose group. These data suggest both a response rate and a survival advantage over the radiation alone series (PEREZ et al. 1986). However, the number of patients entered in these studies is too small to permit meaningful statistical analysis and definitive conclusions.

Analysis of the results according to cell type confirmed the findings of other authors concerning local response and survival (KYRIAZIS et al. 1983; PEREZ et al. 1986; The Lung Cancer Study Group 1986), in that squamous cell carcinoma was found to be locally less responsive than adenocarcinoma and large cell carcinoma. However, since adenocarcinoma and large cell carcinoma metastasize more often, the survival results are still better in squamous cell carcinoma patients. These findings indicate that with a further increase in the complete response rate, especially in squamous cell carcinoma, and increase in survival may be seen.

The toxicity rate in our study was quite acceptable with both intermediate and low dose infusion of cisplatin during radiation therapy. None of the patients had to interrupt treatments because of nausea, renal toxicity, or esophagitis. This is in contrast to other series, where close to 40% of patients receiving high dose cisplatin as i.v. bolus experienced such side-effects. We believe that the $20 \, mg/m^2/24 \, h$ dose as concomitant infusion therapy during the 1st and 4th weeks of radiation therapy is well tolerated. Further, the results appear to be superior as compared with the use of low dose cisplatin or weekly cisplatin by i.v. bolus or short infusion to accompany radiation (COUGHLIN et al. 1986; SCHAAKE-KONING et al. 1983) or the use of radiation alone. In view of the small number of patients entered in these nonrandomized series, no statistical significance can be attributed to our data; however, these results warrant a larger randomized trial.

References

Cade IS, McEwen JB (1978) Clinical trials of radiotherapy in hyperbaric oxygen at Portsmouth, 1964–1976. Clin Radiol 29: 333–338

Choi N, Doucette J (1981) Improved survival of patients with unresectable non small cell bronchogenic carcinoma by an innovated high-dose en-bloc radiotherapeutic approach. Cancer 48: 101–109

Coughlin CT, Delprete SA, Grace MP et al. (1986) Definitive radiation therapy of locally advanced squamous cell carcinoma of the lung. Cancer Treat Rep 70: 643–645

Cox J, Komaki R, Eisut D (1980) Irradiation for inoperable carcinoma of the lung and high performance status. JAMA 244: 1931–1933

Double EB, Richmond RC (1978) Platinum complexes as radiosensitizers of hypoxic mammalian cells. Br J Cancer 37: 98–102

Holmes CE (1988) Current status of adjuvant chemotherapy in the treatment of non small cell lung cancer. In: Devita VT, Hellman S, Rosenberg SA (eds) Important advances in oncology 1988. Lippincott, Philadelphia, pp 259–272

Katz H, Alberts R (1983) A comparison of high dose continuous and split course irradiation in non oat cell carcinoma of the lung. Am J Clinical Oncol 6: 445–457

Katz HR (1983) The effects of resection on local failure in irradiated non oat cell carcinoma of the lung. Int J Radiat Oncol Biol Phys 9: 1793–1805

Kyriazis AP, Yagoda A, Kereiaskes JG, Kiriazis AA, Whitmore W (1983) Experimental studies of the radiation modify in effects of Cis-diaminedi chloroplatinum (CDDP) in human bladder carcinoma grown in nude mice. Cancer 52: 452–457

Leichman C, Steiger Z, Seydel HG et al. (1984) Preoperative chemotherapy and radiation therapy for patients with cancer of the esophagus: a potentially curative approach. J Clin Oncol 2: 75–79

Perez CA, Stanley K, Rubin P et al. (1980) A prospective randomized study of various irradiation doses and fractionation schedules in the treatment of inoperable non oat cell carcinoma of the lung. Cancer 45: 2744–2753

Perez CA, Stanley K, Grundy G et al. (1982) Impact of irradiation technique and tumor extent in tumor control and survival of patients with unresectable non oat cell carcinoma of the lung. Cancer 50: 1091–1099

Perez CA, Bauer M, Edelstein S, Gillespie BW, Birch R (1986) Impact of tumor control on survival in carcinoma of the lung treated with irradiation. Int J Radiat Oncol Biol Phys 12: 539–547

Perez CA, Pajak TF, Rubin P et al. (1987) Long term observations of the patterns of failure in patients with unresectable non-oat cell carcinoma of the lung treated with definitive radiotherapy. Cancer 59: 1874–1881

Reimer RR, Gahbauer R, Bukowski RM et al. (1981) Simultaneous treatment with cisplatinum and radiation therapy for advanced solid tumors: A pilot study. Cancer Treat Rep 65: 219–222

Rosenthal CJ, Rotman MZ, Choi K, Sand J (1986) Cisplatin by continuous infusion with concomitant radiation in malignant tumors (a phase I-II study). In: Rosenthal JC, Rotman M (eds) Clinical applications of continuous infusion chemotherapy and concomitant radiation therapy. Plenum, New York, pp 177–180

Schaake-Koning C, Schuster O, Herhoeve L, Hart G, Gonzalez DG (1983) Prognostic factors of inoperable localized lung cancer treated by high dose radiotherapy. Int J Radiat Oncol Biol Phys 9: 1023–1028

Sealy R, Lagakos S, Bartley T, Ryall R, Tucker R, Lee R, Ehlers G (1982) Radiotherapy of regional epidermoid carcinoma of the lung: a study in fractionation. Cancer 49: 1338–1345

Shah K, Olson M, Ray P, Wright A (1981) Comparison of dose-time-fractionation schemes in non-oat cell lung cancer. Cancer 48: 1127–1132

Showell JL, Murthy AK, Hutchinson LD, Caldarelli DE, Taylor SS (1983) Synchronous radiation therapy and cisplatinum 5-FU chemotherapy in advanced head and neck cancer. Proc. 2nd Europ. Conf. Clinical Oncology (Abs) 162

Silowberg E, Lubera JA (1989) Cancer statistics, 1989. CA 39: 3–20

Simpson J, Perez C, Phillips T, Concannon J, Carella R (1982) Large fraction radiotherapy plus misonidazole for treatment of advanced lung cancer. Int J Radiat Oncol Biol Phys 8: 303–308

Simpson JR, Francis ME, Perez-Tamayo R, Marks RD, Rao DU (1985) Palliation radiotherapy for inoperable carcinoma of the lung: final report of a RTOG multiinstitutional trial. Int J Radiat Oncol Biol Phys 11: 751–758

Stanley K, Cox J, Petrovich Z, Paig C (1981) Patterns of failure in patients with inoperable carcinoma of the lung. Cancer 47: 2725–2729

The Lung Cancer Study Group (1986) Effects of postoperative mediastinal radiation on completely resected stage II and stage III epidermoid cancer of the lung. N Engl J Med 315: 1377–1381

Wodinsky I, Swiniarski J, Kensler CI, Verditi JM (1974) Combination radiotherapy and chemotherapy for P388 lymphographic leukaemia in vivo. Cancer Treat Rep 4: 73–76

Section V
Radiopotentiation by Combined Cisplatin
and Continuous Infusion 5-Fluorouracil

27 Head and Neck Cancer

SAMUEL G. TAYLOR, IV and KATHERINE GRIEM

CONTENTS

27.1 Introduction

Cisplatin has been an important addition to the treatment of head and neck cancer. It is the only drug to have been proven to cause a survival benefit when compared with supportive care alone in the palliative management of advanced head and neck cancer (MORTON et al. 1985). It has interesting radiation-sensitizing properties in some systems and it is part of the most active drug combination in head and neck cancer when combined with 5-fluorouracil infusion. In comparison with the newer analogs of carboplatin and iproplatin, cisplatin has the highest tumor cell uptake of the platinates when given parenterally (HECQUET et al. 1987).

27.2 Biology of Cisplatin as a Radiation Sensitizer

The combination of cisplatin and radiation therapy is currently being tested in several clinical

protocols designed to exploit the potential for cisplatin to act as a radiosensitizer. The biological rationale for this combination dates from 1971, when ZAK and DROBNIK first observed a change in mouse survival after whole–body irradiation with the addition of cisplatin. RICHMOND and POWERS (1976) demonstrated an increase in radiation-induced killing of bacterial spores with the addition of cisplatin, most pronounced under hypoxic conditions. Potentiation of radiation effects by cisplatin has also been demonstrated in cultured mammalian cells and human cancer nodules in vitro.

In vitro studies have found radiopotentiation with the administration of cisplatin both before and after radiation therapy. The mechanisms of each type of interaction are incompletely understood at present. Radiopotentiation by cisplatin after radiation therapy is thought to be due to inhibition of repair of radiation damage. Split-dose experiments have shown a partial or complete inhibition of sublethal damage repair by the addition of the drug (DRITSSCHILO et al. 1979). Cisplatin also inhibits potentially lethal damage repair in plateau phase cells. The enhanced cell killing when cisplatin is administered before radiation therapy is thought to be due to the activity of cisplatin as a hypoxic cell sensitizer. Some cell lines have shown radiosensitization to cisplatin only under hypoxic conditions, though other cell lines have shown the effect under well-oxygenated conditions (ALVAREZ et al. 1978).

Animal studies have also demonstrated enhanced control of transplanted tumors when cisplatin is combined with radiation therapy. DOUPLE and RICHMOND (1979) found a supra-additive effect of cisplatin and radiation therapy in murine tumors using a tumor latency assay. The decrease in cell survival with the administration of cisplatin following radiation therapy was greater than that expected from adding both agents alone.

Cross-resistance to cisplatin and radiation therapy has been observed clinically. SCWARZ and col-

SAMUEL G. TAYLOR IV, MD, Professor of Medicine, Section of Medical Oncology, KATHERINE GRIEM, MD, Assistant Professor of Therapeutic Radiology, Rush-Presbyterian-St. Luke's Medical Center, 1725 W. Harrison St., Chicago, IL 60612, USA

leagues (1988) have found radioresistance to be associated with cisplatin resistance in several early passage human tumor cell lines, suggesting an inherent cellular resistance to both agents. WALLNER and LI (1987), however, found no increased radiation resistance in cisplatin-resistant Chinese hamster fibroblasts and no altered capacity for radiation therapy damage repair in these cells.

Cisplatin is usually administered by rapid i.v. infusion. Few clinical studies have been done with prolonged i.v. infusion of cisplatin. It has been given as a 24-h infusion in head and neck cancer with reduced gastrointestinal toxicity (JACOBS et al. 1978). The popularity of this approach has waned due to lack of evidence for improved efficacy and the development of more effective antiemetics. FORESTIERE and colleagues (1988) have performed pharmacological studies on serum levels of platinum derivatives in patients receiving five daily injections or continuous infusion. They noted higher peak serum levels with injection, but a larger area under the concentration – time curve

with infusion therapy. This may have accounted for the greater toxicity with this method of administration (FORESTIERE et al. 1988). It is not clear from this experiment, however, which method of administration would result in greater tumor cell concentration. It is possible that peak serum levels (first passage) may be more important than concentration – time factors with a drug that is so strongly protein bound.

27.3 Concomitant Cisplatin and Radiation

These considerations make cisplatin a very attractive drug to combine with radiation therapy due to its individual effectiveness and radiation – sensitizing properties. Table 27.1 summarizes many such studies in head and neck cancer. Most of these have combined conventionally fractionated radiation with low dose repetitive treatments with cis-

Table 27.1. Phase II studies of concomitant cisplatin and radiation therapy in head and neck cancer

Schedule	Number of pts	Stage	Percentage CR	CR + PR	Months survival	Reference
100 mg/m² d1, 22, 43 1.8–2 Gy/d to 70 Gy	124	22 III, 102 IV	69%	NS	55% at 24 mo	AL-SARRAF et al. 1987
20 mg/m² d1–4, 22–25ᵃ 45 Gy over 5 weeks	43	14 III, 28 IV, 1 NS	49%	NS	12	CHANG et al. 1988
10–20 mg/m² d1–5ᵇ 4 Gy d1–5	38	6 III 32 IV	18%	82%	11.2	McDONALD et al. 1987
15 mg/m² d1–5, 22–26 2 Gy/d to 60–66 Gy	36	36 IV	25%	81%	CR = 15 PR = 7	SNYDERMANN et al. 1986
20 mg/m² d1–5, 22–26 1.8–2 Gy/d	34	1 III 28 IV 5R	53%	85%	CR = 13 mo NS	BLOOM et al. 1985
20 mg/m² d1–5, 28–32 2 Gy/d to 60–70 Gy	32	32 III/IV	69%	NS	76% at	HIGH et al. 1983
20 mg/m²/weekᶜ 2 Gy/ to 48 Gyᵈ	21	9 III 12 IV	52%	100%	14 months	COUGHLIN and RICHMOND 1985
10 mg/ for 6 weeks 2 Gy/d to 60 Gy	19	1 II 18 III/IV	47%	84%	NS	TOBIAS et al. 1987
20 mg/m² d1–4, 22–25 1.8 Gy/d to 45 Gyᵈ	18	12 III 6 IV	72%	89%	NS	SLOTMAN et al. 1986
40 mg/m² d1–5, 29–33, 57–61 1.8 Gy/d to 60 Gy	17	5 III, 12 IV	100%	–	71% at 9 mo	WHEELER et al. 1988
20 mg/m²/week 1.8 Gy/d to 60 Gy	16	3 III 13 IV	75%	100%	NS	ZERILLO et al. 1986

Abbreviations: CR, complete response; PR, partial response; NS, not stated
ᵃ Followed by surgery or further cisplatin/radiation therapy and by cisplatin/5-FU as adjuvant
ᵇ Responders continued cisplatin 10 mg/m² and 3.2 Gy three times weekly to 38.4 Gy
ᶜ All patients received cisplatin 100 mg/m² dl and 21 prior to cisplatin/radiation therapy
ᵈ Followed by surgery

platin. A 4- to 5-day schedule of cisplatin 15–20 mg/m^2/day repeated every 3–4 weeks has been most frequently used. This schedule and the next most common one of 20 mg/m^2 weekly have not produced substantial improvement in the expected survival from radiation or surgery and radiation alone. These studies usually consist of unresectable stage III/IV patients and have median survivals of approximately 12 months. In support of limited benefit from this approach are the results of the randomized Intergroup trial of weekly cisplatin (20 mg/m^2) during radiation. This trial showed a small increase in the total response rate, but no survival benefit (HASELOW 1988).

These studies do establish that cisplatin can be combined with radiation without undue toxicity. Early studies had discouraged further use of concomitant cisplatin and radiation because of poor tolerance and prolonged cachexia following radiation (CREAGAN et al. 1981). With the use of high dose antiemetics this complication has not been a problem in subsequent studies. No increase in mucositic or normal tissue reactions has been observed to date.

Use of higher intermittent dosage of cisplatin may be more effective during radiation. The Radiation Therapy Oncology Group's phase II trial of 100 mg/m^2 every 3 weeks was thought to show benefit over historical data in the complete response rate and survival (AL-SARRAF et al. 1987). One–year survival was 66% and median survival was just past 2 years. This was a large, multi-institutional study with 82% of patients stage IV, but it compared favorably with smaller single institution studies using fractionated doses of 15–20 mg/m^2. The highest complete response rates were in patients with nasopharyngeal or poorly differentiated lesions.

WHEELER et al. (1988) have piloted a small group of patients receiving high dose cisplatin (40 mg/m^2 days 1–5 for three cycles) during radiation therapy. They reported complete responses in all patients treated, again suggesting dose may be important for cisplatin synergy with radiation. Unfortunately, this study was reported with limited follow-up available.

Another schedule in a limited number of patients is one giving cisplatin daily with radiation. TOBIAS et al. (1987) have reported preliminary results using a fixed dose of 10 mg/day in 19 patients. This dose would be in excess of 25 mg/m^2 weekly for most patients. The authors noted that all 16 patients completing treatment responded, but

renal toxicity was high. Response duration and survival were not stated.

One needs to conclude from the above that, although an interaction between radiation and cisplatin has been recognized for almost two decades and cisplatin is one of the most active drugs in head and neck cancer treatment, the value of concomitant cisplatin and radiation remains undefined. While preliminary results of one randomized trial, not yet reported in the peer-review literature, were disappointing (HASELOW 1988), the optimal schedule of cisplatin may not have been used. In many fewer years than cisplatin has been available, five randomized studies have been completed with the (inactive) radiation sensitizer, misonidazole, in over 700 patients. It seems far more rational to spend clinical research energies and dollars on exploring the combination of radiation therapy with currently available radiation sensitizers, such as cisplatin and/or other chemotherapeutic agents, that also have independent antineoplastic activity.

27.4 Concomitant Cisplatin, 5-Fluorouracil, and Radiation

In 1981, after AL-SARRAF had described early results with cisplatin and 5-fluorouracil infusion, achieving twice the complete response rate of any previously reported regimen (AL-SARRAF et al. 1980), we began evaluating this combination with radiation therapy. BYFIELD et al. (1980) had published the rationale for an alternating weekly schedule of radiation integrated with 5-fluorouracil infusion in other cancers which allowed for repeated doses of chemotherapy and radiation. We discovered very early that continuous daily fractionation of radiation during the "off-week" of chemotherapy resulted in prohibitive mucositis, preventing further chemotherapy and mandating prolonged interruption in radiation. With an alternating weekly schedule, we used a modification of dose of the AL-SARRAF regimen, giving cisplatin 60 mg/m^2 day 1 and 5-fluorouracil 800 mg/m^2 continuous infusion days 1–5 every other week. This allowed a dose equivalent of 90 mg/m^2 for cisplatin and 6.0 g/m^2 for 5-FU administered every 3 weeks, quite comparable to the AL-SARRAF regimen.

In our initial experience with this regimen, we were very impressed with the durability of responses and excellent regional control (TAYLOR et al. 1985). Our subsequent experience has supported this observation. We have recently analyzed results in the first 53 patients treated with this regimen who had not had prior radiation therapy or M_1 disease (TAYLOR et al., 1989a). Follow-up ranged from 12 to 83 months (median 41 months). This population included patients with stage III (8, 15%), stage IV (36, 68%), and recurrent disease (9, 17%). Thirty-two percent had N_3 disease and 51% T_4 primaries. Based on the data from numerous pilot studies with cisplatin and radiation, this patient distribution would be expected to have a survival of approximately 12 months.

The complete response rate of 55% for this series was unremarkable. The remaining patients, however, with the exception of one who had a severe cerebral vascular accident during the second cycle and was never reassessed, had partial responses consisting usually of more than 75% reduction in tumor bulk. Five of nine patients with clinically assessed partial responses who underwent surgery or biopsy had no microscopic evidence of cancer. Four of six complete responders who underwent surgery or biopsy were histologically negative. This experience indicated to us the unreliability of clinical assessment of response with this program of combined chemotherapy and radiation.

The subsequent long-term follow-up of all patients reinforced the unreliability of clinical assessment of response. Whereas with induction cisplatin and 5-fluorouracil the median survival was 37 months for complete responders and only 8 months for partial responders to the chemotherapy, giving a highly significant difference (JACOBS JR et al. 1987), with concomitant treatment the survival of all patients was 37 months, with 52 months for complete responders and 30 months for partial responders. This difference was not significant and the trend could be explained by the more advanced patient population in the partial response group. These patients had bulky nodes, bone erosion, and sinus opacification that tended not to normalize within 6 weeks of ending treatment at the time of response assessment.

The durability of response was reflected in the pattern of failure. Only 27% of patients had a regional failure. None of eight stage III patients failed. Of 23 stage IV patients without N_3 disease, seven (30%) failed at any site. Median survival of each group had not been reached out to 5 years or beyond.

27.4.1 Toxicity of Treatment

The most severe toxicities were weight loss, mucositis, and leukopenia. Average weight loss was 10% (range + 3% to −21%). Grade 3 or worse mucositis occurred in 52%. Leukopenia less than $2000/mm^3$ occurred in 29%, but in only two patients was hematological toxicity considered life threatening (leukocytes less than $1000/mm^3$ or platelets less than $20000/mm^3$). No routine nutritional intervention to bypass oral feeding was done, but five patients (9%) required forced feeding supplementation.

Nine patients (17%) had major treatment interruptions. Four patients died during treatment of apparently nontoxic deaths, although two were probably cardiac in origin. A cerebral vascular accident and traumatic vertebral fracture in an elderly patient, and two patients refusing further therapy led to four other early terminations. The one final patient had chemotherapy stopped due to acute renal failure from cisplatin; however, radiation only was continued.

Toxicity of concomitant chemotherapy and radiation is of major concern. Indeed, concern over toxicity is the major reason for the reluctance of many investigators to use concomitant treatment. To address this concern, TAYLOR et al. have compared toxicity from (a) their concomitant treatment with cisplatin, 5-fluorouracil infusion, and radiation and (b) induction treatment with the same drugs followed by radiation in a randomized study (TAYLOR et al., 1989b). Mucositis and leukopenia were the main dose-limiting toxicities. Severe mucositis was similar between the two regimens (44% for sequential and 40% for concomitant treatment). Weight loss during treatment measured a combination of mucositis coupled with nausea, vomiting, anorexia, and loss of taste. Mean weight loss from concomitant treatment was 11% and from sequential therapy, 7%. While not significant, this did indicate a trend towards more severe nutritional depletion during concomitant therapy. However, the concomitant treatment used a lower dose of chemotherapy per cycle and this appeared to result in fewer untoward events, including cerebral vascular accident, sudden death, myocardial infarction, and gastrointestinal problems (12% vs 34%, difference not significant). While toxicities of both regimens are challenging in this difficult patient population, we have not found evidence for a substantial worsening of toxicity with concomitant treatment.

Table 27.2. Phase II studies of concomitant cisplatin, 5-fluorouracil, and radiation in head and neck cancer

Dose and schedule	Number of		Disease stage	Percentage		Months survival	Reference
	Cycles	Pts		CR	CR + PR		
DDP 75 mg/m² dl, 43 5-FU 1 g/m² d1–4, 43–46 CI RT 2 Gy d1–5 × 3 weeks	2	54	6 I/II, 21 III 25 IV, 2R	94%	100	64% at 21 months	ADELSTEIN et al. 1988
DDP 60 mg/m² dl 5-FU 800 mg/m² d1–5, CI RT 2 Gy d1–5	7	53	8 III, 36 IV, 9R	55%	98%	37	TAYLOR, to be published, a
DDP 15 mg/m² dl, 2, 5–7 5-FU 350 mg/m² d1–7 RT 4 Gy d3, 4	3¹	40	10 III, 17 IV 3M1	51%	78%	20% at 36 months	DIONET et al. 1988
DDP 20 mg/m² dl, 2, 5, 6 5-FU 400 mg/m² for 2 h, d1–6 RT 3 Gy d3, 4	3¹	36	36 IV	31%	61%	38% at 12 months	BOLLA et al. 1988
DDP 20 mg/m² d1–5 5-FU 200 mg/m² d1–5 RT 2 Gy d8–12, 15–19	3	34	17 IV 17R	41%	76%	10.8	MERLANO et al. 1988b
DDP 60 mg/m² dl, CIᵇ 5-FU 350 mg/m² d2–5, CIᵇ RT 1.8 Gy b.i.d. d2–10	3	34	6 III 28 IV	82%	94%	58% at 24 months	WENDT et al. 1987

Abbreviations: DDP, cisplatin; 5-FU, 5-fluorouracil; CI, continuous infusion; RT, radiation therapy; CR, complete response; PR, partial response
ᵃ Followed by conventional radiation to full dosage
ᵇ With leucovorin 100 mg/m₂ d2–5, CI

27.4.2 Comparative Results

Table 27.2 summarizes our results and those of several other investigators using various schedules of cisplatin, 5-fluorouracil, and radiation. The follow-up on most of these studies is limited, however. Two groups have used cisplatin and 5-fluorouracil infusion with radiation that was continued for an additional 1–2 weeks after the 1st week of concomitant treatment (ADELSTEIN et al. 1988; WENDT et al. 1987). Both of these programs used prolonged breaks between chemotherapy cycles, with that by Wendt et al. substantially reducing the dose of 5-fluorouracil and adding leucovorin. Both programs had high response rates and excellent survival results. All three regimens using some form of split-course fractionation and concomitant cisplatin/5-fluorouracil chemotherapy had median survivals in excess of 2 years, although the study by ADELSTEIN et al. included some relatively early stage patients.

This latter program noted a high complete response rate after just one course (30 Gy) of treatment. Patients in this study had an option of undergoing surgery between chemotherapy and radiation cycles. Twenty-four patients actually underwent surgery, with the investigators withholding surgery in several patients, as they gained confidence in the concomitant treatment regimen. This study emphasizes the potential of concomitant cisplatin, 5-fluorouracil, and radiation to avoid surgery in consideration of the excellent regional control achieved without it.

Others have studied induction chemotherapy as a means of avoiding surgery in good risk patients defined as complete resonders to chemotherapy (JACOBS C et al. 1987). Approximately 40% of advanced disease patients were able to avoid surgery with this approach. The VA Study Group has compared surgery plus radiation with induction cisplatin and 5-fluorouracil followed by radiation as a means of avoiding laryngectomy (HONG WK et la. 1989). They found, in their randomized study, that induction chemotherapy enabled avoidance of surgery in 61% of patients. The survival of this group of patients was equivalent to that of patients treated with surgery and radiation therapy, although follow-up is still limited (HONG WK et al. 1989). While these results with induction chemotherapy are promising, concomitant chemotherapy and radiation may enable a higher percentage of patients to achieve regional control without surgery.

TAYLOR et al. (1989a) have examined their series of patients to cvaluate the effect of concomitant chemotherapy and radiation on the preservation of speech and swallowing function. As all patients were deemed inoperable, this analysis is hypothetical. Twenty-eight patients with T_3 or T_4 tongue, hypopharyngeal, or laryngeal lesions would have required more than a hemiglossectomy or a laryngectomy for surgical management (12 tongue, 10 hypopharynx, and 6 laryngeal lesions). Two of these patients had surgery on the primary immediately following treatment, one with and one with no residual malignancy histologically. A third patient required a delayed laryngectomy due to repeated aspirations from an incompetent larynx due to prior tumor destruction, but with no residual tumor found. A fourth patient had a salvage laryngectomy 18 months later for recurrence. Six other patients failed regionally. Thus, 64% retained tongue and laryngeal function with regional control. Median survival, based on Kaplan-Meier estimate, was 45 months for all 28 patients. These results compare favorably with those of the VA Study Group and indicate concomitant chemotherapy and radiation may also be a substitute for surgery in selected situations.

Two European studies have used cycles of cisplatin/5-fluorouracil chemotherapy with high dose fractions of radiation in the middle of each cycle (DIONET et al. 1988; BOLLA et al. 1988). Each treated very advanced cancers which even included patients with distant metastases. Comparison of results is consequently hazardous, but the response rates, durability of response, and survival did not appear to be cleary different over that expected from radiation alone. Use of high dose radiation fractions along with a more concentrated drug delivery schedule, given concomitantly, may be more promising.

Another schedule integrating chemotherapy with radiation has been the use of an alternating schedule of chemotherapy and radiation. MERLANO and colleagues used the chemotherapy combination of bleomycin, methotrexate, and vincristine with success. They found this alternating schedule, with split-course radiation, to be more effective than induction chemotherapy followed by radiation given by conventional fractionation (MERLANO et al. 1988a). The same investigators have used a similar sequence of cisplatin/5-fluorouracil injection for 1 week followed by 2 weeks of radiation in an alternating schedule (MERLANO et al. 1988b). This combination was piloted in a very advanced group of patients, making conclusions indefinite concerning survival results.

27.5 Conclusions

While none of the above pilot studies offer definitive results, they do seem to support the basic biological principles originally observed by BAGSHAW (1961) and BYFIELD et al. (1982) that maximal benefit from 5-fluorouracil and radiation depends on a high concentration of 5-fluorouracil and exposure over 24 h after each radiation treatment. In addition, they support the suggestion, based on studies with cisplatin and radiation, that high intermittent dosage of cisplatin may be the optimal way to integrate cisplatin into concomitant therapy. This is by no means established, however, and further work with prolonged infusion of cisplatin would be of interest. Our results and those by ADELSTEIN et al. (1988) suggest durable response rates and a survival advantage not previously described with other regimens or with induction chemotherapy. They appear to allow the substitution of chemotherapy for surgery in situations where surgery would produce significant morbidity.

These principles have yet to be tested in definitive randomized studies, but the above pilot studies at least offer promising directions which such future studies might explore.

References

Adelstein D, Sharan V, Earle A et al. (1988) Simultaneous radiotherapy and chemotherapy with 5-fluorouracil and cisplatin for locally confined squamous cell head and neck cancer. NCI Monogr 6: 347–351

Al-Sarraf M, Weaver A, Peppard S et al. (1980) High dose cis-platinum and 5-fluorouracil infusion as part of a multidisciplinary therapeutic approach for advanced previously untreated epidermoid cancers of the head and neck. In: Abstracts, International Head and Neck Oncology Research Conference, vol II. Natl Cancer Inst, Rosslyn, VA, p 15

Al-Sarraf M, Pajak TF, Marcial VA et al. (1987) Concurrent radiotherapy and chemotherapy with cisplatin in inoperable squamous cell carcinoma of the head and neck. Cancer 59: 259–265

Alvarez MV, Cobreeros G, Heras A et al. (1978) Studies on cis-dichlorodiammineplatinum (II) as a radiosensitizer. Br J Cancer 37: 68–72

Bagshaw MA (1961) Possible role of potentiators in radiation therapy. AJR 85: 822–833

Bloom EJ, Green MD, Cooper JS et al. (1985) Concomitant use of cis-platinum (CDDP) chemotherapy and radiation therapy (RT) in the treatment of advanced head and neck cancer. In: Foti M, Mennite MA, Pusztay HM (eds) Proc Am Soc Clin Oncol. Waverly, Baltimore, p 137

Bolla M, Borgel J, Guenoun A et al. (1988) Chemotherapy with low doses of radiation followed by definitive radiotherapy for advanced unresectable carcinoma of the head and neck. NCI Monogr 6: 357–359

Byfield JE, Barone RM, Mendelsohn J (1980) Infusional 5-fluouracil and x-ray therapy for non-resectable esophageal cancer. Cancer 45: 703–708

Byfield JE, Calabro-Jones PM, Klisak I et al. (1982) Pharmacologic requirements for obtaining sensitization of human tumor cells in vitro to combined 5-fluorouracil or ftorafur and x-rays. Int J Radiat Oncol Biol Phys 8: 1923–1933

Chang H, Leone LA, Tefft M, Nigri PT (1988) Advanced head and neck cancer: response to and toxicity of multimodality therapy. Radiology 168: 863–867

Coughlin CT, Richmond RC (1985) Platinum based combined modality approach for locally advanced head neck carcinoma. Int J Radiat Oncol Biol Phys 22: 915

Creagan ET, Fountan KS, Frytak S et al. (1981) Concomitant radiation therapy and cis-diamminedichloroplatinum (II) in patients with advanced head and neck cancer. Med Pediatr Oncol 9: 119–120

Dionet C, Rozan R, Achard JL et al. (1988) Sequential combination of 5-fluorouracil, cis-platinum and irradiation: advanced head and neck cancers. Radiat Oncol 11: 123–131

Douple EB, Richmond RC (1979) Radiosensitization of hypoxic tumour cells by cis- and trans-dichlorodiammineplatinum (II). Int J Radiat Oncol Biol Phys 5: 1369–1372

Dritsschilo A, Piro AJ, Kelman AD (1979) The effect of cis-platinum on the repair of radiation damage in plateau phase Chinese hamster (V-79) cells. Int J Radiat Oncol Biol Phys 5: 1345–1349

Forestiere AA, Belliveau JF, Goren MP et al. (1988) Pharmacokinetic and toxicity evaluation of five-day continuous infusion versus intermittent bolus cis-diamminedichloroplatinum (II) in head and neck cancer patients. Cancer Res 48: 3869–3874

Haselow RE, (1988) Presentation on integrated chemotherapy-radiation therapy to the Second Int Conf Head and Neck Cancer. DR Goffinet, moderator. Boston, MA

Hecquet B, Caty A, Fournier C et al. (1987) Comparison of platinum concentrations in human head and neck tumors following administration of carboplatin, iproplatin, or cisplatin. Bull Cancer 74: 433–436

High M, Heuser L, Schmidt CH et al. (1983) Simultane cisplatin- und bestrahlungstherapie lokal fortgeschrittener plattenepithelkarzinome der Kopf-Hals-Region. Dtsch Med Wochenschr 46: 1743

Hong WK, Wolf GT, Fisher S et al. (1989) Laryngeal preservation with induction chemotherapy and radiotherapy in the treatment for advanced laryngeal cancer: fnterim survival data of vacsp 268, VA laryngeal cancer study group. Am: Soc Clin Oncol 8: 167

Jacobs C, Bertino JR, Goffinet DR et al. (1978) Twenty-four-hour infusion of cis-platinum in head and neck cancer. Cancer 42: 2135–2140

Jacobs C, Goffinet DR, Goffinet L et al. (1987) Chemotherapy as a substitute for surgery in the treatment of advanced head and neck cancer. Cancer 60:1178–1183

Jacobs JR, Weaver A, Ahmed K et al. (1987) Protochemotherapy in advanced head and neck cancer. Head Neck Surg 10: 93–98

McDonald S, Mills EED, van der Merwe AM et al. (1987) Simultaneous radiation therapy and cisplatin chemotherapy in advanced cancer of the head and neck. Am J Clin Oncol (CCT) 10: 410–416

Merlano M, Rosso R, Sertoli MR et al. (1988a) Sequential versus alternating chemotherapy and radiotherapy in stage III-IV squamous cell carcinoma of the head and neck: a phase III study. J Clin Oncol 6: 627–632

Merlano M, Grimaldi A, Benasso M et al. (1988b) Alternating cisplatin–5-fluorouracil plus radiation in head and neck cancer. NCI Monogr 6: 343–345

Morton RP, Rugman F, Dorman EB et al. (1985) Cisplatinum and bleomycin for advanced or recurrent squamous cell carcinoma of the head and neck: a randomised factorial phase III controlled trial. Cancer Chemother Pharmacol 15: 283–289

Richmond RC, Powers EL (1976) Radiation sensitization of bacterial spores by cis-dichlorodiammineplatinum (II). Radiat Res 68: 20–23

Schwarz JL, Rotmensch J, Beckett MA et al. (1988) x-ray and cis-diamminedichloroplatinum (II) cross-resistance in human tumor cell clones. Cancer Res 48: 5133–5135

Slotman GJ, Cummings FJ, Glicksman AR et al. (1986) Preoperative simultaneously administered cis-platinum plus radiation therapy for advanced squamous cell carcinoma of carcinoma of the head and neck. Head Neck Surg 8: 159–164

Snydermann NL, Wetmore SJ, Suen JY (1986) Cisplatin sensitization to radiotherapy in stage IV squamous cell carcinoma of the head and neck. Arch Otolaryngol Head Neck Surg 112: 1147–1150

Taylor SG IV, Murthy AK, Showel JL et al. (1985) Improved control in advanced head and neck cancer with simultaneous radiation and cisplatin/5-FU chemotherapy. Cancer Treat Rep 69: 938–939

Taylor SG IV, Murthy AK, Caldarelli DD et al. (1989) Combined, simultaneous cisplatin/5-FU infusion chemotherapy and split course radiation in head and neck cancer. J Clin Oncol, 7: 846–856

Taylor SG IV, Murthy AK, Showel JL et al. Comparison of toxicity in a randomized trial of sequential vs. simultaneous cisplatin/5-FU infusion and radiation therapy in head and neck cancer. Proc Am Soc Clin Oncol, 8: 175, 1989

Tobias JS, Smith BJ, Blackman G, Finn G (1987) Concurrent daily cisplatin and radiotherapy in locally advanced squamous carcinoma of the head-and-neck and bronchus. Radiother Oncol 9: 263–268

Wallner KE, Li GC (1987) Effect of cisplatin resistance on cellular radiation response. Int J Radiat Oncol Biol Phys 13: 587–591

Wendt TG, Wustrow TPU, Hartenstein RC et al. (1987) Accelerated split-course radiotherapy and simultaneous cis-dichlorodiammine-platinum and 5-fluorouracil chemotherapy with folinic acid enhancement for unresectable carcinoma of the head and neck. Radiother Oncol 10: 277–284

Wheeler R, Salter M, Stephens S et al. (1988) Simultaneous therapy with high-dose cisplatin and radiation for unresectable squamous cell cancer of the head and neck: a phase I-II study. NCI Monogr 6: 339–341

Zak M, Drobnik J (1971) Effects of cis-dichlorodiammineplatinum (II) on the post-irradiation lethality in mice after irradiation with x-rays. Strahlentherapie 142: 112–115

Zerillo G, Cupido G, Ardizzone S et al. (1986) Funzione radio-sensibilizzante del cis-platino nei carcinomi avanzati della largine. Protocollo combinato chemioradioterapico. Oto-Rino-Laringolia 36: 11–14

28 Combined Cisplatin and Concomitant Continuous Infusion 5-Fluorouracil and Accelerated Radiation in Advanced Head and Neck Cancer

Jadranka Dragovic

CONTENTS

28.1 Introduction

Advanced, unresectable stage III and IV squamous cell carcinoma of the head and neck has a 2-year mortality of over 70% when standard treatment with conventional radiation therapy is employed (Million et al. 1984; Marcial et al. 1985). The control of locoregional disease remains a major therapeutic challenge since morbidity and mortality relate primarily to local invasion and lymph node metastases. Among the various new approaches that are being explored in an effort to improve the therapeutic ratio, combinations with adjunctive chemotherapy have attracted major interest.

28.2 Background

While sequential combinations employing neoadjuvant chemotherapy have been associated with high rates of response, most randomized controlled clinical trials have shown no survival benefit (Tannock and Browman 1986). Administration of chemotherapy concurrently with radiation has in-

dicated significant improvement in response and survival (Lo et al. 1976, Clifford et al. 1982), but also prohibitive toxicity (Fu et al. 1979). The work of Byfield (Byfield et al. 1982) and excellent results with infusional 5-fluorouracil (5-FU)/ mitomycin C in anal carcinoma (Nigro et al. 1981) have set the scene for renewed interest in infusional chemotherapy in head and neck cancer. In an uncontrolled study of simultaneous radiation therapy and cisplatin/5-FU chemotherapy (Taylor et al. 1985), improved tumor control was associated with increased toxicity. In order to reduce the acute toxicity, 1-week breaks between treatment cycles were introduced (Murthy et al. 1987). A potential disadvantage of such a regimen is the increased probability of tumor cell repopulation during the protracted course of radiation therapy, which might not be countered by the synergistic effect. To address this particular problem, our group set out to explore an alternative way of administration of radiation therapy, which would eliminate the treatment protraction but at the same time retain the breaks necessary for normal tissue recovery. It was apparent that some form of multiple daily fractionation with treatment acceleration would best fit the requirement.

In an accelerated fractionation regimen, radiation therapy is given two or more times a day and the overall treatment time is significantly reduced (Withers 1985). A decrease in overall treatment time reduces the opportunity for tumor cells to repopulate during the treatment course and therefore increases the probability of tumor control for a given dose level compared with conventional fractionation. Overall treatment time, on the other hand, has very little influence on the probability of late normal tissue injury provided the size of the dose per fraction is not increased above conventional and the time interval between fractions is sufficiently long (i.e., >4 h) to allow repair of sublethal damage in normal tissue.

Large total daily doses with reduced interfraction time and marked shortening of overall treat-

Jadranka Dragovic MD, FRCP (C), Henry Ford Hospital, Dept. of Radiation Oncology, 2799 West Grand Boulevard, Detroit, MI 48202-2689, USA

ment time have been shown to result in marked depletion of both acute and late responding tissues (PARECCHIA and SALTI 1981, NGUYEN et al. 1988). In an attempt to decrease the acute toxicity and yet preserve the shortening of overall treatment time, accelerated fractionation regimens have been modified by introducing breaks during the treatment course (WANG 1988; VIKRAM 1987). The breaks are not considered to be detrimental (even though some tumor cell repopulation may occur) as long as the overall duration of the treatment course is reduced in comparison to the conventional radiotherapy to the same dose level.

28.3 Concomitant Chemotherapy and Accelerated Fractionation Radiotherapy in Advanced, Unresectable Head and Neck Cancer

The potential advantages of a combination of interrupted accelerated multiple fraction-per-day radiotherapy with simultaneous infusional chemotherapy are threefold: (a) radiosensitizing properties of 5-FU and cisplatin can lead to increased effect on tumor through synergism; (b) acceleration of radiotherapy can lead to increased effect on tumor through decreased tumor cell repopulation; and (c) the rest intervals between treatment cycles can allow for normal tissue to recover, leading to decreased acute mucosal toxicity.

28.3.1 Methods and Materials

With the above-described background we have designed a treatment program consisting of accelerated, interrupted, twice-a-day radiation therapy concomitant with 5-FU and cisplatin (treatment schema shown in Fig. 28.1). It consists of three 5-day treatment cycles repeated every 14 days. Each cycle consists of cisplatin 60 mg/m² given on day 1, and 5-FU 800 mg/m² per day given as a continuous infusion concurrently with twice-a-day radiation therapy at 2 Gy per fraction, on days 1 through 5. The two daily fractions are given at least 5 h apart. The total radiation dose is 60–70 Gy in 5–5½ weeks (33–38 elapsed days). This is a reduction of 1–2 weeks in comparison to a conventionally fractionated regimen to the same total dose level. When 70 Gy is delivered, the last 10 Gy in five

fractions over 2½ days is given to a reduced field, following the third treatment cycle without a break (other than the weekend), and without concomitant chemotherapy. The spinal cord is shielded after 40 Gy and a shrinking field technique is employed. The volumes and techniques are similar to conventional treatment regimens and electrons are used for posterior neck irradiation.

Prior to study entry, patients undergo a thorough pretreatment evaluation and are considered eligible if they have biopsy documented stage III or IV unresectable squamous cell carcinoma of the oral cavity, oropharynx, nasopharynx, paranasal sinuses, larynx, or hypopharynx, with adequate bone marrow, renal, and hepatic function, age of 75 years or less, and ECOG performance status of 0–3. The characteristics of the first fifteen patients treated on this protocol are presented in Table 28.1.

28.3.2 Preliminary Results

The objectives of this ongoing study are to determine tumor response, acute and late treatment related morbidity, and survival and locoregional control at 2 years. The follow-up duration to date is very brief, ranging from 2 months to 27 months, allowing for evaluation of acute treatment morbidity and tumor response, but not of survival or late tissue effects.

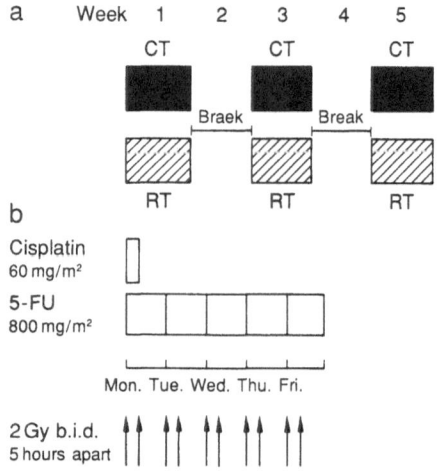

Fig. 28.1 a, b. Concomitant cisplatin/5 FU infusion and accelerated twice-a-day radiotherapy treatment schema. a Concomitant chemoradiotherapy is administered in three cycles separated by 1-week breaks. b Chemotherapy and radiotherapy scheduling in each cycle (days 1–5, 15–19, and 29–33)

Table 28.1. Patient characteristics

Patient	Age (years)	Sex	Tumor site	Stage (TNM)	Outcome
1	36	M	Maxillary sinus	$T_4N_0M_0$	NED[a] @ 27 months
2	60	M	Oropharynx	$T_4N_0M_0$	Expired during treatment (MI[b])
3	45	M	Hypopharynx	$T_2N_{2a}M_0$	NED @ 18 months
4	70	F	Maxillary sinus	$T_4N_0M_0$	Expired @ 8 months (primary recurrence)
5	74	M	Pharynx	$T_4N_0M_0$	Alive, with disease, @ 14 months (primary recurrence and lung metastases)
6	38	M	Oral tongue	$T_XN_2M_0$	NED @ 12 months
7	38	M	Hypopharynx	$T_4N_3M_0$	Expired @ 9 months (free of disease, hemorrhage)
8	37	M	Nasopharynx	$T_4N_3M_0$	Alive, with disease, @ 15 months (liver metastases, primary under control)
9	35	M	Nasopharynx	$T_2N_1M_0$	NED @ 12 months
10	75	F	Maxillary sinus	$T_4N_0M_0$	Expired @ 2 months (massive GI[c] bleed)
11	58	M	Nasopharynx	$T_2N_3M_0$	NED @ 4 months
12	49	F	Oral tongue	$T_4N_3M_0$	NED @ 6 months
13	69	F	Oral tongue	$T_XN_3M_0$	Expired @ 1 month (renal failure)
14	63	F	Nasopharynx	$T_4N_0M_0$	Alive, with PR[d] @ 3 months
15	50	F	Pharynx	$T_4N_0M_0$	NED @ 3 months

[a] no evidence of disease, [b] myocardial infarction, [c] gastrointestinal, [d] partial response

28.3.2.1 Toxicity

Toxicity is summarized in Table 28.2. The majority of patients developed transient grade 3 leukopenia and grade 3 mucositis with dysphagia, most commonly during the second and third treatment cycle. However, no treatment interruptions occurred and only one patient required omission of one chemotherapy cycle due to development of acute non A non B hepatitis with increased hematopoietic toxicity (presumably on the basis of poor clearance of 5 FU received). This was the only patient with grade 4 leukopenia (patient #8). To circumvent nutritional problems secondary to mucositis, most patients had gastrostomy tube placement during the course of therapy.

28.3.2.2 Response and Outcome

One patient was not evaluable for response due to death from myocardial infarction while on treatment (patient #2). Of the remaining fourteen patients, twelve had achieved an unequivocal complete response, one had a partial response of a massive nasopharyngeal tumor with multiple cranial nerve involvement (patient #14) and one

had a residual 1 cm jugulodigastric node which on neck dissection showed only microscopic foci of residual carcinoma (patient #3). An example of the kind of impressive tumor response seen with this treatment combination is depicted in Fig. 28.2 (patient #1).

Outcome is shown in Table 28.2. Seven patients are alive and free of disease with follow-up ranging from 3 months to 27 months; three are alive with persistent, recurrent or metastatic disease and five have expired. Only one death could be directly

Table 28.2. Cisplatin/5-FU + AIBIDRT[a] Toxicity

	Grade				
	0	1	2	3	4
Anemia[b]	3	5	3	4	
Leukopenia[b]	2	1	3	8	1
Thrombocytopenia[b]	11	2	2		
Nausea and vomiting[b]	2	9	3		
Diarrhea[b]	14	1			
Mucositis[c]	1		3	11	
Dysphagia[c]	1		4	10	
Skin reaction[c]	1		8	6	

[a] accelerated interrupted twice-a-day radiation therapy
[b] ECOG toxicity scoring criteria
[c] RTOG acute radiation morbidity scoring criteria

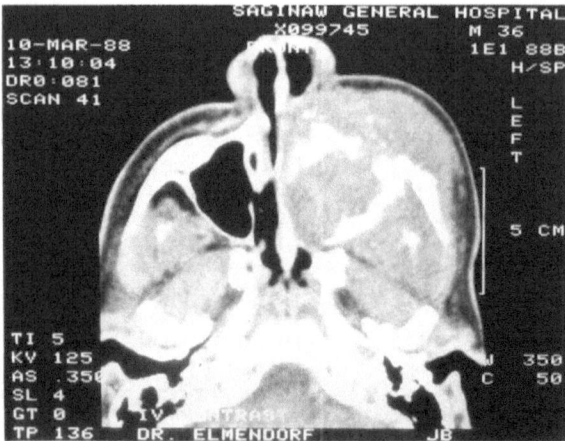

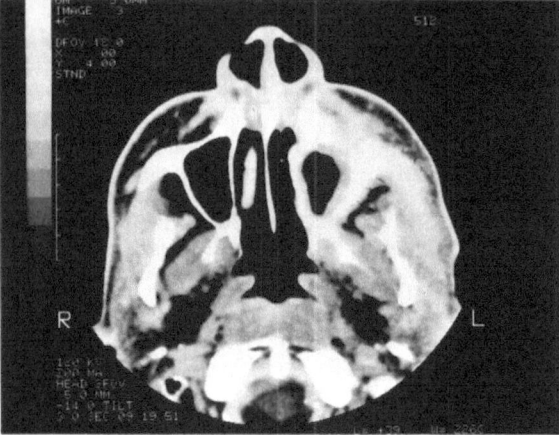

Fig. 28.2. a Pretreatment CT scan of a 36-year-old man with a $T_4N_0M_0$ maxillary sinus carcinoma demonstrating extensive mass with destruction of maxilla and invasion of soft tissues of the cheek. **b** Posttreatment CT scan demonstrating complete resolution of the mass. The residual mild mucosal thickening was biopsied and showed no residual carcinoma

related to treatment (patient #13) and only one patient had evidence of tumor recurrence at the time of demise (patient #4).

28.4 Conclusion

The tolerance to this treatment regimen and the dramatic tumor responses are impressive and encouraging. It remains to be seen if the loco-regional control and survival will be improved without an increase in the late tissue effects, as we continue to accrue and study patients on this protocol.

References

Byfield JE, Calabro-Jones P, Klisak I, Kulhanian F (1982) Pharmacologic requirements for obtaining sensitization of human tumor cells in vitro to combined 5-fluorouracil or ftorafur and x-rays. Int J Radiat Oncol Biol Phys 8: 1923–1933

O'Connor D, Clifford P, Dally VM, Durden-Smith DJ, Edwards WG, Hollis BA (1979) Advanced head and neck cancer treated by combined radiotherapy and VBM cytotoxic regimen-four year results. Clin Otol 4: 329–337

Fu KK, Silverberg IJ, Phillips TL, Friedman MA (1979) Combined radiotherapy and multidrug chemotherapy for advanced head and neck cancer: results of a Radiation Therapy Oncology Group pilot study. Cancer Treat Rep 63: 351–357

Lo TCM, Wiley AL Jr., Ansfield FJ et al. (1976) Combined radiation therapy and 5-fluorouracil for advanced squamous cell carcinoma of the oral cavity and oropharynx: a randomized study. AJR 126: 229–235

Marcial VA, Pajak TF (1985) Radiation therapy alone or in combination with surgery in head and neck cancer. Cancer 55: 2259–2265

Million RR, Casisi NJ (1984) Management of head and neck cancer. A multidisciplinary approach. Philadelphia, Lippincott

Murthy AK, Taylor SG, Showel J et al. (1987) Treatment of advanced head and neck cancer with concomitant radiation and chemotherapy. Int J Radiat Oncol Biol Phys 13: 1807–1813

Nguyen TD, Panis X, Froissart, D, Legros M, Coninx P, Loirette M (1988) Analysis of late complications after rapid hyperfractionated radiotherapy in advanced head and neck cancers. Int J Radiat Oncol Biol Phys 14: 23–25

Nigro MD, Vaitkevicius VK, Buroker T, Bradley GT, Considine B (1981) Combined therapy for cancer of the anal canal. Dis Colon Rectum 24: 73–75

Parecchia G, Salti C (1981) Radiotherapy with thrice-a-day fractionation in a short overall time: clinical experiences. Int J Radiat Oncol Biol Phys 7: 99–104

Tannock I, Browman G (1986) Lack of evidence for a role of chemotherapy in the routine managment of locally advanced head and neck cancer. J Clin Oncol 4: 1121–1126

Taylor SG, Murthy AK, Showel JL et al. (1985) Improved control in advanced head and neck cancer with simultaneous radiation and cisplatin/5 FU chemotherapy. Cancer Treat Rep 69: 933–939

Vikram B (1987) Accelerated, interrupted, twice-a-day (AIBID) radiation therapy decreases acute mucosal toxicity. Int J Radiat Oncol Biol Phys 13: 1971–1972

Wang CC (1988) Local control of oropharyngeal carcinoma after two accelerated hyperfractionation radiation therapy schemes. Int J Radiat Oncol Biol Phys 14: 1143–1146

Withers HR (1985) Biologic basis for altered fractionation schemes. Cancer 55: 2086–2095

29 Toxicity of Combined Cisplatin, Infusional 5-Fluorouracil and Concomitant Radiotherapy in Advanced Head and Neck Cancer

ALFRED DiSTEFANO, SAMUEL L. JAMPOLIS, GEORGE R. BLUMENSCHEIN, BARRY A. FIRSTENBERG, JOHN P. KELLY, and JOSE E. GOMEZ-YEYILLE

CONTENTS

29.1 Introduction

Advanced head and neck cancer is well suited to clinical protocols that utilize concomitant administration of radiotherapy and chemotherapy. Both therapeutic modalities yield high response rates when given individually. There is also a large body of data documenting the radiosensitizing effects of various chemotherapeutic agents. While many side-effects of concomitant therapy are not overlapping, augmented toxicity is a problem in many tissues. Hematological, infectious, and gastrointestinal toxicities are frequently additive. Our approach to concomitant therapy in patients with advanced head and neck cancer has been directed towards administration of maximum therapeutic dose of radiation and chemotherapy, while using recent technological advances to support the patient during treatment.

29.2 Materials and Methods

Eighteen consecutive patients with advanced head and neck cancer were treated (Table 29.1). The patients with primary cancer were treated with

ALFRED DiSTEFANO, MD, SAMUEL L. JAMPOLIS, MD, GEORGE R. BLUMENSCHEIN, MD, BARRY A. FIRSTENBERG, DO, JOHN P. KELLY, MD, JOSE E. GOMEZ-YEYILLE, MD, Arlington Cancer Center, 906 W. Randol Mill Road, Arlington, TX 76012, USA

twice-a-day fractionated radiation to approximately 72 Gy and continuous infusion 5-fluorouracil (5-FU) and bolus cisplatin (Table 29.2). The median dose of 5-FU was $600 \, mg/m^2$ for 5 days by continuous infusion. The last seven patients received $1000 \, mg/m^2$ for 5 days. Patients with recurrent cancer received twice-a-day fractionated radiation to approximately 25 Gy in combination with interstitial hyperthermia and the same chemotherapy agents. Radiation therapy was individualized in all patients. Suitable patients received boost to areas of bulk disease with iridium 192 brachytherapy. All patients underwent placement of vascular access catheters before beginning therapy.

Parenteral hyperalimentation was administered at the discretion of the attending physician when the patient was unable to swallow or when the patient had lost 3%–5% of body weight and further weight loss was anticipated. Standard formulations were used to deliver between 1400 and 3900 calories.

Parenteral antibiotics were prescribed upon suspicion or documentation of serious infection and were administered using an ambulatory automated programmable drug delivery system (Inteliject Pump, Intelligent Medicine, Englewood, Co.). Multiple parenteral antibiotics could easily be given using this system.

29.3 Results

All 18 patients were in complete remission at the conclusion of therapy. At a median follow-up of 12 months, 15 patients remain cancer-free. Two patients died in remission and one died of pulmonary metastasis (Fig. 29.1).

Table 29.3 demonstrates the toxicity seen in the study patients. Hematological toxicity was mild. Stomatitis was severe in eight patients. Infection was severe in six patients. Weight loss was maintained at a minimal level by liberal use of hyper-

Table 29.1. Characteristics of 18 treated patients

Male	16
Female	2
Median age in years (range)	65 (27–77)
Number with untreated cancer	15
Number with recurrent cancer	3
Squamous cancer	17
Adenocarcinoma	1
Primary site	
Oral cavity	10
Nasophayrnx	2
Larynx	3
Salivary gland	1
Maxillary sinus	1
Lacrimal duct	1
Stage III cancer	5
T_2N_1	1
T_3N_0	4
Stage IV cancer	10
T_2N_3	1
T_3N_2	2
T_3N_3	6
T_4N_0	1

Table 29.2. Treatment Schema

Radiation therapy:
  Twice-a-day fractionation
  72–76 Gy final tumor dose
  1.2 Gy–4-h interval – 1.2 Gy
Chemotherapy:
  5-Fluorouracil (median dose 600 mg/m^2/24 h × 5 days)
  Cisplatin (median dose 80 mg/m^2 × 1 day)   14 pts.
  Other   4 pts.

Table 29.3. Grade of toxicity in 18 study patients

	Grade				
	0	1	2	3	4
Hematological	10	3	5	0	0
Stomatitis	0	2	8	4	4
Nausea/emesis	2	5	6	4	1
Infection	9	0	3	3	3
Weight loss[a]	5	12	1	0	0

[a] Median weight loss 3.6 kg (5.1% body weight) (12 patients required hyperalimentation)

alimentation. No patient had therapy interrupted because of toxicity.

29.4 Discussion

Table 29.4 shows the modalities used in the management of toxicity. Many topical solutions were administered in the treatment of mucositis; however, they were largely ineffective and 12 patients required parenteral nutrition due to mucositis and inability to eat. Nausea and emesis were related to cisplatin administration. The combination of haloperidol, lorazepam, and diphenhydramine with or without metoclopramide was effective when given parenterally using the programmable infusion pump.

Weight loss was kept to a minimum by careful monitoring of nutritional status and early use of parenteral nutrition. Infectious episodes were successfully managed with outpatient antibiotics. One patient died of a second episode of aspiration pneumonia in complete remission 5 months after diagnosis.

Figure 29.2 shows the clinical course of a patient

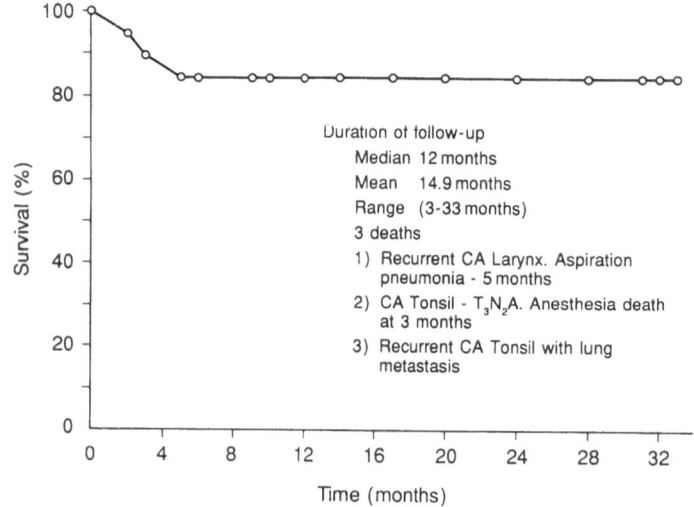

Duration of follow-up
  Median 12 months
  Mean   14.9 months
  Range (3-33 months)
  3 deaths
  1) Recurrent CA Larynx. Aspiration pneumonia - 5 months
  2) CA Tonsil - T_3N_2A. Anesthesia death at 3 months
  3) Recurrent CA Tonsil with lung metastasis

Fig. 29.1. Disease-free survival of 18 patients treated with concomitant radiation therapy and chemotherapy

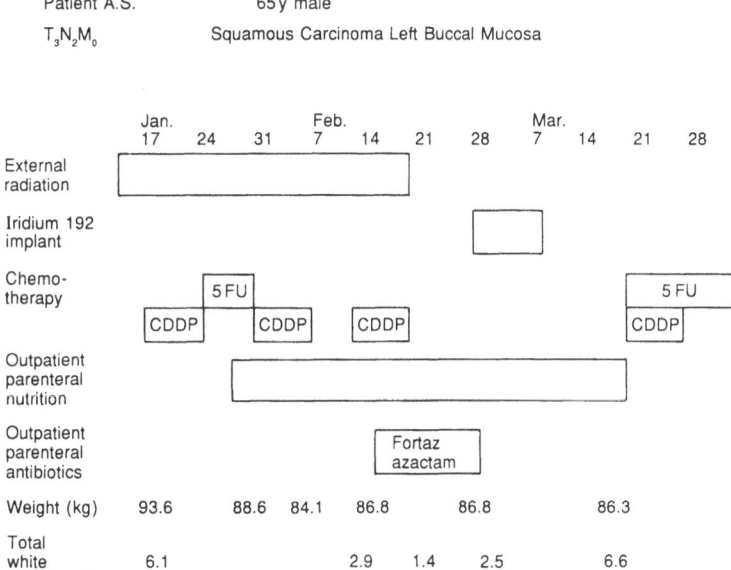

Fig. 29.2. Example of anticipated management of toxicity of concomitant radiation therapy and chemotherapy

Table 29.4. Management of toxicity

Management of stomatitis:
Clotrimazole troches
Nystatin suspension
Chlorhexidine gluconate 0.12% (Peridex)
Parenteral nutrition

Management of nausea/emesis:

Haloperidol	0.25 mg	Parenteral
Lorazepam	0.5 mg	Administration
Diphenhydramine	25 mg	With programmable
Metoclopramide	30 mg	Drug delivery system

Management of weight loss:
Intravenous hyperalimentation

TPN A	*TPN B*	*TPN C*
1400 calories	2840 calories	3970 calories
42.5 g protein	85 g protein	42.5 g protein

Management of infection:
Outpatient administration of multiple parenteral antibiotics
using a programmable drug delivery system

with advanced squamous carcinoma of the buccal mucosa ($T_3N_2M_0$). This patient demonstrates the integration of radiation therapy (external irradiation and an interstitial boost) with continuous infusion 5-FU and bolus cisplatin. Parenteral nutrition was started when the patient developed grade 3 mucositis and demonstrated weight loss.

Outpatient parenteral antibiotics were administered during a period of neutropenic fever. The patient required hospitalization only for the iridium implant.

Our approach to the patient with advanced head and neck cancer is one in which the therapeutic dose of radiation is maximized through twice-a-day fractionation, individualization of therapy, and concomitant use of chemotherapy. Rather than alter therapy to eliminate toxicity, we have chosen to support the patient during periods of toxicity. This approach has demonstrated excellent tumor control and patient acceptance. We plan to explore escalation of the dose of chemotherapy and consider protracted drug infusion.

References

DiStefano A, Blumenschein G, Fanning J et al. (1989) Outpatient administration of multiple antibiotics to neutropenic and non-neutropenic cancer patients using an automatic programmable drug delivery system. Proc ASCO 8: 324 (abstr 1331)

Jacobs C, Goffinet DR, Goffinet L, Kohler M, Fee WE (1987) Chemotherapy as a substitute for surgery in the treatment of advanced resectable head and neck cancer. Cancer 60: 1178–1183

30 Esophageal Carcinoma

MADHU J. JOHN

CONTENTS

30.1 Introduction

Carcinoma of the esophagus is a relatively uncommon malignancy in the United States. An incidence rate of 1.2–4.1 per 100 000 population in the United States differs sharply from endemic areas in Iran and China, where corresponding rates of over 200 per 100 000 population are reported (FRANK-STROMBORG 1989).

The major etiological factors in esophageal cancer of alcohol ingestion, cigarette smoking, and various nutritional factors have been established for some time (WYNDER and MABUCHI 1973). Nevertheless, the incidence and mortality of this disease have been virtually unchanged (SILVERBERG et al, 1990).

Major breakthroughs in the management of esophageal cancer have come through two environmentally and culturally diverse areas of the world – from China and North America. In China, where this disease is endemic in certain provinces, the major advance has been in the form of presymptomatic cytological screening

which has resulted in quantum improvements in survival rates in that country (HUANG 1981). In the United States and Canada the major potential breakthrough in managing this disease has been through a combination of chemotherapy and radiotherapy in more advanced disease. We will address this modality of chemoradiation, as it is often called, with a description of our own 7-year experience with chemoradiation in esophageal carcinoma at the University of California, San Francisco – Fresno program. This experience will be described in the overall context of the historical rationale, survival results, toxicity, and controversies of chemoradiation in the North American experience.

30.2 Material and Methods

Between January 1982 and June 1989 a total of 49 patients with esophageal carcinoma were treated with progressively intensive courses of chemoradiation at the University of California, San Francisco – Fresno program. All these patients had biopsy – proven squamous cell carcinoma or adenocarcinoma without evidence of distant metastases. They were staged by a modified American Joint Committee on Cancer (AJCC) clinical-diagnostic staging system described previously (JOHN et al. 1989a).

Patients were treated in three separate protocols combining radiotherapy and chemotherapy in chronologically intensified doses. The first 14 patients received an average of three courses of alternating 5-fluorouracil (5-FU) + mitomycin C and 5-FU + cisplatin (CDDP) with 41.4 Gy radiotherapy directed to the primary tumor over 7 weeks (group A). This protocol and its preliminary results were described in 1987 by JOHN et al. Subsequently, 22 patients received chemoradiation in the form of an average of 50.4 Gy to the primary and four courses of chemotherapy includ-

MADHU J. JOHN, MD, Director Radiation Oncology, Kaweah Delta Cancer Care Center, 248 S. Floral, Visalia, CA 93291 and Associate Clinical Professor, University of California, San Francisco, CA 94143, USA

Table 30.1. Chemoradiation for esophageal carcinoma in group C patients

Week	RT dose (Gy)	Accumulated RT dose (Gy)	Chemotherapy
1	2.2 daily	11	5-FU: 1000 mg/m^2/24 h for 96 h Mito C: 10 mg/m^2 day 1
2–3	1.8 daily	29	–
4	1.8 daily	38	5-FU: same as week 1 CDDP: 75 mg/m^2/ day 1 of 5-FU
5–7	Rest		Rest
8	1.8 daily	47	MTX: 200 mg/m^2 i.v. 5-FU: 600 mg/m^2 1 h after MTX LCR: 10 mg/m^2 q 6 h × 5, 6 h after MTX
9–10	Rest		Rest
11	HDR 7 at 1 cm	54	Same as week 8
12	Rest		Rest
13	Same as week 11	61	Same as week 8

Abbreviations: RT, radiotherapy; 5-FU, 5-fluorouracil; mito C, mitomycin C; CDDP, cisplatin; MTX, methotrexate; LCR, leucovorin; HDR, intraluminal high dose rate radiotherapy

Table 30.2. Descriptive characteristics of patients with esophageal cancer treated by three chemoradiation protocols

	Group A	Group B	Group C
Median age	71	67	67
Sex (M:F)	1.8:1	2.1:1	1.6:1
Mod. AJCC stage (%)			
I	0	5	15
II	36	32	23
III	64	63	62
Histology			
Poorly differentiated squamous cell carcinoma	28	27	54
Adenocarcinoma (%)	7	27	23
Primary site			
Upper (%)	29	18	23
Middle (%)	64	36	54
Lower (%)	7	46	23

ing one cycle of methotrexate (MTX) + 5-FU + leucovorin combination in addition to the previously mentioned drugs (group B). Part of this experience and its preliminary results have been described previously (JOHN et al. 1989). Since May 1988, we have added two doses of intraluminal high dose rate treatments (for a total of 61 Gy) to the primary tumor site and one additional course (cycle #5) of MTX + 5-FU + leucovorin to the above regimen. The preliminary results of this experience were reported recently (JOHN et al., 1989b) on ten patients. This regimen (Table 30.1) was employed in 13 consecutive patients with nonmetastatic disease (group C).

The patient characteristics of groups A, B, and C are described in Table 30.2. The median age and sex distribution were not significantly different in these three groups when classified according to the modified AJCC clinical system. Patients with stage III disease predominated in all three groups (62%–64%). Patients with stage II and III combined composed 80%–100% of the three groups. With regard to histological classifications, it could be said that there appeared to be more awareness and detailed reporting regarding differentiation and glandular origin of tumor in later years. Primary tumors designated to have originated in the upper and middle third of the esophagus constituted the majority of cases (54%–93%) in the three groups. In group B, notably, there was a 46% incidence of tumors originating from the lower third of the esophagus.

30.3 Treatment Particulars

30.3.1 Radiotherapy

As described previously, conventional radiotherapy fields were abandoned in favor of limited fields excluding significant pulmonary tissues and grossly uninvolved lymphatic drainage sites (JOHN et al. 1987, 1989a). Initial anterior–posterior fields up to 30.6138 Gy measured 6.5–7 cm in width and extended 3 cm beyond gross disease vertically as seen on esophagograms, endoscopy, and CT scan. Subsequent reduced fields employed only a 1- to 1.5-cm margin beyond original disease. These were usually two posterior wedged oblique fields acutely angled off the median to minimize radiation doses to both the spinal cord and hitherto untreated pulmonary tissues. Lung inhomogeneity corrections were always employed. External radiotherapy fractionation schedules were always 1.8 Gy daily 5 times per week with one exception. In group C, 2.2 Gy was delivered daily during week 1 of external radiotherapy.

Two doses of intraluminal high dose rate (HDR) brachytherapy were delivered as follows: The patients underwent endoscopy on an outpatient basis and an esophageal catheter was placed against and beyond the original tumor mapped out as seen on original endoscopy, esophagogram, and CT scan. The catheter was connected to an HDR iridium applicator system, the MicroSelectron. A dose of 7 Gy was delivered at a distance of 1 cm from the center of the catheter through a distance of 1–2 cm beyond the original tumor in the craniocaudal direction. This entire process of endoscopy, treatment planning, and delivery took an average of 1 1/2 h. This treatment was then repeated 2 weeks later. Endoscopy during this second treatment included multiple biopsies and brushings from the original tumor site(s). Both treatments were immediately followed by outpatient chemotherapy. Four patients had positive biopsies during the second endoscopy–HDR procedure. These patients underwent repeat endoscopies and frozen-section biopsy 2 weeks later with plans to deliver a third dose of chemoradiation. But all these biopsies turned out to be negative and none of these four patients required further treatment.

30.3.2 Chemotherapy

The drug regimens employed for groups A and B have been described previously (JOHN et al. 1987, 1989a). In group A, alternating cycles of 5-FU + mitomycin C and 5-FU + CDDP for a total of three to four cycles were planned. In group B, we substituted an MTX + 5-FU + leucovorin combination for the last course of 5-FU + CDDP in the first 16 patients. In the last six patients of this group the MTX + 5-FU + leucovorin combination was given instead of the second cycles of 5-FU + mitomycin C and 5-FU + CDDP (as given to group A). Chemotherapy for group C patients differed in that three courses of outpatient chemotherapy with MTX + 5-FU + leucovorin were delivered and only one course each of 5-FU + mitomycin C and 5-FU + CDDP were given. The MTX + 5-FU + leucovorin combination was administered during the last week of external radiotherapy and immediately after the two intraluminal HDR treatments (JOHN et al., 1989b).

30.4 Patient Evaluation

30.4.1 Pretreatment Workup

Patients were staged clinically with complete blood count, platelet count, blood chemistries, chest x-ray, esophagogram or barium swallow, endoscopy–biopsy of primary tumor, and CAT scan of the mediastinum, liver, and celiac axis. Additional tests such as bone and liver scans and pulmonary function tests were done only on clinical suspicion or evidence of distant metastases or severe chronic obstructive pulmonary disease. Patients were only staged clinically per modified AJCC system previously described (JOHN et al. 1989).

30.4.2 Evaluation During Treatment

Complete blood and platelet counts were obtained weekly throughout the treatment course. Endoscopy was done during the two HDR procedures in group C patients or 4 weeks after completion of the treatments in group A and B patients.

Patients in group C were considered for a third endoscopy and HDR treatment if biopsy during the second endoscopy showed residual malignancy.

30.4.3 Posttreatment Evaluation

Patients underwent follow-up physical evaluations and routine blood tests every 2–4 months following completion of planned treatment. Karnofsky status and the presence or absence of dysphagia were recorded. Endoscopy with/without biopsies was carried out every 4–6 months in asymptomatic patients and earlier in symptomatic patients.

30.5 Results

30.5.1 Therapeutic Results

Treatment results for the three groups of patients are tabulated in Table 30.3. These results are set against the average radiotherapy dose and number of chemotherapy cycles actually given to each group of patients. An escalation of actual

Table 30.3. Dose response and patterns of failure with three different chemoradiation schedules

	Group A (n = 14)	Group B (n = 22)	Group C (n = 13)
Planned RT dose (Gy)	41.4	50.4	61
Average RT dose (Gy)	39.7	49.9	61
Planned # chemo. cycles	3–4	4	5
Average # chemo. cycles	2.8	3.3	4.7
Complete response rate (%)	57	72	100
Median survival (mo)	11	21	–[a]
1-year survival (%)	50	68	–[a]
2-year survival (%)	35	50	–[a]
Follow-up range (mo)	1–81	5–42	5–18
Local failure only (%)	50	14	15
Local + distant mets. (%)	21	18	8
Distant mets. only (%)	7	18	15

[a] Too early for analysis; median follow-up 11 months

Table 30.4. Grade 3 and 4 toxicities in three groups of patients with esophageal carcinoma

Toxicity	Group A	Group B	Group C
Hematological			
WBC			
Grade 3	3	3	1
Grade 4	0	0	0
Platelets			
Grade 3	3	2	2
Grade 4	2	2	0
Pancytopenia	1	0	1[a]
Nonhematological			
Esophagitis			
Grade 3	1	2	2
Grade 4	0	0	0
Esophageal stricture			
Grade 3	1	2	1
Pulmonary fibrosis			
Grade 3	0	1	0
Grade 4	0	0	0
Pericarditis			
Grade 3	1	0	0
Fistula			
Grade 4	0	1	1
Stomatitis			
Grade 3	2	3	2
Grade 4	1	1	0
Acute renal failure	0	1	0

[a] Secondary to accidental nonprotocol chemotherapy

radiotherapy and chemotherapy doses is accompanied by progressive improved complete response rates from 57% to 100%. It is too early to know whether this trend will translate to improved survival since the pertinent data from group C are not available at this time. However, it is evident that the median survival and 1- and 2-year survival rates have improved significantly in group B patients compared with group A. The median survival of group C has not been reached, though median follow-up for this group is 11 months.

In addition, even though the available data in group C may be premature, there is some indication that the incidence of local failure, alone or in combination with distant metastases, may decline with increasing chemoradiation doses (from 71% to 23%).

30.5.2 Toxicity

Treatment toxicity was predominantly hematological (Table 30.4). However, no significant treatment delay was noted secondary to such toxicity with three exceptions. Two patients in group A had 27- and 31-day treatment interruptions for leukopenia and thrombocytopenia, having received three courses of 5-FU and mitomycin C consecutively since renal functions did not allow for CDDP administration. One patient in group C received an accidental high dose of Alkeran

instead of mitomycin C, resulting in a 60-day interruption of treatment secondary to pancytopenia. Thus there was an overall 11% (5/45) of grade 4 but transient hematological toxicity which did not result in mortality secondary to speticemia or bleeding. Also there appeared to be no evidence of increased hematological toxicity as the number of chemotherapy cycles and radiotherapy dose were escalated over the three regimens.

Nonhematological toxicity was comparatively minimal. The incidence of pulmonary fibrosis or acute respiratory distress syndrome does not appear to be a major problem with increasing chemoradiation. Aside from the unconventional radiation fields used, the decreased use of mitomycin C in group C patients may be another reason for decreased pulmonary toxicity. The single incidence of fistula formation in group B was secondary to recurrent local disease. The patient in group C had actually a blind diverticula or pouch which appeared closed off from the adjacent trachea on esophagogram with Gastrografin 2 months following treatment completion. This patient with an extensive primary (over 13 cm in length) died with no evidence of disease at autopsy and with no detectable reason for his death. The incidence of grade 3 or 4 esophagitis and esophageal stricture did not appear to increase significantly with intraluminal HDR treatment.

30.6 Discussion

The history of treatment of esophageal carcinoma in this century could be described as uniformly dreary were it not very occasionally alleviated by a few results of long-term cure for very early disease treated by surgical resection in some countries or by radiotherapy in Scotland (HUANG 1981; ENDO et al. 1982; SKINNER 1981; BORST et al. 1981; PEARSON 1969). The central fact of the presence of locally advanced or disseminated disease at initial diagnosis in the vast majority of patients with esophageal cancer has been the main reason for the lack of progress in the management of this disease until recently. The successful use of cytological screening in presymptomatic populations in endemic areas of China cannot realistically be expected to be considered as standard care in other parts of the world (HUANG 1981).

The net experience of modern surgery and megavoltage radiotherapy until 1979 was compiled by EARLAM and CUNHA-MELO (1980a, b). The verdict on both modalities was resoundingly clear and painful. Over 80000 patients treated by surgery alone averaged 18%, 9%, and 4% survival rates at 1, 2, and 5 years, respectively. A 29% mean surgical mortality was the clincher. Over 8000 patients treated by radiotherapy alone fared no better with 18%, 8%, and 6% 1-, 2-, and 5-year survival rates, respectively. It was evident, however, that patients treated with radiotherapy were mainly surgical rejections due to unresectability or inoperability and yet suffered no significant treatment mortality. Integrating these two modalities served to marginally increase survival rates with no palpable impact on the above surgical mortality (DOGGETT et al. 1970; NAKAYAMA and KINOSHITA 1974).

In 1981, STEIGER et al. reported on a prototype preoperative chemoradiation protocol for esophageal cancer using either 5-FU + mitomycin C or 5-FU + CDDP and 30 Gy of radiotherapy. Only one chemotherapy cycle was concomitantly given with radiotherapy. One- and 2-year survival rates of 52% and 30% were reported – a radical departure then from the litany of poor results with surgery or radiotherapy alone. Since then, numerous studies using various drug combinations with varying doses radiotherapy, with or without surgery, have been reported with more or less similar results (POPLIN et al. 1987; RICHMOND et al. 1987; KEANE et al. 1985; LEICHMAN et al. 1987). Until this report, the sole exception has been the experience of Coia et al. (1989), who achieved 47% and 34% 2- and 5-year survival rates primarily with stage I and II patients. With a median survival of 21 months, group B patients in the current series (predominantly stage III) have a 50% 2-year survival.

Even so, whereas a dose–response relationship to radiotherapy has been established in esophageal cancer (DOGGETT et al. 1970; NEWAISHY et al. 1982; BEATTY et al. 1979), the relationship between chemoradiation doses and the disease response is not established (JOHN et al. 1987). Most noncohort studies from various institutions use 30–60 Gy of radiotherapy with varying chemotherapy combinations culminating in almost identical results. The current study from a single institution employing a three-tiered *quantitative* escalation in radiation and chemotherapy doses may provide some clues regarding dose relationship. On the other hand, the data here are partly flawed in that the results of treatment of group C patients are immature. Though there appears to be a trend in increasing complete response rates from groups A to C, this may not translate to better survival rates with group C. Secondly, there has been a *qualitative* change in the treatment given to group C patients in that (a) the external radiotherapy fractionation for week 1 was changed to 2.2 Gy daily from 1.8 Gy daily, (b) the biological compatibility of conventional and HDR radiotherapy is currently unknown, and (c) the institution of three cycles of MTX + 5-FU + leucovorin and consequent sacrifice of one cycle each of 5-FU + mitomycin C and 5-FU + CDDP in the group C regimen, while decreasing hospitalization and increasing patient acceptability, may translate to decreased efficacy in eradicating tumor.

Over the last decade, along with these chemoradiation protocols, there have been some studies primarily from Memorial Sloan-Kettering Cancer Center relating their experience with preoperative chemotherapy (KELSEN 1981, 1984; KELSEN et al. 1983, 1986; ROTH et al. 1988; HILGENBERG et al. 1988). These studies generally use one to two cycles of CDDP-based two- to three-drug combinations prior to planned esophagectomy. Complete response rates seen at surgery are usually less than 10%. The surgical mortality in these series matches that of surgery alone during this decade, averaging around 9%. The best results appear to be from KELSEN (1986), who reported 25% and 18% 2- and 5-year survival rates, and from HILGENBERG et al. (1988), who reported a 60% 2-year survival rate from patients who were able to undergo resection (46% if all potentially resectable patients are included). With few exceptions, most of these series employ radiotherapy for residual disease, positive margins, or involved lymph nodes.

From this spate of multimodality protocols for esophageal carcinoma, two major trends seem to have gradually evolved. These involve the use of the systemic modality of chemotherapy with either surgery or radiotherapy. The scenario is now strikingly similar to the pre-1970s, when surgery alone and radiotherapy alone were dominant modalities. The difference is that preoperative chemotherapy now consistently provides about a 25%–30% 2-year survival rate and about a 9% surgical mortality (KELSEN 1984; KELSEN et al. 1986; ROTH et al. 1988; HILGENBERG et al. 1988). Chemoradiation alone (without surgery) provides a similar 30% 2-year survival rate, with 1%–2% mortality for a population of patients with more advanced disease than those treated by preoperative chemotherapy alone (RICHMOND et al. 1987; KEANE et al. 1985; LEICHMAN et al. 1987; COIA 1989; JOHN et al. 1989a). The question as to which combination of modalities is optimal for most patients with esophageal carcinoma should be settled by various research groups over the next decade.

References

Beatty JD, DeBoer G, Rider WD (1979) Carcinoma of the esophagus: pre-treatment assessment, correlation of radiation treatment parameters with survival and identification and management of radiation treatment failure. Cancer 43: 2254–2267

Borst HG, Dragojevic C, Peck W (1981) Carcinoma of the esophagus. Results of resection and reconstruction. In: Stipa S, Belsey RHR, Moraldi A (eds) Medical and surgical problems of the esophagus. Proceedings of the Serono Symposium, vol 43. Academic, New York, pp 345–352

Coia LR (1989) Esophageal cancer: Is esophagectomy necessary? Oncology 3(4): 101–110

Doggett RLS, Guernsey JM, Bagshaw MA (1970) Combined radiation and surgical treatment of carcinoma of the thoracic esophagus. Radiat Ther Oncol 5: 147–154

Earlam R, Cunha-Melo JR (1980a) Oesophageal squamous

cell carcinoma: I. A critical review of surgery. Br J Surg 67: 381–390

Earlam R, Cunha-Melo JR (1980b) Oesophageal squamous cell carcinoma. I. A critical review of radiotherapy. Br J Surg 67: 457–451

Endo M, Kinoshita Y, Yamada A et al. (1982) Surgical treatment of thoracic esophageal cancer, including clinical evaluation of early esophageal cancer. In: Pfeiffer CJ (ed) Cancer of the esophagus, vol II. CRC, Boca Raton, pp 57–69

Frank-Stromborg M (1989) The epidemiology and primary prevention of gastric and esophageal cancer. A worldwide perspective. Cancer Nursing 12(2): 53–64

Hilgenberg AD, Carey RW, Wilkins EW, Choi NC, Mathisen DJ, Grillo HC (1988) Preoperative chemotherapy, surgical resection, and selective postoperative therapy for squamous cell carcinoma of the esophagus. Ann Thorac Surg 45: 357–363

Huang KC (1981) Diagnosis and surgical treatment of early esophageal carcinoma. In: Stipa S, Belsey RHR, Moraldi A (eds) Medical and surgical problems of the esophagus. Proceedings of the Serono Symposium, vol. 43. Academic, New York pp 296–299

John M, Flam M, Wittlinger P, Mowry PA (1987) Inoperable esophageal carcinoma: results of aggressive synchronous radiotherapy and chemotherapy. A pilot study. Am J Clin Oncol (CCT) 10: 310–316

John MJ, Flam MS, Mowry PA, Podolsky WJ, Xavier AM, Wittlinger PS, Padmanabhan A (1989a) Radiotherapy alone and chemoradiation for nonmetastatic esophageal carcinoma. A critical review of chemoradiation. Cancer 63: 2397–2403

John MJ, Wong DS, Flam MS, Wittlinger PS (1989b) Esophageal carcinoma: A three-tiered study of progressively aggressive chemoradiation therapy. Radiology 173(P): pp 39. (Abst. 67)

Keane TJ, Harwood AR, Elhaleim T, Rider WD, Cummings BJ, Ginsberg RJ, Cooper JC (1985) Radiation therapy with 5-fluorouracil infusion and mitomycin C for oesophageal squamous carcinoma. Radiother Oncol 4: 205–210

Kelsen D (1981) Treatment of advanced esophageal cancer. Cancer 50: 2576–2581

Kelsen D (1984) Chemotherapy of esophageal cancer. Semin Oncol 11: 159–168

Kelsen D, Hilaris B, Coonley C et al. (1983) Cisplatin, vindesine and bleomycin chemotherapy of local-regional and advanced esophageal carcinoma. Am J Med 75: 645–652

Kelsen DP, Hilaris B, Martini N (1986) Neoadjuvant chemotherapy and surgery of cancer of the esophagus. Semin Oncol 2: 170–176

Leichman L, Herskovic A, Leichman CG et al. (1987) Nonoperative therapy for squamous-cell cancer of the esophagus. J Clin Oncol 5: 365–370

Nakayama K, Kinoshita Y (1974) Surgical treatment combined with preoperative concentrated irradiation. In: Rubin P (ed) Cancer of the gastrointestinal tract. Esophagus: treatment – local and advanced. JAMA 227: 178–181

Newaishy GA, Read GA, Duncan W, Kerr GR (1982) Results of radical radiotherapy of squamous cell carcinoma of the esophagus. Clin Radiol 33: 347–352

Pearson JG (1969) The value of radiotherapy in the management of esophageal cancer. Am J Roentgenol Radium Ther Nucl Med 105: 500–513

Poplin E, Fleming T, Leichman L et al. (1987) Combined therapies for squamous cell carcinoma of the esophagus, a Southwest Oncology Group Study (SWOG-8307). J Clin Oncol 5: 622–628

Richmond J, Seydel HG, Bae Y, Lewis J, Burdakin J, Jacobsen G (1987) Comparison of three treatment strategies for esophageal cancer within a single institution. Int J Radiat Oncol Biol Phys 13: 1617–1620

Roth JA, Pass HI, Flanagan M, Graeber GM, Rosenberg JC, Steinberg S (1988) Randomized clinical trials of preoperative and postoperative adjuvant chemotherapy with cisplatin, vindesine and bleomycin for carcinoma of the esophagus. J Thorac Cardiovasc Surg 96: 242–248

Silverberg E, Boring C. Squires T. Cancer statistics 1990. CA 40(1): 9–26

Skinner DB (1981) Mediastinectomy for esophageal carcinoma. In: Stipa S, Belsey RHR, Moraldi A (eds) Medical and surgical problems of the esophagus. Proceedings of the Serono Symposium, vol 43. Academic, New York, pp 331–334

Steiger Z, Franklin R, Wilson RF et al. (1981) Complete eradication of squamous cell carcinoma of the esophagus with combined chemotherapy and radiotherapy. Am Surg 47: 95–98

Wynder EL, Mabuchi K (1973) Etiological and environmental factors. Cancer of the gastrointestinal tract. B. Esophagus: detection and diagnosis. JAMA 226: 1546–1548

31 Adenocarcinoma of the Gastroesophageal Junction: Preoperative Cisplatin and Concomitant Continuous Infusion 5-Fluorouracil and Radiation Therapy

GARY V. BURTON, WALTER G. WOLFE, IAN CROCKER, HILLIARD F. SEIGLER, LEONARD R. PROSNITZ, and JEFFREY CRAWFORD

CONTENTS

31.1 Introduction

The results of multimodal approaches to esophageal carcinoma suggest an improved patient outcome as compared with historical patients (POPLIN et al. 1987). Adenocarcinomas of the gastroesophageal junction (GEJ) are often included in multimodal reports. However, the different tumor histology, site of disease, and patient outcome suggest that these tumors should be considered separately (FEIN et al. 1985; MAHONEY and CONDON 1987; TURNBULL and GOODNER 1969). We initiated a multimodal protocol for the treatment of adenocarcinomas involving the GEJ using a debulking course of cisplatin (CDDP) and 5-fluorouracil (5-FU) chemotherapy prior of two courses of concomitant chemotherapy with radiotherapy. The rationale for debulking chemotherapy included: a means to evaluate response to the chemotherapy alone, an attempt to reduce tumor burden and thus allow for improved oral intake and nutrition prior to beginning radiotherapy, and an attempt to reduce the tumor mass and improve tumor oxygenation prior to initiating radiotherapy. Concomitant chemotherapy was administered to exploit the radiosensitizing potential of both CDDP (RICHMOND et al. 1977) and 5-FU (BYFIELD et al. 1982; VIETTI et al. 1971). Multimodal patients were compared with a historical control group treated initially with surgery and/or radiotherapy with chemotherapy at time of relapse.

GARY V. BURTON, MD, Department of Medicine, Louisiana State University Medical Center, P.O. Box 33932, Shreveport, LA 71130–3932, USA

WALTER G. WOLFE MD, Department of Surgery, IAN CROCKER, MD, Department of Medicine, HILLIARD F. SEIGLER, MD, Department of Surgery, LEONARD R. PROSNITZ, MD, Professor and Chairman, Department of Radiation Oncology, JEFFREY CRAWFORD, MD, Department of Medicine, Duke University Medical Center, Durham, NC 27710, USA

31.2 Methods

Twenty-one consecutive patients seen at Duke University Medical Center between April 1985 and September 1987 with stage II and III adenocarcinoma involving the GEJ were entered on a multimodal protocol (Table 31.1). Chemotherapy consisted of 5-FU 1000 mg/m^2/day continuous 24 h infusion and CDDP 20 mg/m^2/day over 1 h infusion daily for 5 days repeated every 21–28 days for three courses. Radiotherapy began on day 1 of chemotherapy course number 2 at 2 Gy daily 5 days/week to a total of 45 Gy in 25 fractions using parallel opposed fields with minimum 5-cm margins. Chemotherapy course number 3 was administered during the last week of radiotherapy. The patients underwent an esophagogastrostomy 28–42 days following completion of all therapy. Pretherapy and presurgical staging studies included esophagoscopy, barium swallow, chest and abdomen CT, bone scan, and chest x-ray. Limited staging prior to chemotherapy course number 2 consisted of barium swallow, esophagoscopy, and chest x-ray. The treatment program was evaluated for response to chemotherapy course number 1, concomitant chemo/radiotherapy, weight gain, toxicity, pathological findings at surgical resection, disease-free survival, sites of recurrence, and overall survival.

The multimodal group was compared with 21 consecutive patients with stage II/III adenocarcinoma of the GEJ treated at Duke University

Table 31.1. Patient populations

	Multimodal patients	Historical controls
Patient number	21	21
Age (range)	59 (28–74)	66 (35–81)
Sex (male:female)	19:2	20:1
Race		
White	21	20
Black		1
Stage[a]		
IIA	9	10
IIB	6	5
III	6	6
Tumor grade		
Well differentiated	1	
Moderately well differentiated	14	
Poorly differentiated	6	
Tumor size		
<5 cm	2	5
≥5 cm	19	16

[a] American Joint Committee on Cancer

between January 1980 and March 1985 (Table 31.1).

31.3 Results

Twenty-one patients entered the study with 17 completing chemotherapy and radiotherapy. Sixteen patients underwent resection (including one patient who refused radiotherapy). Reasons for not completing therapy included: noncompliance (two patients), comorbid condition (two), arterial thrombosis (one), and progressive disease (one).

Toxicity: Myelosuppression was common. The first chemotherapy course (21 patients) resulted in mild leukopenia ($<3.0 \times 10^9$/l) in 24% and mild thrombocytopenia ($<1.0 \times 10^9$/l) in 10%. Concomitant chemotherapy and radiotherapy (18 patients) resulted in increased myelosuppression with mild leukopenia in 30% and severe leukopenia ($<1.0 \times 10^9$/l) in 24%. Mild thrombocytopenia was seen in 35%. There were no infectious complications. Grade 1 or 2 mucositis was seen in seven patients. Esophagitis was common during radiotherapy (14 of 18 patients) although major breaks were not necessary. One patients developed radiation pericarditis requiring a pericardial window. An arterial thrombosis occurred in one patient and a subclavian venous thrombosis occurred in a second.

The first "debulking" course of chemotherapy provided subjective swallowing improvement in 15 of 19 evaluable patients. Nine patients had an increase in weight (>1.5 kg), five maintained their weight, and five lost weight. Objective radiographic improvement was seen in 13 of 19 patients although most responses were minor (one complete remission, four partial remissions, eight minor responses, one progressive disease). Concomitant chemotherapy and radiotherapy was associated with weight loss in most patients (11 lost weight, three were stable, and three gained weight). Objective radiographic improvement was seen in 16 of 17 evaluable patients (six complete remissions, ten partial remissions, and one progressive disease).

Sixteen patients underwent esophagogastrostomy without significant surgical morbidity or mortality. Surgical pathology revealed no tumor in five, microscopic foci or minimal disease in six, and gross disease in five. Positive lymph nodes were found in only two patients. Surgical pathological findings were not predictive of outcome. Three of five patients with no residual tumor, two of six with minimal tumor, and three of five with gross residual tumor remain disease-free.

The multimodal group was compared with 21 consecutive historical patients treated initially with surgery (17) and/or radiotherapy (6) with chemotherapy on relapse (18). Survival was inferior to the multimodal group (Fig. 31.1).

Despite the improved survival in the multimodal group, several late relapses have occurred. Relapses have involved the anastomosis in four patients.

31.4 Discussion

Multimodal therapy in adenocarcinoma of the GEJ appears superior to surgery and/or radiotherapy as assessed by reference to recent historical patients. Although comparison between these two populations may not be completely valid, a randomized study of two radically different therapeutic approaches is unlikely to be undertaken.

Debulking chemotherapy appears to be successful at both predicting tumor response and improving oral intake as evidenced by weight gain in the majority of patients.

Concomitant chemotherapy and radiotherapy may have improved local tumor response. Myelo-

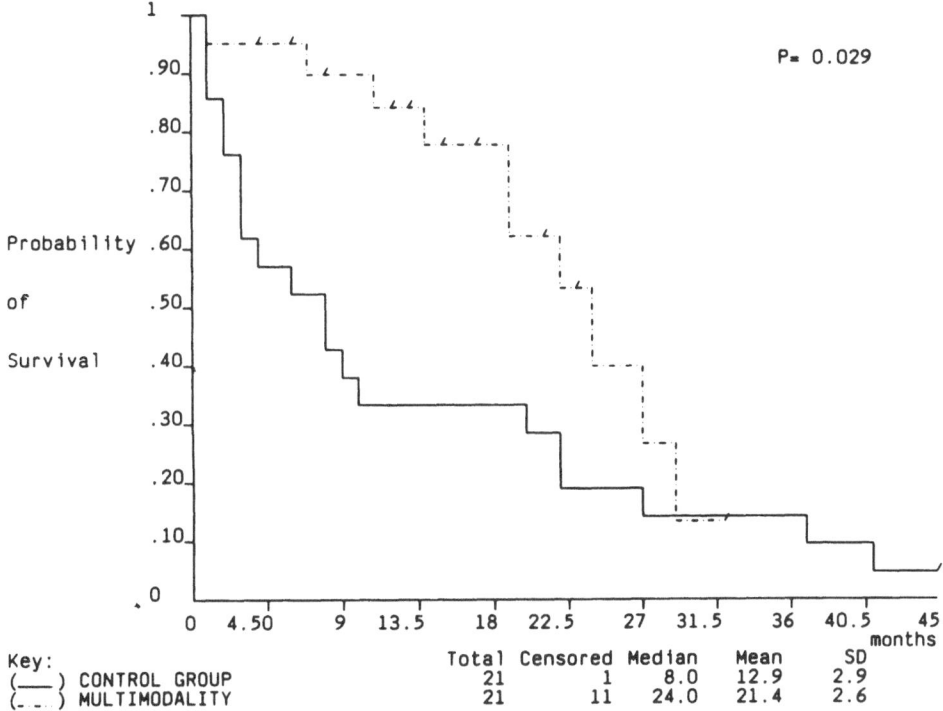

P= 0.029

Key:	Total	Censored	Median	Mean	SD
(——) CONTROL GROUP	21	1	8.0	12.9	2.9
(_ _ _) MULTIMODALITY	21	11	24.0	21.4	2.6

suppression, although increased, was acceptable. Esophagitis was seen in all patients, but was also acceptable. Late local relapse was seen in several patients, which suggest local therapy was inadequate. Possible solutions include total gastric radiotherapy or total gastrectomy.

This multimodal program for GEJ adenocarcinoma provides improved survival as compared with historical controls. Late relapse continues to be a problem, which suggests that alternative approaches should be used in future trials.

Fig. 31.1. Survival curves comparing multimodal patients and historical control patients

References

Byfield J, Calabro-Jones P, Klisak I, Kulhanian F (1982) Pharmacologic requirements for obtaining sensitization of human tumor cells in vitro to combined 5-fluorouracil and x-rays. Int J Radiat Oncol Biol Phys 8: 1923–1933

Fein R, Kelsen D, Geller N, Bains M, McCormack P, Brennan M (1985) Adenocarcinoma of the esophagus and gastroesophageal junction. Cancer 56: 2512–2518

Mahoney J, Condon R (1987) Adenocarcinoma of the esophagus. Ann Surg 205: 557–562

Poplin E, Fleming T, Leichman L et al. (1987) Combined therapies for squamous-cell carcinoma of the esophagus, a Southwest Oncology Group study. J Clin Oncol 5: 622–628

Richmond R, Zimbrick J, Hykes D (1977) Radiation induced DNA damage and lethality in *E. coli* as modified by the antitumor agent cis-dichlorodiammineplatinum(II). Radiat Res 71: 447–460

Turnbull A, Goodner J (1969) Primary adenocarcinoma of the esophagus. Cancer 22: 915–917

Vietti T, Eggerding F, Valeriote F (1971) Combined effect of x-radiation and 5-fluorouracil on survival of transplanted leukemic cells. JNCI 47: 865–870

32 Efficacy of 5-Fluorouracil by Continuous Infusion and Other Agents as Radiopotentiators for Gynecological Malignancies

PERRY W. GRIGSBY and CARLOS A. PEREZ

CONTENTS

32.1 Introduction

Failure to control tumor in the pelvis occurs in about 60% of patients dying of cervical cancer (BRADY et al. 1988; PEREZ et al. 1988b). Local control is also a significant problem in patients with advanced carcinoma of the vulva, vagina, and endometrium (PAO et al. 1988; PEREZ et al. 1988a; GRIGSBY et al. 1987). Modifications of conventional irradiation with misonidazole (MEOZ et al. 1983), hyperbaric oxygen (BRADY et al. 1981), neutrons (MORALES et al. 1981), altered fractionation schedules (WANG 1987), hydroxyurea (PIVER et al. 1987b), and chemotherapy (LIPSZTEIN et al. 1987) have had limited success in increasing pelvic control rates of patients with advanced gynecological malignancies.

5-Fluorouracil (5-FU) has been demonstrated to be an effective radiopotentiator in animal studies (VIETTI et al. 1971; LOONEY et al. 1979). This drug has also been shown to have limited effectiveness

PERRY W. GRIGSBY, MD, Associate Professor, Radiation Oncology Center, CARLOS A. PEREZ, MD, FACR, Professor, Director, Radiation Oncology Center, Mallinckrodt Institute of Radiology, Washington University School of Medicine, 510 S. Kingshighway, St. Louis. MO 63110, USA

when used as single-agent chemotherapy for patients with advanced or recurrent gynecological tumors (DEVITA et al. 1976; WASSERMAN and CARTER 1977).

Cisplatin has also been shown to be a radiation sensitizer. It is also effective as single-agent therapy for advanced or recurrent carcinoma of the cervix (THIGPEN et al. 1981). Cisplatin combined with other chemotherapeutic agents has also been shown to be an effective method of treating advanced cervical carcinoma (ROSENTHAL et al. 1983).

Patients with carcinoma of the cervix treated with irradiation alone have a greater local tumor control and a decreased incidence of distant metastasis when a complete tumor response following initial therapy is achieved in the pelvis (PEREZ et al. 1988b). The rationale for the use of 5-FU and other agents combined with pelvic irradiation is to enhance local tumor control and thereby increase overall cure rates. There is also a potential direct effect of chemotherapy on micrometastatic disease. In this chapter we will review the results of the use of 5-FU (with and without other drugs) by continuous infusion as a radiopotentiator.

32.2 Overview of Treatment Schemas

Multiple treatment schemas have been developed for using 5-FU as a radiopotentiator (Table 32.1). Only two studies, SMITH et al. (1972) and MALKASIAN et al. (1977), have employed irradiation and 5-FU alone for patients with cervical carcinoma. Most investigators have used this combination in conjunction with cisplatin or mitomycin C. As shown in Table 32.1, the most prevalent dose of 5-FU administered in recent studies is 1000 mg/m^2/day by continuous infusion for 1–4 days and for one to three cycles. Mitomycin C is given at 6–10 mg/m^2 as a bolus injection for one or two cycles. Cisplatin was given in only the Mallinckrodt

Table 32.1. Schema for concomitant 5-FU and radiotherapy

Authors	Pelvic irradiation	Intracavitary irradiation	Chemotherapy	
			5-FU	Other agents
SMITH et al. 1972	50 Gy/5 wks	No	10 mg/kg/d d 1–15 1 cycle	No
THOMAS et al. 1984	45.6 Gy/28 Fx or, 45.6 Gy/28 Fx + 3600/24 Fx to para-aortic nodes	× 1	1000 mg/m² /d i.v. d 1–4, d 35–38	Mitomycin C 6 mg/m² i.v. d 1, d 35
JOHN et al. 1987	36 Gy/20 Fx	× 2, 200 mgh ea	1000 mg/m² /d i.v. d 1–4 (of weeks 2 and 7)	Mitomycin C 10 mg/m² d 1 (of wk 2) Cisplatin 75 mg/m² d 2 (of wk 7)
EVANS et al. 1988	50 Gy/5 wks	× 1	1000 mg/m² i.v. d 1–4 1 cycle	Mitomycin C 10 mg/m² i.v. d 1
LUDGATE et al. 1988	46–50 Gy/5–6 wks	× 1	1000 mg/m² /d d 2–5, d 21–24	Mitomycin C 10 mg/m² d 1
KUSKE et al. 1989	50–60 Gy/6–7 wks	× 2	750 mg/m² /d d 1–5, d 22–26, d 43–47	Cisplatin 75 mg/m² d 1, d 22, d 43
GRIGSBY and PEREZ Present series	50–60 Gy/6–7 wks	× 2	100 mg/m² /d d 1–4, d 22–25, d 43–46	Cisplatin 100 mg/m² d 1, d 22, d 43
ROBERTS et al. 1989	45 Gy/5 wks	× 2	1000 mg/m² /d d 1–4, d 29–32, d 57–60	Cisplatin 50 mg/m² d 1, d 29, d 57

series, initially at 50 mg/m² as a drip infusion for three cycles then subsequently increased to 75 mg/m² per cycle.

Misonidazole has been administered at 4 g/m² 4–6 h prior to single-fraction irradiation (10 Gy) and repeated at 3-week intervals for a total of three courses (MEOZ et al. 1983). Oral hydroxyurea is usually administered at 80 mg/kg every 3 days during irradiation (PIVER et al. 1985; MADOC-JONES et al. 1980; STEHMAN et al. 1988).

In the randomized Radiation Therapy Oncology Group (RTOG) study, LEIBEL and co-workers (1987) randomized patients with stage III-B or IV-A squamous cell carcinoma of the cervix or irradiation alone or irradiation and misonidazole (400 mg/m² daily 2–4 h prior to radiation therapy). The Gynecologic Oncology Group (GOG) administered hydroxyurea (80 mg/kg every 3 days, 2 h before irradiation) or misonidazole (1 g/m² every 3 days, 4 h before irradiation) to patients with stage II-B, III, or IV-A cervical carcinoma (STEHMAN et al. 1988).

Cisplatin has been employed weekly during irradiation at 20–25 mg/m² (TWIGGS et al. 1986; LIPSZTEIN et al. 1987). Twice weekly cisplatin at 25 mg/m² during irradiation has also been investi-

gated (WONG et al. 1989). Concomitant weekly cisplatin and irradiation has been followed by prolonged combination chemotherapy consisting of cisplatin (40 mg/m²), Adriamycin (40 mg/m²), and cyclophosphamide (400 mg/m²) at monthly intervals (PIVER et al. 1987a) or cisplatin (50 mg/m²) plus cyclophosphamide (400 mg/m²) at monthly intervals (HAIE et al. 1988). Concomitant weekly cisplatin (25 mg/m²) with irradiation has been preceded by combination chemotherapy consisting of cisplatin (50 mg/m², q 3 weeks x 2), vincristine (1 mg/m², q 3 weeks x 2), mitomycin C (10 mg/m² x 1), and bleomycin (10 units, q week x 6) (LIPSZTEIN et al. 1987). Combination chemotherapy during irradiation consisting of cisplatin (100 mg/m² q 3 weeks x 3), bleomycin (30 mg/m² q 3 weeks x 3), and mitomycin C (6 mg/m² q 6 weeks x 2) has been attempted in a limited number of patients (GORDON and LYNCH 1988).

32.3 Toxicity

The intra-arterial administration of 5-FU with pelvic irradiation by SMITH et al. (1972) resulted in severe toxicity in 35% (6/17) of their patients. The planned course of therapy was completed in 84%. Hematological toxicity was not reported separately and most of the toxicity was related to the placement of the intra-arterial catheter.

Thomas et al. (1984, 1987) treated 35 patients with concurrent irradiation, mitomycin C, and 5-FU for advanced or recurrent cervical carcinoma. Transient leukopenia and/or thrombocytopenia occurred in 31% (11/35). Sigmoid strictures occurred in two patients (one requiring surgery), and another patient died following a sigmoid perforation. Severe or life-threatening neutropenia developed in 12% (3/25) of the patients reported by Evans et al. (1988). The incidence of severe non-hematological toxicity in their report was 28% (7/25).

Ludgate et al. (1988) have distinguished those patients having acute versus chronic severe non-hematological toxicity and reported the incidence of toxicity to be 3% (1/38) and 5% (2/38), respectively. In a recent update, John et al. (1989) reported an 11% (4/36) incidence of grade 3 non-hematological toxicity and an 11% incidence of reversible grade 4 hematological toxicity. No deaths were reported to be related to toxicity.

A prospective study currently in progress at the Mallinckrodt Institution of Radiology, Radiation Oncology Center, employs definitive irradiation and concurrent cisplatin and 5-FU. In the initial phase of the study the first 23 patients received three courses of chemotherapy (3 weeks apart) consisting of a drip infusion of cisplatin at 50 mg/m^2 and a 5-day infusion of 5-FU at 750 mg/m^2 (Kuske et al. 1989). Only 18 of 23 patients completed therapy, with one-half having a delay in either irradiation or chemotherapy. Grade 2 and 3 sequelae consisted of a pulmonary embolus in two cases (one fatal), and one case of severe proctitis, vesicovaginal fistula, bowel obstruction, lower extremity edema, nausea and vomiting, hypocalcemia, and leukopenia. The overall severe complication rate was 35% (8/23) with a minimum follow-up of 1 year. In the second phase of the study the cisplatin dose was increased to 75 mg/m^2 and the 5-FU dose was changed to 1000 mg/m^2 (for 4 days continuous infusion). In this second group 17 of 24 completed therapy and one-third had a delay in therapy of 1 week or longer. Three patients developed leukopenia (granulocytes <1000/mm^3). Additional severe complications occurred in nine patients, with one having diarrhea, one perirectal ulcers and diarrhea, one small bowel obstruction, two a rectovaginal fistula, one a vesicovaginal fis-

tula, and three moist desquamation. The overall severe complication rate in this second group was 46% (11/24, some with more than one complication) with 0.5–1.7 years' follow-up. An additional six patients with less than 6 months' follow-up have been treated, with one dying from severe leukopenia and pneumonia.

The toxicity of combined misonidazole and single-fraction irradiation (10 Gy q 3 weeks x 3) was severe nausea and vomiting in 27%, neurotoxicity in 23%, and 27% with severe gastrointestinal, genitourinary, and gynecological complications (Meoz et al. 1983).

In the RTOG study for stages III-B and IV-A cervical cancer (Leibel et al. 1987) grades 3 and 4, complications from misonidazole were noted in only 5% (3/58), a rate not significantly different from that in patients receiving irradiation alone.

Of 157 patients receiving misonidazole q 3 days, 17 (11%) suffered grade 3 or 4 toxicity which was mostly gastrointestinal (Stehman et al. 1988). Hydroxyurea administered at 80 mg/kg q 3 days caused severe toxicity in 15%–24% of patients and was primarily gastrointestinal (Piver et al. 1983, 1985, 1987b; Stehman et al. 1988). At the Mallinckrodt Institute of Radiology only one of 28 patients with advanced cervical cancer who were randomized to receive hydroxyurea completed the drug regime per protocol. Of those not completing the protocol 12 had severe gastrointestinal or bone marrow toxicity, 12 had dose reductions due to gastrointestinal and bone marrow toxicity, and three refused to take the drug (Madoc-Jones et al. 1980).

Weekly cisplatin at 20–25 mg/kg is associated with a severe toxicity rate of about 10% (Monyak et al. 1988). When concurrent irradiation and weekly cisplatin was followed by combination chemotherapy, the toxicity rate was about 20% at 4 years after completion of therapy (Haie et al. 1988). Piver et al. (1987a) treated nine patients with concurrent weekly cisplatin and pelvic and para-aortic irradiation followed by cisplatin, Adriamycin, and cyclophosphamide. Acute toxicity occurred in two and none developed long-term complications. In the randomized study by Wong et al. (1989) there was a significantly higher severe complication rate in those receiving irradiation and chemotherapy than in those receiving irradiation alone. Severe leukopenia causing a delay in radiotherapy occurred in 12/39 (31%), and 7/39 (18%) developed severe anemia (Hgb <89%) in the combined therapy group. None of the patient treated with irradiation alone developed severe leukopenia or anemia. One patient treated with radiotherapy alone had proctitis and one developed a vesicovaginal fistula. Only one of five patients treated with combined irradiation and cisplatin, bleomycin, and mitomycin C developed a severe complication in the series reported by GORDON and LYNCH (1988).

32.4 Clinical Response and Survival

32.4.1 Primary Cervical Cancer

Table 32.2 is a summary of the results of treatment of patients with previously untreated advanced cervical cancer. In most studies the follow-up time is limited and, therefore, 5-year survival data are unavailable. Control rates in the pelvis as well as the rates of distant metastasis are variable due to the limited follow-up time. Combining all patients, Table 32.2 shows a 61% (93/153) progression-free survival rate, 12% (18/153) alive with tumor, and 25% (39/153) dead of disease. Death due to com-

plications of therapy occurred in 2% (3/153). A total of 53 patients had a recurrence; 40% failed in the pelvis alone, 42% failed with only distant metastasis, and 19% failed with both local recurrence and distant metastasis.

The RTOG studied the use of radiotherapy alone versus radiotherapy plus misonidazole for patients with stage III-B or IV-A cervical cancer (LEIBEL et al. 1987). The median survival was 1.9 years for those receiving radiotherapy alone versus 1.6 years for those receiving radiotherapy plus misonidazole (Table 32.3).

The use of palliative large-fraction irradiation and misonidazole was also studied by the RTOG (MEOZ et al. 1983). Of four patients with advanced cervical cancer there was one with a complete response, one with a partial response, and two with no response in the pelvis.

Multiple randomized and nonrandomized studies have used concomitant irradiation and hydroxyurea (Table 32.3). HRESHCHYSHYN (1979) reported the results of GOG #4, in which patients with stage III-B or IV-A cervical cancer were

Table 32.2. Results of radiotherapy and concomitant 5-FU for patients with advanced cervical cancer

Authors	No. of patients	Disease	Follow-up time	Status				Death due to complication	Site of recurrence		
				NED	AWD	DID	DOD		Pelvis only	Pelvis + DM	DM only
SMITH et al. 1972	17	Advanced cervix	2–5 yrs	7	3	–	7	–	7	–	2
THOMAS et al. 1984	27	Advanced cervix	4–24 mo	16	5	–	5	1	7[a]	1	2
JOHN et al. 1987	10	Advanced cervix	6–37 mo	8	1	–	1	–	–	1	1
EVANS et al. 1988	10	Advanced cervix	7–38 mo	7	–	–	3	–	1	–	2
LUDGATE et al. 1988	38	Advanced cervix	5–36 mo	26	1	–	10	1	3	2	6
KUSKE et al. 1989	15	Advanced cervix	12–36 mo	8	2	–	4	1	2[a]	1	4
ROBERTS et al. 1989	18	Advanced cervix		9	4	–	5	–	1	3	1
GRIGSBY and PEREZ Present series	18	Advanced cervix	6–20 mo	12	2	–	4	–	–	2	4
Total	153			93 (61%)	18 (12%)		39 (25%)	3 (2%)	21 (14%)	10 (7%)	22 (14%)

Abbreviations: NED, no evidence of disease; AWD, alive with disease; DID, dead of intercurrent disease; DOD, dead of disease; DM, distant metastasis
[a] One patient NED after pelvic exenteration

Table 32.3. Results of radiotherapy and concomitant misonidazole or hydroxyurea for patients with cervical cancer

Authors	No. of patients	Stage	Follow-up time	Status				Death due to complication	Site of recurrence		
				NED	AWD	DID	DOD		Pelvis only	Pelvis + DM	DM only
PIVER et al. 1983											
RT	20	II-B	5–9 yrs	8	–	1	9	2	Data not available		
RT + hydroxyurea	20	II-B	5–9 yrs	12	–	3	1	4	Data not available		
PIVER et al. 1985	20	II-B	6–83 mo	17	1	1	1	–	–	1	1
PIVER et al. 1987											
RT	25	III-B		52% 5-yr progression-free					Data not available		
RT + hydroxyurea	20	III-B		60% 5-yr progression-free					Data not available		
STEHMAN et al. 1988											
Hydroxyurea	139	II-B–IV-A		43 months median progression-free interval					37 Data not available		
Misonidazole	157	II-B–IV-A		40 month median progression-free interval					25 Data not available		
LEIBEL et al. 1987	61	III-B–IV-A	Median 33 months	25	–	–	36	–	11	17	6[a]
RT	58	III-B–IV-A	Median 33 months	20	–	–	38	–	14	13	8[a]
RT + misonidazole											
HRESHCHYSHYN 1979											
RT	46	III-B–IV-A		7.6 month median progression-free interval							
RT + hydroxyurea	51	III-B–IV-A		13.6 month median progression-free interval							

[a] Site unknown in five patients

randomized to receive radiation and hydroxyurea or radiation and placebo. The complete response rate in the pelvis was 68% (32/47) for hydroxyurea compared with 49% (21/43) for placebo. The overall and disease-free survivals were significantly improved for those patients receiving hydroxyurea. The median survival for the hydroxyurea patients was 19.5 months versus 10.7 months for those receiving the placebo.

After completion of the above study a second GOG study randomized patients with stage II-B to IV-A cervical cancer to receive radiotherapy and hydroxyurea or radiotherapy and misonidazole (STEHMAN et al. 1988). In that study there was no difference in the progression-free survival by treatment group. The median survival was 42.9 months for hydroxyurea and 40.4 months for misonidazole. The pelvic failure rate was 18.0% for hydroxyurea and 23.6% for misonidazole.

PIVER et al. (1983) reported on a prospective study of patients with stage II-B cervical cancer with negative para-aortic lymph nodes by pretherapy staging laparotomy. The 5-year progression-free survival was 94% for those receiving hydroxyurea versus 53% for those given a placebo ($P = 0.06$) (PIVER et al. 1983). In a second study by PIVER et al. (1985) stage II-B patients without a pretherapy staging laparotomy (but negative lymphangiograms) all received radiotherapy plus hydroxyurea. The 5-year progression-free survival was 92%. A further study was performed by PIVER et al. (1987b) in stage III-B cervical carcinoma where patients with negative para-aortic lymph nodes (by staging laparotomy) were randomized to receive radiotherapy with hydroxyurea or placebo. The 5-year progression-free survival was 60% for the hydroxyurea arm and 52% for the placebo arm ($P = 0.49$).

The use of weekly cisplatin combined with irradiation has been reported by several investigators. The results of these studies are summarized in Table 32.4. There is no apparent advantage to the use of weekly cisplatin combined with irradiation in these studies. There is only one randomized study comparing weekly cisplatin, twice weekly cisplatin, and irradiation alone (WONG et al. 1989). This study showed no significant difference in progression-free survival between the three study arms ($P = 0.83$). However, MONYAK et al. (1988) did report an impressive 2-year survival of 59% in their patients with positive para-aortic nodes.

32.4.2 Recurrent Cervical Cancer After Primary Surgery

Table 32.5 demonstrates the short-term results of concomitant irradiation and chemotherapy for patients with a pelvic recurrence after a hysterectomy for primary cervical cancer. A summary for these patients shows 52% (14/27) to be alive with-

out evidence of disease and 48% to be dead of recurrent disease. Of the 13 patients wtih recurrent disease, 11 failed in the pelvis (with or without distant disease) and eight failed with distant metastasis (with or without a pelvic recurrence).

32.4.3 Other Gynecological Malignancies

Only a few patients with advanced or recurrent carcinoma of the vagina, vulva, or endometrium have been treated with irradiation and continuous infusion 5-FU. Table 32.6 summarizes the results of therapy for this group of patients. Combining the series, analysis shows three of seven with vaginal carcinoma to be free of disease, four of seven with vulvar carcinoma to be alive without tumor, two patients with endometrial cancer to be dead of disease, and one patient with endometrial cancer to be dead of intercurrent disease. All three patients with vaginal cancer and all three patients with vulvar cancer who failed, did so only in the

Table 32.4. Results of radiotherapy and concomitant weekly cisplatin for patients with cervical cancer

Authors	No. of patients	Stage	Follow-up time	Status				Death due to complication	Site of recurrence		
				NED	AWD	DID	DOD		Pelvis only	Pelvis + DM	DM only
LIPSZTEIN et al. 1987	2	I-B (barrel)		2	–	–	–	–	–	–	–
	5	II-B	11–26 mo	4	1	–	–	–	–	1	–
	3	III-B		1	1	–	1	–	1	–	–
PIVER et al. 1987a	9	Paraaortic nodes positive	12–25 mo	2	2	–	5	–	2	–	5
MONYAK et al. 1988	11	I-B	6 mo–	52%	3-year	relapse-free	–		–	–	–
	13	II-B	4 yrs	survival							
	11	III									
	3	IV-A		1	–	–	2	–	–	–	–
	11	IV-B		–	–	–	11	–	–	–	–
HAIE et al. 1988	24	III		44% 4-year overall survival				–	56% 4-year locoregional ± DM		
	1	IV-A		28% 4-year overall survival				–	83% 4-year locoregional		
	11	IV-B							± DM failure rate		
WONG et al. 1989											
RT only	15	II-B		13	–	–	12	–	4	5	3
	10	III-B									
RT + wkly cisplatin	17	II-B		10	1	–	11	–	4	4	4
	2	III-A									
	3	III-B									
RT + twice wkly cisplatin	13	II-B		10	1	–	6	–	3	3	1
	1	III-A									
	3	III-B									

Table 32.5. Results of radiotherapy and concomitant 5-FU for patients with recurrent cervical cancer following primary surgery

Authors	No. of patients	Disease	Follow-up time	Status				Death due to complication	Site of recurrence		
				NED	AWD	DID	DOD		Pelvis only	Pelvis + DM	DM only
THOMAS et al. 1987	17	Recurrent cervix	21–58 mo	8	–	–	9	–	4	4	1
KUSKE et al. 1989	4	Recurrent cervix	12–36 mo	3	–	–	1	–	–	–	1
ROBERTS et al. 1989	2	Recurrent cervix		–	–	–	2	–	1	1	–
GRIGSBY and PEREZ Present series	4	Recurrent cervix	6–17 mo	3	–	–	1	–	–	1	–
Total	27			14 (52%)			13 (48%)		5 (19%)	6 (22%)	2 (7%)

Table 32.6. Results of radiotherapy and concomitant 5-FU for patients with carcinoma of the vagina, vulva, and endometrium

Authors	No. of patients	Disease	Follow-up time	Status				Death due to complication	Site of recurrence		
				NED	AWD	DID	DOD		Pelvis only	Pelvis + DM	DM only
EVANS et al. 1988	7	Advanced vagina	8–39 mo	3	1	1	2	–	3	–	–
EVANS et al. 1988	4	Advanced vaulva	8–29 mo	2	1	–	1	–	2	–	–
KUSKE et al. 1989	2	vulva	12–36 mo	1	1	–	–	–	1	–	–
GRIGSBY and PEREZ Present series	1	Recurrent vulva	6 mo	1	–	–	–	–	–	–	–
KUSKE et al. 1989	2	Endo-metrium	12–36 mo	–	–	1	1	–	–	1	–
GRIGSBY and PEREZ Present series	1	Endo-metrium	7 mo	–	–	–	1	–	–	1	–

pelvis. Both patients with endometrial cancer who failed had distant metastasis in addition to a pelvic failure.

32.5 Current Clinical Trials

Only a limited number of clinical trials are currently available in the United States for patients with advanced or recurrent gynecological malignancies which involve the use of 5-FU as a radio-potentiator. The RTOG recently closed its study [RTOG-85-15, Phase II Nonrandomized Infusion Chemotherapy (5-FU, Mitomycin C, Cisplatin) and Radiotherapy for Advanced Carcinoma of the Cervix]. The study accrued 50 patients and only the preliminary toxicity results have been reported (JOHN et al. 1989).

A review of the National Cancer Institute PDQ database discloses only one current nationally funded phase III protocol, which is sponsored by the GOG (GOG-85) and is a randomized comparison of 5-FU and cisplatin versus hydroxyurea as potentiators of radiotherapy in patients with stage II-B, III, or IV-A carcinoma of the uterine cervix with negative para-aortic lymph nodes by staging laparotomy. Approximately 300 patients have been entered into this protocol and the results are pending.

The Radiation Oncology Center, Mallinckrodt Institute of Radiology, has accrued a total of 52 patients with advanced or recurrent carcinoma of the cervix, vulva, vagina, and endometrium to a study in progress using 5-FU and cisplatin as radio-potentiators. The University of Virginia Medical Center is also continuing its nonrandomized study (Evans et al. 1988) of irradiation plus continuous infusion 5-FU and bolus mitomycin C for patients with advanced gynecological malignancies.

32.6 Summary

Pelvic recurrence is a significant problem for patients with advanced carcinoma of the cervix, vagina, vulva, and endometrium. In this chapter we have presented a summary of the results of therapy for these patients. Most studies employing radiotherapy and concomitant 5-FU also utilize cisplatin and/or mitomycin C. These combinations result in a severe toxicity rate in the range of 30% – 40%, which is 10% – 20% higher than historical results for patients treated with radiotherapy alone for advanced cervical cancer (Perez et al. 1986; Montana et al. 1986; Souhami et al. 1987). Short-term survival results for those with advanced or recurrent cervical cancer are slightly higher than expected when compared with historical studies (Perez et al. 1986; Larson et al. 1988). These survival results may decrease with longer follow-up. There are no currently available randomized clinical trials comparing irradiation alone and irradiation plus concomitant 5-FU for patients with advanced gynecological malignancies. Misonidazole combined with irradiation offers no survival advantage over radiotherapy alone or radiotherapy plus hydroxyurea. Hydroxyurea appears to increase the pelvic control rate compared with irradiation alone and may provide an improved progression-free and overall survival. Weekly cisplatin with or without other agents does not appear to be more effective than radiotherapy alone.

References

Brady LW, Plenk HP, Hanley JA, Glassburn JR, Kramer S, Parker RG (1981) Hyperbaric oxygen therapy for carcinoma of the cervix – stages IIB, IIIA, IIIB and IVA: results of a randomized study by the Radiation Therapy Oncology Group. Int J Radiat Oncol Biol Phys 7: 991–998

Brady LW, Markow AM, DeEulis T, Lewis GC (1988) Gynecology: combined radiotherapy and chemotherapy in gynecologic oncology. Int J Radiat Oncol Biol Phys 14: S203–S209

DeVita V, Wasserman T, Young R, Carter S (1976) Perspectives on research in gynecologic oncology. Cancer 38: 509–525

Evans L, Kersh C, Constable W, Taylor P (1988) Concomitant 5-fluorouracil, mitomycin-C and radiotherapy for advanced gynecologic malignancies. Int J Radiat Oncol Biol Phys 15: 901–906

Gordon AN, Lynch GR (1988) Multi-agent chemotherapy in combination with fractioned radiation therapy for advanced carcinoma of the cervix: acute toxicity. Eur J Gynaecol Oncol 9: 351–354

Grigsby PW, Perez CA, Kuske RR, Kao MS, Galakatos AE (1987) Results of therapy, analysis of failures, and prognostic factors for clinical and pathologic stage III adenocarcinoma of the endometrium. Gynecol Oncol 27: 44–57

Haie C, George M, Pejovic MH et al. (1988) Feasibility study of an alternating schedule of radiotherapy and chemotherapy in advanced uterine cervical carcinoma. Radiother Oncol 12: 121–127

Hreshchyshyn MM (1979) Hydroxyurea or placebo combined with radiation to treat stages IIIB and IV cervical cancer confined to the pelvis. Int J Radiat Oncol Biol Phys 5: 317–322

John M, Cooke K, Flam M, Padmanabhan A, Mowry P (1987) Preliminary results of concomitant radiotherapy and chemotherapy in advanced cervical carcinoma. Gynecol Oncol 28: 101–110

John M, Flam M, Sikic B et al. (1989) Preliminary results of concurrent radiotherapy and chemotherapy in advanced cervical carcinoma: a phase II prospective intergroup NCOG-RTOG study. Proc ASCO 8: 157

Kuske R, Perez C, Grigsby P, Lovett R, Jacobs A, Galakatos A, Camel H, Kao M (1989) Phase I/II study of definitive radiotherapy and chemotherapy (cisplatin and 5-fluorouracil) for advanced or recurrent gynecologic malignancies, preliminary report. Am J Clin Oncol (CCT) 12: 467–473

Larson D, Copeland L, Stringer C, Gershenson D, Malone J, Edwards C (1988) Recurrent cervical carcinoma after radical hysterectomy. Gynecol Oncol 30: 381–387

Leibel S, Bauer M, Wasserman T et al. (1987) Radiotherapy with or without misonidazole for patients with stage IIIB or stage IVA squamous cell carcinoma of the uterine cervix: preliminary report of a Radiation Therapy Oncology Group randomized trial. Int J Radiat Oncol Biol Phys 13: 541–549

Lipsztein R, Kredenster K, Dottino P, Goodman H, Dalton J, Bloomer W, Cohen C (1987) Combined chemotherapy and radiation therapy for advanced carcinoma of the cervix. Am J Clin Oncol (CCT) 10: 527–530

Looney WB, Hopkins HA, MacLeod MS, Ritenour R (1979) Solid tumor models for the assessment of different treatment modalities, XII. Combined chemotherapy-radiotherapy: variation of time interval between time of administration of 5-fluorouracil and radiation and its effects on the control of tumor growth. Cancer 44: 437–445

Ludgate S, Crandon A, Hudson C, Walker Q, Langlands A (1988) Synchronous 5-fluorouracil, mytomycin-C and radiation therapy in the treatment of locally advanced carcinoma of the cervix. Int J Radiat Oncol Biol Phys 15: 893–899

Madoc-Jones H, Perez C, Camel M, Jennings F (1980) Preliminary experience in a prospective randomized trial to assess the value of hydroxyurea in addition to conventional radiotherapy in the management of advanced stages of carcinoma of the uterine cervix. Int J Radiat Oncol Biol Phys 6: 1430

Malkasian GD, Decker DG, Jorgensen EO (1977) Chemotherapy of carcinoma of the cervix. Gynecol Oncol 5: 109–120

Meoz RT, Spanos WJ, Doss L, Johnson R, Wasserman TH (1983) Misonidazole combined with large-fraction pelvic irradiation in the treatment of patients with advanced pelvic malignancies, preliminary report of an ongoing RTOG phase I-II study. Am J Clin Oncol 6: 417–422

Montana G, Fowler W, Varia M, Walton L, Mack Y, Shemanski L (1986) Carcinoma of the cervix, stage III: results of radiation therapy. Cancer 57: 148–154

Monyak DJ, Twiggs LB, Potish RA et al. (1988) Tolerance and preliminary results of simultaneous therapy with radiation and cisplatin for advanced cervical cancer. NCI Monogr 6: 369–373

Morales P, Hussey DH, Maor MH, Hamberger AD, Fletcher GH, Wharton JT (1981) Preliminary report of the M.D. Anderson Hospital randomized trial of neutron and photon irradiation for locally advanced carcinoma of the uterine cervix. Int J Radiat Oncol Biol Phys 7: 1533–1540

Pao WM, Perez CA, Kuske RR, Sommers GM, Camel HM, Galakatos AE (1988) Radiation therapy and conservation surgery for primary and recurrent carcinoma of the vulva: report of 40 patients and a review of the literature. Int J Radiat Oncol Biol 14: 1123–1132

Perez C, Camel H, Kuske R, Kao MS, Galakatos A, Hederman M, Powers W (1986) Radiation therapy alone in the treatment of carcinoma of the uterine cervix: a 20-year experience. Gynecol Oncol 23: 127–140

Perez CA, Camel HM, Galakatos AE, Grigsby PW, Kuske RR, Buchsbaum G, Hederman MA (1988a) Definitive irradiation in carcinoma of the vagina: long-term evaluation of results. Int J Radiat Oncol Biol Phys 15: 1283–1290

Perez CA, Kuske RR, Camel HM, Galakatos AE, Hederman MA, Kao M-S, Walz BJ (1988b) Analysis of pelvic tumor control and impact on survival in carcinoma of the uterine cervix treated with radiation therapy alone. Int J Radiat Oncol Biol Phys 14: 613–621

Piver MS, Barlow JJ, Vongtama V, Blumenson L (1983) Hydroxyurea: a radiation potentiator in carcinoma of the uterine cervix. Am J Obstet Gynecol 147: 803–808

Piver MS, Krishnamsetty RM, Emrich LJ (1985) Survival of nonsurgically staged patients with negative lymphangiograms who had stage IIB carcinoma of the cervix treated by pelvic radiation plus hydroxyurea. Am J Obstet Gynecol 151: 1006–1008

Piver MS, Lele SB, Malfetano JH (1987a) Cis-diamminedichloroplatinum II based combination chemotherapy for the control of extensive paraaortic lymph node metastasis in cervical cancer. Gynecol Oncol 26:71–76

Piver M, Vongtama V, Emrich L (1987b) Hydroxyurea plus pelvic radiation versus placebo plus pelvic radiation in surgically staged stage III-B cervical cancer. J Surg Oncol 35: 129–134

Potish RA, Twiggs LB, Adcock LL, Savage JE, Prem, KA, Levitt SH (1986) Effect of cis-platinum on tolerance to radiation therapy in advanced cervical cancer. Am J Clin Oncol (CCT) 9: 387–391

Roberts WS, Kavanagh JJ, Greenberg H et al. (1989) Concomitant radiation therapy and chemotherapy in the treatment of advanced squamous carcinoma of the lower female genital tract. Gynecol Oncol 34: 183–186

Rosenthal CJ, Kulpateea N, Boyce J, Mehrotra S, Tamarin S (1983) Effective chemotherapy for advanced carcinoma of the cervix with bleomycin, cisplatin, vincristine, and methotrexate. Cancer 52: 2025–2030

Smith JP, Randall GE, Castro JR, Lindberg RD (1972) Hypogastric artery infusion and radiation therapy for advanced squamous cell carcinoma of the cervix. AJR 114: 110–115

Souhami L, Melo J, Pareja G (1987) The treatment of stage III carcinoma of the uterine cervix with telecobalt irradiation. Gynecol Oncol 28: 262–267

Stehman FB, Bundy BN, Keys H, Currie JL, Mortel R, Creasman WT (1988) A randomized trial of hydroxyurea versus misonidazole adjunct to radiation therapy in carcinoma of the cervix. Am J Obstet Gynecol 159: 87–94

Thigpen T, Vance RB, Balducci L, Blessing J (1981) Chemotherapy in the management of advanced or recurrent cervical and endometrial carcinoma. Cancer 48 [Suppl]: 658–665

Thomas G, Dembo A, Beale F et al. (1984) Concurrent radiation, mitomycin C and 5-fluorouracil in poor prognosis carcinoma of cervix: preliminary results of a phase I-II study. Int J Radiat Oncol Biol Phys 10: 1785–1790

Thomas G, Dembo A, Black B et al. (1987) Concurrent radiation and chemotherapy for carcinoma of the cervix recurrent after radical surgery. Gynecol Oncol 27: 254–260

Twiggs LB, Potish RA, McIntyre S, Adcock LL, Savage JE, Prem KA (1986) Concurrent weekly cis-platinum and radiotherapy in advanced cervical cancer: a preliminary dose escalating toxicity study. Gynecol Oncol 24: 143–148

Vietti T, Eggerding F, Valeriote F (1971) Combined effect of x radiation and 5-fluorouracil on survival of transplanted leukemic cells. JNCI 47: 865–870

Wang CC (1987) Altered fractionation radiation therapy for gynecologic cancers. Cancer 60: 2064–2067

Wasserman J, Carter S (1977) The integration of chemotherapy into combined modality treatment of solid tumors. Cancer Treat Rev 4: 25–46

Wong LC, Choo YC, Choy D, Sham JST, Ma HK (1989) Long-term, follow-up of potentiation of radiotherapy by cis-platinum in advanced cervical cancer. Gynecol Oncol 35: 159–163

**Section VI
Efficacy of Continuous Infusion Adriamycin
as a Radiation Potentiator**

33 Concomitant Continuous Infusion Adriamycin and Radiation: Evidence of Synergistic Effects in Soft Tissue Sarcomas

C. Julian Rosenthal and Marvin Rotman

CONTENTS

33.1 Introduction

The current lack of effective therapy against most malignant tumors in advanced stages is due, primarily, to its lack of specific cytotoxicity for neoplastic cells. In order to circumvent this problem various chemotherapeutic agents have been used in combinations aiming to increase their overall therapeutic index.

Potentiation of antineoplastic effects has also been sought from the combined administration of chemotherapy agents and radiation therapy (D'Angio et al. 1959). The benefit of radiation enhancement by chemotherapy agents has been described as additive or synergistic (Phillips al. and Fu 1976). The latter refers to a situation in which the effect of the combined treatment is greater than the sum of the cell kill expected from the two modalities administered alone. A para-meter termed the dose effect factor (DEF), defined as the ratio of radiation dose required in the absence of a drug to the radiation dose required to cause the same level of damage in its presence, was introduced to assess the sensitizing effect of various agents (Phillips et al. 1975; Byfield 1974). Among all antineoplastic agents the anthracyclines have the higher DEF for both neoplastic cells and normal tissues; consequently, their combination with radiation to large areas or vital structures could be lethal. However, preliminary clinical studies (Byfield et al. 1975; Chan et al. 1976) showed that single pulses of Adriamycin in conventional doses ($40-60$ mg/m^2 q 3 weeks) or in lower doses (12 mg/m^2) administered concurrently with radiation therapy were well tolerated.

In vitro studies (Shimoyama 1975) showed that increased exposure of tumor cells to Adriamycin yielded equal cytotoxic effect at one thousand fraction of the usual dose. Further, Adriamycin administered by continuous intravenous infusion for up to 96 h at a dose of 20 mg/m^2/24 h was found to have significantly less cardiotoxic effects (Legha et al. 1982). Based on these data, we postulated that concomitant administration of low dose Adriamycin in continuous infusion with daily pulses of radiotherapy to metastatic, recurrent, or unresectable malignant lesions could improve the therapeutic index of these two modalities of treatment.

At the time this study was started there were no clinical data concerning the use of Adriamycin in continuous infusion nor any reported clinical experience with the concomitant use of this drug in infusion and radiation therapy. For this reason this investigation was initially developed as a phase I study with three objectives: (a) to establish the dose and the duration of administration of Adriamycin infusion having the best therapeutic index; (b) to determine the dose of radiation which in combination with the optimal dose of Adriamycin administered by continuous infusion would have the best therapeutic index; (c) to establish the nature and the incidence of side-effects of these

C. Julian Rosenthal, MD, Professor of Medicine and Oncology, Marvin Rotman, MD, Professor and Chairman, Department of Radiation Oncology, SUNY Health Science Center at Brooklyn, 450 Clarkson Avenue, Brooklyn, NY 11203, USA

combined modalities of therapy. The therapeutic effect of the optimal Adriamycin infusion dose in combination with concomitant radiotherapy was then assessed in a preliminary phase II study; it was found to have a significant enhancing effect in a few cases of hepatoma and in most of the cases of recurrent and metastatic soft tissue sarcoma.

33.2 Materials and Methods

33.2.1 Patient Population

Thirty-six patients were entered in this study over a period of 36 months; 13 received Adriamycin infusion alone, and 23 received Adriamycin infusion and concomitant irradiation to some of the measurable lesions. Seven of 13 patients also had measurable lesions that did not receive radiation therapy; this permitted a comparison of the effect of combined modality treatment with that of Adriamycin infusion alone in the same patient. Active infections, cardiac arrhythmia, cardiac failure, and bone marrow suppression (platelet count $<10^5/\mu l$ and WBC count $<4 \times 10^3/\mu l$) were contraindications for entering patients in this study. There were 16 females and 20 males varying in age be-

tween 16 and 75 years. All patients had advanced metastatic and/or recurrent locoregional disease measurable by palpation, x-ray, or computerized tomography scan. All patients had pretreatment staging workup and had advanced metastatic or recurrent disease of various histologies and grades, with invasion of regional lymphatics or of neighboring structures (Table 33.1). Several patients had been treated previously by bolus injections of Adriamycin or had received limited radiation therapy >3 months prior to entry in this study to lesions that subsequently showed an unequivocal increase in size.

33.2.2 Therapeutic Regimen

Adriamycin was either (a) dissolved in 1000 ml of 5% dextrose solution in 0.5 N saline and delivered at a constant rate through silicone elastomer catheters (Deseret-Parke-Davis, Sandy, UT) inserted in the superior vena cava via the external jugular vein or (b) mixed with 60 ml of normal saline and delivered slowly into the subclavian vein through a Hickman catheter (CHAN et al. 1976) connected to a battery-activated pump (Cormed, Medina, NY).

Initially in the phase I study, Adriamycin was given at a dosage of 9 mg/m^2 per day, which had

Table 33.1. Patients' characteristics

Patient No.	Diagnosis	Primary site	Metastasis	Recurrence	Stage or grade	Performance status, (ECOG Scale)
1	Liposarcoma	Right arm	Lung		3	2
2	Synovial STS	Retroperitoneum	Lung, bones		3	2
3	Poorly different. STS	Retroperitoneum		×	3	2
4	Leiomyosarcoma	Left psoas	Liver		2	1
5	Leiomyosarcoma	Retroperitoneum		×	3	1
6	Leiomyosarcoma	Duodenum	Liver		2	0
7	Fibrosarcoma	Right Arm	Right axilla		3	1
8	Fibrohistiocytoma	Paraspinal area	Ribs, retroperitoneum		2	2
9	Leiomyosarcoma	Righ Thigh	Lung, mediastinum		3	1
10	Rhabdomyosarcoma	Thigh	Lungs	+	3	1
11	Fibrohistiocytoma	Retroperitoneum	Lung		3	2
12	Adenocarcinoma	Stomach	Abdominal wall		IV	2
13	Adenocarcinoma	Stomach	Abdominal wall		IV	3
14	Adenocarcinoma	Colon	Omentum		D	3
15	Adenocarcinoma	Colon	Pelvis, bones, thigh		D	2
16	Breast cancer	Breast	Breast, lung		IV	3
17	Breast cancer	Breast		×	IV	1
18	Breast cancer	Breast	Bones	×	IV	
19	Transitional cell ca.	Bladder	Pelvis, bones, thigh		D	3
20	Hepatoma	Liver		×	II	1
21	Hepatoma	Liver		×	I	1
22	Hepatoma	Liver	Omentum		III	1
23	Hepatoma	Liver	Omentum	×	II	2

been found to be appropriate in a prior study (Rosen et al., 1975) when given by continuous intraarterial infusion for 5 days and repeated every 3–4 weeks as soon as the bone marrow recovered. The dose was escalated every cycle until toxic effects developed. The number of cycles for each dose increment and the toxic effects of Adriamycin infusion are shown in Table 33.2. Statistical considerations have indicated that the repeated transient but severe leukopenia resulting from six consecutive cycles of Adriamycin at a dosage of 15 mg/m^2 per day was sufficient to determine that the lower dosage of 13 mg/m^2 per day was the maximum tolerable dosage.

In the second part of the phase I study, radiation therapy was given and Adriamycin was administered by continuous 5-day infusion at a dosage of 12 mg/m^2 per day. Irradiation was initially delivered in five daily fractions of 1 Gy per session to three patients and was repeated each time Adriamycin was administered (every 3–4 weeks). The radiation dosage was escalated for each new 5-day cycle by increments of 0.3–0.5 Gy per daily session until daily conventional radiation dosages of 1.5 Gy per session for the trunk lesions and 2 Gy per session for the extremity lesions were reached.

33.2.3 Monitoring Response and Toxicity

All patients had a complete pretreatment staging workup except for laparotomy. The irradiated palpable lesions were measured before treatment and every week during and after therapy was administered. When radiological tests were required to measure the lesions, they were repeated every 6–8 weeks.

Objective responses to treatment were defined using customary criteria. Patients were monitored for cardiotoxicity. The ventricular ejection fraction was calculated initially by echocardiography, more recently by technetium 99 pool multiple-gated acquisition scan.

Complete blood counts and differential counts, liver function tests, blood urea nitrogen, and creatinine values were obtained at appropriate time intervals.

33.2.4 Pharmacokinetics of Adriamycin

The Adriamycin levels in serum and urine were determined in three patients by a solid-phase radioimmunoassay (RIA) (van Vunak's et al., 1974) using the commercially available ^{125}I-labeled Adriamycin RIA kit (Diagnostic Biochemicals, San Diego, CA), and were expressed in nanograms per milliliter. The Adriamycin levels determined by RIA represent the amounts of Adriamycin and its immediate metabolites, adriamycinol and deoxyadriamycinol aglycones, with which the anti-Adriamycin antibody has a strong cross-reaction (Russell et al. 1981).

33.3 Results

33.3.1 Toxicity and Optimal Dose of Adriamycin by Continuous Infusion

In nine patients in whom escalating doses of Adriamycin were administered the limiting factor was represented by bone marrow suppression (Table 33.2).

At an Adriamycin dose of 15 mg/m^2/day administered for 5 consecutive days, severe leukopenia (550 ± 120 cells/µl) developed; its nadir was reached between the 10th and 15th day from the start of the infusion. This was accompanied by

Table 33.2. Toxicity of escalating doses of Adriamycin by continuous infusion

Dose of Adriamycin (mg/m²/dx5)	Nadir counts		Mucositis	Skin erythema	Ventricular ejection fraction (gated pool scanning)	
	WBC (x10³/µl)	Platelets (x10³/µl)			Direct (nl: 57% ± 8%)	After exercise (nl: 71% ± 8%)
9	3.6 ± 0.85	135 ± 42	0	0	55%	74%
11	3.1 ± 0.52	120 ± 25	0	0	ND	ND
13	2.2 ± 0.75	82 ± 35	+	0	53%	72%
15	0.55 ± 0.72	35 + 14	+ +	0	52%	61%

nl, normal; ND, not determined

moderate to severe thrombocytopenia (35 000 ± 14 000 platelets/µl) (Table 33.2) and moderate mucositis, especially glossitis. On one occasion a patient developed sepsis which responded to antibiotic therapy. Patients' ventricular ejection fraction had only a modest decrease after exercise (by 11%). At a lower dose of Adriamycin, 13 mg/m^2/day (Table 33.2), the nadir of the WBC was at 2200 ± 750 cells/µl, that of the platelet count at 82 000 ± 35 000/µl, and no other side-effects were noted. For this reason when Adriamycin was administered alone, this dose was then used in all patients who entered the study. The WBC and platelet counts were back to normal by the 18th–21st day from the start of the infusion, which led to a repeat of the infusion cycle every 3 weeks. The number of cycles administered was related to the total dose of Adriamycin the patient had received during the course of his disease. In three cases the cycles were repeated until a decrease of more than 20% in the ventricular ejection fraction after exercise was noted. This was reached at cumulative doses of Adriamycin of 820, 860, and 850 mg/m^2 (average 840 mg/m^2). Based on this result it was decided to stop the administration of 120-h infusion of Adriamycin at a cumulative dose of 840 mg/m^2.

33.3.2 Kinetics of Adriamycin by Continuous Infusion

The values of Adriamycin serum level determined by RIA represent the amount of Adriamycin as well as that of its immediate metabolites, adriamycinol and deoxyadriamycinol aglycone, with which the anti-Adriamycin antibody strongly cross-reacts (VAN VUNAKIS et al. 1974; BACHUR et al. 1976).

As seen on Fig. 33.1, after starting the Adriamycin infusion at a rate of 12 mg/m^2/day, its serum level had a rapid rise to 20 ng/ml, followed by a 16-h plateau. Thereafter, there was an almost exponential increase to 60 ng/ml for another 24 h, followed by a steady plateau at that level until the infusion was terminated. The disappearance of Adriamycin and adriamycinol to 20% of the previously achieved steady level followed a first order kinetics curve. This was succeeded by a much slower disappearance phase lasting 48 h. From the disappearance curve (Fig. 33.1) the mean half-life of Adriamycin and its metabolites was calculated as 20.5 h, while the half-time of the short disappearance curve was only 2.5 h. The Adriamycin excretion in the urine (Fig. 33.1, bottom graph) averaged 20 µg/h during the first 8 h of infusion and increased to 40 µg/h during the following 16 h; then it continued to rise slowly up to an average of 80 µg/h during the last 2 days of infusion. There-

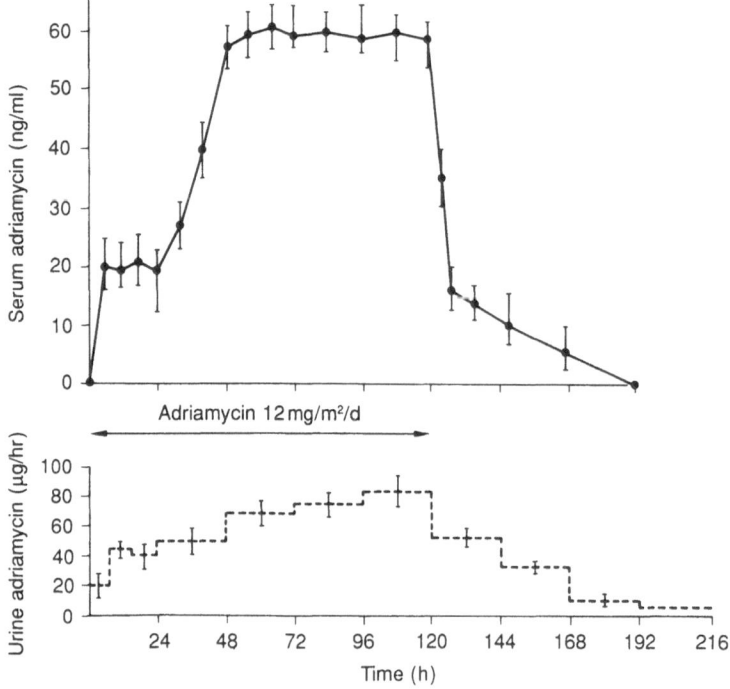

Fig. 33.1. Kinetics of doxorubin (Adriamycin) administered by 5-day continuous infusion. Serum levels are marked on upper graph as mean values of 3 different determinations at same time intervals from the start of infusion. Lower graph depicts rate of urinary excretion of doxorubicin during same period, represented by average hourly excretion calculated in each of the 3 studies

after, the Adriamycin excretion decreased first rapidly to a mean of 53 µg/h on the day following the termination of the infusion, and then at a slower pace; it was still excreted in the urine (average 9 µg/h) on the 4th postinfusion day. The cumulative urinary excretion of Adriamycin and its immediate metabolites represented 9.7% of the total Adriamycin dose administered during the 5-day infusion.

33.3.3 Optimal Radiation Dose and Toxicity of the Concomitant Administration of Continuous Adriamycin Infusion with Radiation

Based on previous data, an Adriamycin dose of 12 mg/m^2/day was chosen for administration with concurrent radiation therapy for 5 consecutive days every 3 weeks.

The effects of escalating doses of radiation (starting at 1 Gy/day) were assessed on the first six patients entered in this study. No severe side-effects were noted (Table 33.3). Skin erythema and nonpitting edema developed 5 days after a daily dose of 2 Gy was administered for 5 consecutive days; because of this reaction the following cases entered in this study received daily doses of 1.5 Gy to measurable lesions in their chest and abdominal cavity and 1.8 Gy to those in their limbs and head and neck region in cycles of 5 days every 3 weeks with concurrent administration of Adriamycin. At this dose local skin reaction at the site of administration of radiation consisted of hyperemia, noted after the administration of at least 10 Gy, followed by hyperpigmentation, which became apparent 5–6 weeks later; in patients receiving a total dose greater than 25 Gy a slight degree of skin induration and thickening became apparent 3 months later.

One patient developed a more intense erythema with nonpitting edema over the irradiated area of his left lower abdominal quadrant 3 days after the first cycle. This patient had received 40 Gy radiation therapy to the same region 3 months prior to his concomitant radiation–Adriamycin regimen. Therapy with prednisone administered orally at a daily dose of 60 mg abated the pain within 48 h and resolved the erythema within 5 days. During the following cycle this patient was started on prednisone at the beginning of the cycle, which prevented the recurrence of most of this local reaction.

Another patient developed pulmonary fibrosis with retraction of the right hilum 4 months after receiving the combined modality treatment with the radiation delivered to the mediastinum and the right hilum. In this case, however, the radiation dose was much higher (45 Gy) than that given in all other cases and it was delivered during as well as after the Adriamycin infusion, at variance with our original protocol.

Alopecia was universally encountered, usually after the second cycle of therapy.

Moderate mucositis with dysphagia or diarrhea, due at least in part to candida infection, developed only in five patients (Table 33.4) who had the lower third of the esophagus or the small bowel included in the radiation ports. It remitted after 2 weeks' therapy with mycostatin.

Ventricular ejection fraction decreased in only one case at rest (by 15% of the initial value); this was the patient who received 45 Gy to the mediastinum. One other patient presented a reduction of the ventricular ejection fraction after exercise, following the administration of a total dose of Adriamycin of 840 mg/m^2.

Moderate bone marrow suppression developed in most of the cases (Table 33.4), as reflected by moderate pancytopenia corresponding to that expected after the administration of Adriamycin infusion alone.

One patient (JE) with a previous history of peptic ulcer had transient gastrointestinal bleeding

Table 33.3. Toxicity of limited field radiation and concomitant continuous Adriamycin infusion

Dose			Nadir counts		Mucositis	Skin erythema	Ventricular ejection fraction (gated pool scanning)	
Adriamycin (mg/m^2/dx5)	+	RT (Gy/dx5)	WBC ($\times 10^3$/µl)	Platelets ($\times 10^3$/µl)			Direct (nl: 57% ± 8%)	After exercise (nl: 71% ± 8%)
12	+	1	2.1 ± 0.8	84 ± 27	+	+	ND	ND
12	+	1.5	2.2 ± 0.65	85 ± 31	+	+	ND	ND
12	+	2	2.0 ± 0.72	80 ± 28	++	+++	53%	72%

RT, radiation therapy; nl, normal; ND, not determined

Table 33.4. Side-effects of Adriamycin continuous infusion with concurrent radiation

Side-effect	Incidence	
	% of cycles ($n = 72$)	% of patients ($n = 20$)
Skin erythema	82.8	100
Leukopenia (WBC < 1500 > 3000)	85.5	95
Thrombocytopenia (plts. $> 5 \times 10^4 < 1 \times 10^5$)	62.1	70
Mucositis	28.9	25
Infectious episodes (Rx at home)	24.8	50
Infectious episodes (Rx in hosp.)	4.1	10
Cardiac arrhythmias	4.1	15
Decreased ventricular ejection fraction after exercise	2.7	10
Decreased ventricular ejection fraction at rest		5
Cholestasis	1.3	5
GI bleeding	1.3	5
Pulmonary fibrosis	–	5
Alopecia	–	100

from a duodenal ulcer area which was not included in the radiation port.

One patient (MH) with hepatoma and liver cirrhosis had a transient rise of the direct bilirubin to 2.8 mg/dl at the end of the first cycle of combined radiation–Adriamycin infusion. It remitted after 5 days and did not recur with the second cycle of therapy. No other hepatic toxicity was noted in any other patient.

33.3.4 Antitumor Activity of Concomitant Radiation Therapy and Adriamycin Infusion

There were 19 evaluable patients who received the previously described concurrent radiation–Adriamycin infusion treatment; their response to the combined modality treatment, reflected by the status of their irradiated lesions, is summarized in Table 33.5 and listed in more detail in Table 33.6.

Four patients, all with soft tissue sarcoma, achieved complete remission (CR) (Table 33.5). Six patients (three with soft tissue sarcoma and two with hepatoma) reached partial remission (PR); in ten, disease remained stable (SD) and in three patients tumor progressed during radiation and concomitant Adriamycin infusion.

The seven patients with metastatic adenocarci-

noma of the stomach, colon, and breast and the patient with metastatic transitional cell carcinoma of the bladder showed only a modest response: a reduction by less than 20% of the irradiated masses in five patients and just a softening of the radiated mass in three others. This stabilization of their disease lasted a mean of 8 ± 3 weeks.

Among the four patients with hepatoma entered in this study, two (OV and BH) with localized metastatic lesions in the right lobe achieved partial remissions.

The tumor responses of the sarcoma patients were much more remarkable. Complete responses were achieved after only 15 Gy to the right arm lesion of patient EW with liposarcoma, after 25 Gy to the right axillary lesion of patient BF with fibrosarcoma, after 20 Gy to the retroperitoneal lesion of patient FD with leiomyoscircoma and after 24 Gy to the left iliac lesion of patient ME with undifferentiated sarcoma. In the latter CR was achieved after no response was seen following 40 Gy radiation administered alone and two chemotherapeutic regimens. Because of this prior therapy, induration of the skin with subcutaneous fibrosis developed. Five needle biopsies of the indurated, fibrotic areas showed the absence of any malignant cell. In four other patients the radiated lesions achieved partial responses (decrease in size by more than 50%) after the administration of a dose of radiation significantly lower than the one causing similar responses in historical controls receiving radiation without concomitant Adriamycin infusion. In order to better illustrate this difference we introduced a parameter termed dose efficacy ratio (DER) which is calculated by dividing the standard radiation dose by the dose inducing the same response in the presence of concomitant Adriamycin infusion. The DER in all responders had a mean of 2.4 ± 0.8 with a range of 2.1–3.5. In one case of leiomyosarcoma with liver metastases no significant decrease in the size of the hepatic lesions was noted after the administration of 25 Gy. Nonetheless, these lesions have not increased in size and the patient has remained asymptomatic for the last 27 weeks.

Overall, the duration of the response of the radiated sarcoma lesions, which remitted after receiving combined modality therapy, was longer than 66 ± 30 weeks for complete responders and longer than 27 ± 8 weeks for partial responders. In fact, in none of the responders, to date, has a relapse occurred at the radiated site despite the low dose of radiation administered. Two of them,

Table 33.5. Response rate (DER)[a] and duration of response in patients receiving Adriamycin infusion and concomitant radiation

Histology	No. pts.	CR		PR		SD		Progression No. pts.
		No. pts.	Weeks	No. pts.	Weeks	No. pts.	Weeks	
Adenocarcinoma of GI tract	4	0	–	0	–	3	8 ± 3	1
Breast carcinoma	3	0	–	0	–	2	8 ± 4	1
Transitional cell carcinoma of bladder	1	0	–	0	–	0	–	1
Hepatocellular Ca.	4	0	–	2	28 ± 6	2	8 ± 3	0
Soft tissue sarcomas	11	4 (2.5)[a]	66 ± 30	4 (2.3)[a]	27 ± 9	3	26 ± 6	0
Total	23	4	66 ± 30	6	27 ± 8	10	·12 ± 9	3

CR, complete response; Adriamycin PR, partial response; Adriamycin SD, stable disease
[a] DER (dose efficasy ratio, see text page 12)

Table 33.6. Results of patients' treatment

Patient No.	Diagnosis	Treatment		Response	
		Doxorubicin, Total mg/m²	RT total cGy[b]	Type	Duration wks.
1	Liposarcoma	240	Right arm: 4000 (3000) RUL: 2400 (2400)	CR	35
2	Synovial STS	240	Right hilum: 1500 (1500) LUQ: 2370 (1500)	PR	38
3	Poorly differentiated STS	120	LLQ: 2025 (1500)	CR	188+
4	Leiomyosarcoma	180	Liver: 2750	SD	27+
5	Leiomyosarcoma	240	Retroperitoneum: 2000 (2000)	CR	204+
6	Leiomyosarcoma	180	Liver: 2400 (1500)	PR	18+
7	Firbrosarcoma	240	Right axilla: 3700 (2800)	CR	144+
8	Fibrohistiocytoma	240	Para-aortic mass: 3600 (2850)	PR	28+
9	Leiomyosarcoma	160	Upper mediastinum: 2720	SD	24
10	Rhabdomyosarcoma	156	Lung + Mediast.: 2400 (2400)	SD	26
11	Fibrohistocytoma	180	Retroperiton: 3600 (3000)	PR	46
12	Adenocarcinoma	200	Abdominal wall: 1920	SD	11
13	Adenocarcinoma	180	Abdominal wall: 2340	SD	9
14	Adenocarcinoma	120	Pelvis: 750 Liver: 1320	Prog.	–
15	Adenocarcinoma	120	Pelvis: 2300	SD	5
16	Breast cancer	120	Chest wall: 1800	Prog.	–
17	Breast cancer	180	Breast: 3000	SD	12
18	Breast cancer	120	Breast: 2000	SD	5
19	Transitional cell cancer	240	Left thigh: 4860	Prog.	–
20	Hepatoma	60	Left lobe, liver: 1080	PR	35
21	Hepatoma	120	Right lobe, liver: 1500	PR	22
22	Hepatoma	180	Whole liver: 2150	SD	5
23	Hepatoma	140	Whole liver: 2520	SD	12

with synovial sarcoma and liposarcoma (CT and EW), expired 8 and 10 months after therapy due to progressing metastatic lesions elsewhere in their lungs.

Of the eight patients who achieved complete or partial responses of their solitary recurrent or metastatic lesions, three CR patients are maintaining their response after 188, 204 and 144 weeks and two PR patients are doing likewise after 18 and 28 weeks (Table 33.6).

33.4 Discussion

The most significant results of the present study are the lack of toxicity of Adriamycin administered by protracted infusion with concomitant radiation and its radiation-enhancing effect in 86% of patients with sarcoma and in half of the hepatoma patients entered in this study. Conversely, Adiamycin infusion showed no apparent radiation-enhancing effect in any of the patients with metastatic or recurrent adenocarcinoma of the colon, stomach, or breast who received this regimen.

The radiation-enhancing effect of Adriamycin by continuous infusion was better defined by using a new parameter, the DER calculated by dividing the dose that conventionally is delivered to achieve control of the respective lesion by the radiation dose that induced the lesion's maximum response while Adriamycin was intravenously infused. This DER varied between 2.1 and 4.0 for soft tissue sarcoma lesions, indicating that these tumors are sensitive to the combined modality treatment. This effect was even more remarkable if we take into consideration the fact that almost all sarcoma patients had received Adriamycin and two of them were also irradiated to the same lesions more than 3 months before they entered in this study. These data suggest that Adriamycin may indeed have a radiosensitizing effect. Such an effect was previously recognized in experiments carried out in in vitro cultured human tumor cells (BYFIELD et al. 1975). In other experiments (ROSS et al. 1979) using the intestinal crypt cell assay it was noted that cell survival was reduced by the addition of Adriamycin to 70% of the survival of the crypt cells receiving radiation alone (ROSS et al. 1979). There was no evidence of a time interval yielding enhanced response. Preliminary clinical studies (BYFIELD et al.; CHAN et al. 1976) also indicated that Adriamycin can be safely administered in intermittent single pulses with concomitant conventional radiotherapy as well as with accelerated split-dose radiation therapy or brachytherapy. Side-effects represented by progressive bowel fibrosis, esophagitis, and dermatitis were noted in less than 30% of the cases and have been reversible except for the bowel fibrosis. Similar results and toxicity were found (RUCKDESCHEL et al. 1979) following the administration of sequential radiotherapy and Adriamycin to patients with bronchogenic carcinoma. Favorable results with minimal morbidity were reported in the treatment of localized high grade soft tissue sarcoma (BLUM et al. 1979), in the treatment of patients with limited mesothelioma in whom radiotherapy was sequentially administered with Adriamycin alone or in combination with other drugs (SINOFF et al. 1982),

and in the treatment of transitional cell carcinoma of the bladder with low dose Adriamycin (KAGAWA et al. 1981). However, these data have generally been at variance with most previous reports indicating increased toxicity resulting from the concomitant administration of radiation and pulses of Adriamycin i.v. A skin recall phenomenon (CASSIDY 1975), severe enteritis, esophagitis (PHILLIPS et al. 1975; GRECO et al. 1976), and cardiomyopathy (ROSEN et al. 1975) were reported. There appeared to be an enhanced toxicity when Adriamycin was administered between 2 and 48 h before radiation therapy (PHILLIPS et al. 1975). Some experimental in vivo data (ROWLEY et al. 1979) in hepatoma H-4-II-E bearing rats also showed that Adriamycin administered immediately after tumor irradiation failed to cause additional tumor cell kill. However, the data presented herein indicate that toxicity of the concomitant Adriamycin and radiation therapy is mild when the Adriamycin level in serum does not rise above 60 ng/ml; at this level Adriamycin appears to have an antineoplastic effect synergistic with radiation therapy at least on sarcomas and hepatomas.

The mechanism of the radiosensitizing effect of Adriamycin is still a subject of speculation. It has been reported (BYFIELD et al. 1977a, b; GONSALVES et al. 1974) that Adriamycin is an inhibitor of mitochondrial and tumor cell respiration. This effect could lead to reduced oxygen consumption by cells in the outer layers of the tumor and consequently an improved oxygenation of the centrally located hypoxic cells (DURAND 1976). It is conceivable that radiosensitization requires a minimum steady level of Adriamycin in the serum which is readily achieved by continuous i.v. infusion of Adriamycin rather than with i.v. pulses. After the administration of the commonly recommended Adriamycin bolus dose of 60 mg/m^2 q 3 weeks a plasma level of 500 ng/ml is reached within 5–10 min (BACHUR et al. 1976). Thereafter, there is a biphasic disappearance of Adriamycin from plasma; its level declines to 10% in about 48 h and to 5% within 120 h (ROWLEY et al. 1979). Our kinetic data show that when an equal dose of Adriamycin is infused continuously over a period of 5 days a steady plasma level of approximately 60 ng/ml is maintained for 100 h (Fig. 33.1). Starting with its 36th hour of administration this level becomes higher than the plasma level attained after i.v. pulse administration of an equal amount of Adriamycin. Its disappearance from plasma after the administration of the drug as 120-h infusion also had a biphasic pattern. However, the duration of the rapid disappearance phase is longer (Fig. 33.1) than after an i.v. bolus (BENJAMIN et al. 1973); this could be explained by an overlap of infusion with the release of Adriamycin from tissues in the serum and urine. The amount of Adriamycin and of its immediate metabolites, adriamycinol and deoxydriamycinol, found in the urine represented 9.7% of the total amount infused over the 120 h, which constitutes an increase over the usual 5% urinary excretion following i.v. bolus administration (BENJAMIN et al. 1973). This could be due to an increase in the amount of Adriamycin degraded to metabolites cleared by the kidney due to its prolonged retention by various tissues as a result of its slow and protracted administration. The increased Adriamycin retention by tissues could also explain the 24-h delay in reaching the maximum Adriamycin level in plasma (Fig. 33.1).

Adriamycin side-effects have been generally minor when Adriamycin has been administered by continuous infusion in the schedule and dosage found to have the best therapeutic index (13 mg/m^2 in 5-day cycles every 3 weeks).

Cardiac toxicity as determined by the measurement of the ventricular ejection fraction was minimal and was noted only in patients who reached a total dose of 840 mg/m^2 Adriamycin of which less than half was administered as i.v. pulses prior to their entry in this study. It consisted in the reduction by 25% or less of the ventricular ejection fraction after exercise. A significant decrease in cardiac toxicity induced by Adriamycin when administered by 96-h continuous infusion up to a dose of 60 mg/m^2 per cycle was also recently documented by LEGHA et al. (1982) in an extensive study which included an analysis of endomyocardial biopsies and studies in which Adriamycin was administered through ambulatory pump delivery systems for periods of time longer than 30 days at a daily dose lower than 4 mg/m^2.

The side-effects of the concurrent administration of Adriamycin by continuous infusion and radiation therapy have been essentially identical with those of Adriamycin administered alone by protracted infusion. Most remarkable was the lack of detectable hepatic and cardiac toxicity.

Based on these data it can be concluded that Adriamycin at a serum level close to 60 ng/ml appears to have an enhancing effect on radiation in the treatment of soft tissue sarcomas and, to a lesser extent, of hepatomas.

This new combined modality of treatment warrants more extensive phase II and III clinical trials involving recurrent as well as primary neoplasms which respond poorly to their current treatment.

References

Bachur MR, Riggs CE, Green MR, Langone JJ, Van Vunakis H, Levine L (1976) Plasma adriamycin and daunorubicin levels by fluorescence and radioimmunoassay. Clin Pharmacol Ther 21: 70–72

Benjamin RS, Riggs CE Jr, Bachur NR (1973) Pharmacokinetics and metabolism of adriamycin in man. Clin Pharmacol Ther 14: 592–600

Bjeletich J, Hickman RO (1980) The Hickman indwelling catheter. Am J Nurs 80: 62–65

Blum RH, Greenberger JS, Wilson RE, Carson JM (1979) Feasibility of combined modality therapy for localized high-grade soft tissue sarcomas in adults. Int J Radiat Oncol Biol Phys 5: 1281–1285

Byfield JE (1974) The role of radiation repair mechanism in radiation treatment failures. Cancer Chemother Rep 58: 527–538

Byfield JE, Watring WG, Lemkin SR, Juillard GL, Hauskins LA, Smith ML, Lagasse LD (1975) Adriamycin: a useful adjuvant drug for combination radiation therapy (abstr). Proc Am Assoc Cancer Res – Am Soc Clin Oncol 16: 253

Byfield JE, Lee YC, Tu L (1977a) Molecular interactions between Adriamycin and x-ray damage in mammalian tumor cells. Int J Cancer 19: 194–204

Byfield JE, Lynch M, Kulhaman F, Chan PYM (1977b) Cellular effects of combined Adriamycin and X irradiation in human tumor cells. Int J Cancer 19: 194–204

Cassidy JR (1975) Radiation-Adriamycin interactions: preliminary clinical observations. Cancer 36: 946

Chan YM, Byfield JE, Lemkin SR, Aronstam E (1976) Coincident adriamycin (A) and x-ray therapy in bronchogenic carcinoma: response and cardiotoxicity (abstr). Proc Am Assoc Cancer Res – Am Soc Clin Oncol 17–276

D'Angio GJ, Farber S, Maddock GL (1959) Potentiation of x-ray effects by actinomycin D. Radiology 73: 175–177

Durand RE (1976) Adriamycin: a possible indirect radiosensitizer of hypoxic tumor cells. Radiology 119: 217–222

Garnick MB, Weiss GR, Steele GD Jr, Israel M, Schade D, Sack MJ, Frei E III (1983) Clinical evaluation of longterm, continuous infusion doxorubicin. J Clin Oncol 57: 1–10

Gonsalvez M, Blanco M, Hunter J, Miko M, Chance D (1974) Effects of anti-cancer agents on the respiration of isolated mitochondria and tumor cells. Eur J Cancer 10: 567–574

Greco AA, Brereton HD, Kent H, Zimbler H, Merrill J, Johnson Re (1976) Adriamycin and enhanced radiation reaction in normal esophagus and skin. Ann Intern Med 85: 294–298

Haskell CM, Eilber FR, Morton DL (1975) Adriamycin (NSC-123127) by arterial infusion. Cancer Chemother Rep 6: 187–189

Kagawa S, Maebeyashi K, Kubokawa K, Uyoma T, Moriwaski S (1981) Efficacy of combination therapy with intravesical instillation of doxorubicin and low dose radiation for bladder cancer. Urology 18: 479–481

Kimler BF, Loeper DB (1979) The effect of adriamycin and radiation on G cell survival. Int J Radiat Oncol Biol Phys 3: 1297–1300

Legha SS, Benjamin RS, Mackay B et al. (1982) Reduction of doxorubicin cardiotoxicity by prolonged continuous intravenous infusion. Ann Intern Med 96: 133–139

Lokich J, Bothe A, Zipoli T, Green R, Sonneborn H, Paul S, Phillips D (1983) Constant infusion schedule for adriamycin: a phase I–II clinical trial of a 30 day schedule by ambulatory pump delivery system. J Clin Oncol 1: 24–29

Phillips TL, Fu KK (1976) Quantification of combined radiation therapy and chemotherapy effects on critical normal tissues. Cancer 37: 1186–1200

Phillips TL, Wharam MD, Margolis LW (1975) Modification of radiation injury to normal tissues by chemotherapy agents. Cancer 35: 1678–1684

Rosen G, Tefft M, Martinez A, Cham W, Murphy ML (1975) Combination chemotherapy and radiation therapy in the treatment of metastatic osteogenic sarcoma. Cancer 35: 622–630

Ross GY, Phillips TL, Goldstein LS (1979) The interaction of irradiation and adriamycin in intestinal crypt cells. Int J Radiat Oncol Biol Phys 5: 1313–1315

Rowley R, Bacharach M, Hopkins HA, MacLeod M, Ritenour R, Moore JV, Looney WB (1979) Adriamycin and radiation effects upon an experimental solid tumor resistant to therapy. Int J Radiat Oncol Biol Phys 5: 1291–1295

Ruckdeschel JC, Baster DH, McKneally MF et al. (1979) Sequential radiotherapy and adriamycin in the management of broncogenic carcinomas. The question of additive toxicity. Int J Radiat Oncol Biol Phys 3: 1323–1328

Russell WO, Cohen J, Edmonson JH et al. (1981) Staging system for soft tissue sarcomas. Semin Oncol 8: 156–159

Shimoyama M (1975) The cytocidal action of alkylating agents and anticancer antibiotics against in vitro cultured Yoshida ascites sarcoma cells. Jpn Soc Cancer Ther 10: 63–72

Sinoff C, Falkson G, Sandison AG, DeMuelanaere G (1982) Combined doxorubicin and radiation therapy in malignant pleural mesothelioma. Cancer Treat Rep 66: 1605–1608

Van Vunakis H, Langone JJ, Riceberg LJ, Levine L (1974) Radioimmunoassays for adriamycin and daunomycin. Cancer Res 34: 2546–2550

34 Infusion Adriamycin and Radiation in Hepatomas

RICHARD S. STARK, C. JULIAN ROSENTHAL, and MARVIN ROTMAN

CONTENTS

34.1 Introduction

Hepatocellular carcinoma is a highly malignant tumor with a median survival time of only 4 months from the onset of symptoms and 2 months from the diagnosis (NAGASUE et al. 1984; FALKSON and COETZER 1986). While radiation has some activity, its effectiveness is limited by the liver tolerance (ZUM WINKEL et al. 1986). Cytotoxic chemotherapy has usually produced disappointing results (FALKSON and COETZER 1986). New approaches are needed for the treatment of this disease. One such new approach is the concomitant use of hepatic radiation and chemotherapy. The optimal chemotherapy would be drugs which are both individually active in the treatment of hepatocellular carcinoma as well as having a potential for radiation sensitization.

Adriamycin is one of the more widely studied chemotherapuetic agents for treating hepatocellular cancer. Based upon compiled studies, it pro-

duces a response rate in the 10%–30% range (IHDE et al. 1977; OLWENY et al. 1980; VOGEL et al. 1977; SCIARRINO et al. 1985). Adriamycin is also well recognized to have a locally enhancing effect on radiation (ROSENTHAL et al. 1986). In our phase I study, we established that concomitant administration of Adriamycin given as a continuous infusion with standard fractions of radiation was well tolerated (ROSENTHAL et al. 1986). In several patients with liver tumors, no excessive liver toxicity was seen with this approach. In four patients with hepatocellular cancer, two partial responses were seen. These initial encouraging results prompted a phase II study using concomitant infusion Adriamycin and hepatic radiation for the treatment of hepatocellular cancer. The outcome in 12 patients treated to date forms the basis for this report.

34.2 Materials and Methods

34.2.1 Patient Population

All 12 patients had biopsy-proven hepatoma either by core biopsy or compatible needle biospy in association with an elevated serum α-fetoprotein level. Clinical features are summarized in Table 34.1. Two patients had prior treatment with Adriamycin given as a bolus injection during which there was disease progression. Three additional patients had prior chemotherapy with investigational agents and were placed on this trial at the time of disease progression. Four of the patients had metastatic spread beyond the liver. Informed consent was obtained from all patients prior to the start of therapy.

34.2.2 Therapeutic Regimen

All patients received 12 mg/m²/day of Adriamycin by continuous infusion for 5 days. The infusion

RICHARD S. STARK, MD, Director Medical Oncology, Interfaith Medical Center, 555 Prospect Place, Brooklyn, NY 11238, USA

C. JULIAN ROSENTHAL, MD, Professor of Medicine and Oncology, MARVIN ROTMAN, MD, Professor and Chairman, Department of Radiation Oncology, SUNY Health Science Center at Brooklyn, 450 Clarkson Avenue, Brooklyn, NY 11203, USA

Table 34.1. Clinical characteristics of the 12 patients

Initials	Age	Sex	Race	Metastasis	Cirrhosis	HBsAg	Fetoprotein (ng/ml)
OV	44	f	B, A	–	–	–	436
BM	53	f	B, C	–	+	–	8 000
LM	66	m	W	–	–	–	–
FE	59	m	B, C	–	+	–	55 000
WL	62	m	B, A	Lung	+	–	205 000
DE	58	m	B, C	Lung	–	–	3 280
KR	35	m	B, A	–	–	+	25 000
SA	66	f	B, C	–	–	–	8 000
KJ	21	m	O	Mesentery	–	+	NA
SA	71	m	B, C	–	+	–	NA
BG	44	m	B, C	Chest wall	+	+	63 000

Abbreviations: B, A, black, American born; B, C, black, Caribbean born; W, white; O, oriental; +, present; –, absent; NA, information not available; HBsAg, hepatitis B antigen

Table 34.2. Treatment and treatment response in the 12 patients

Initials	Prior therapy	Adriamycin (mg/m²)	RT (Gy)	Response	Duration (weeks)	Survival (weeks)
OV	RT/Adriamycin	360	22.5	PR	72	72
BM	Adriamycin	120	28	PR	24	24
LM	–	180	21.5	NR	–	16
FE	–	140	25.2	PR	16	24
WL	Platinol	120	15	NR	–	12
DE	Acivicin	60	8	NR	–	8
KR	–	120	28.8	NR	–	12
SA	–	180	27	PR	34	42
KJ	–	120	15	NR	–	8
SA	–	120	14.4	NR	–	6
BG	Deoxydoxorubicin	60	8	NR	–	6
AC	–	180	25.5	SD	32	32+

Abbreviations: RT, radiation; PR, partial response; NR, no response; SD, stable disease

was given either through a central venous catheter placed at the time of hospital admission or through an indwelling Hickman type catheter. The total daily dose of Adriamycin was mixed in 1000 cc dextrose and water or normal saline and delivered over 24 h by an IVAC pump. Radiation was delivered in five consecutive fractions of 1.5–1.8 Gy/day simultaneously with the Adriamycin infusion and repeated each time the Adriamycin was administered. Cycles were repeated every 3–4 weeks for a total of three cycles. The total dose of radiation was to be between 25 and 28 Gy, assuming all three cycles were administered.

34.2.3 Response Criteria

Criteria for determining a response are given in detail in Sect. 34.3. Response duration and survival time were measured from the time of initiation of protocol therapy. Survival times and response durations were measured in weeks rounded to the nearest week.

34.3 Results

34.3.1 Antitumor Activity

A total of 12 patients were entered on study. Seven patients completed a total of three cycles, receiving a mean dose of 160 mg/m² Adriamycin and 25.5 Gy. Three patients received two cycles. In one of these patients, this was because the patient had received prior hepatic radiation. In the other two patients, disease progression occurred after two cycles. Two patients received only one cycle of therapy. In both cases, there was rapid deterioration in performance status secondary to disease progression.

A total of four patients achieved a partial response (Table 34.2). The mean duration of response was 36 weeks and the mean survival was 40 weeks. In patient OV, response was determined by a 30% reduction in liver size. This patient had progressed after receiving 15 Gy to the liver and six bolus injections of Adriamycin given sequentially. The response duration was 72 weeks. With patient BM, response was determined by the near disappearance of a 4- to 5-cm lesion seen on liver scan. The response duration was 24+ weeks with the patient then expiring from an intracranial bleed. A third patient, FE, had a greater than 50% reduction in product of diameters of a palpable abdominal mass. The response duration was 16 weeks, with the patient dying at 24 weeks with disease progression. The fourth responding patient, SA, had near complete resolution of a cluster of small nodules seen on abdominal CT scan in association with a decrease in α-fetoprotein from 8000 to 500 ng/ml. The response duration was 34 weeks, with the patient expiring at 42 weeks from disease progression.

One patient demonstrated disease stabilization. Although there was no decrease in the size of a palpable liver mass, the patient remained asymptomatic without disease progression for 30 weeks. After this, the patient was lost to follow-up. Seven additional patients demonstrated no response and had a mean survival of 10 weeks.

34.3.2 Treatment Toxicity

All patients demonstrated a modest degree of neutropenia with a mean white blood cell nadir of 2200/mm^3 (range 700–3700). There was one episode of sepsis associated with neutropenia. The patient responded to antibiotic treatment. The mean platelet nadir was 102000/mm^3 (range 28000–214000). Five patients experienced moderate nausea and vomiting. There were two episodes of grade 2 mucositis. There were three episodes of catheter-related infections that were not life threatening.

Hepatic toxicity was difficult to document. In two cases there were transient elevations in the bilirubin which returned to normal during a time when the patients were felt to be stable or still responding. Almost all patients had evidence of worsening liver function at the end of their course. This was presumed to be secondary to progression of hepatoma although it was impossible entirely to exclude hepatotoxicity from treatment. One patient died after 72 weeks with clinical evidence of intrahepatic cholestasis. There was no clear evidence for progression of hepatoma.

34.4 Discussion

While an uncommon disease in the United States, on a worldwide basis, hepatocellular cancer is one of the more common malignancies. The prognosis for patients with hepatocellular cancer has been dismal. This is because of a tendency for the disease to remain occult until at more advanced stages and because of the lack of effective therapy. Surgical resection, which offers the sole hope for cure, is only rarely feasible. Because of this, there is a need to explore innovative approaches for the treatment of this disease.

One such approach is the concomitant use of hepatic radiation and infusion chemotherapy. The rationale behind this is to achieve at least an additive effect of two active modalities as well as to take advantage of any radiation–sensitizing effect the chemotherapy may have. This report presents the initial results using a continuous infusion of Adriamycin simultaneously with hepatic radiation. The study demonstrates that this approach is feasible with acceptable toxicity. A response rate of 33% was obtained in the 12 patients treated. If one excludes patients with metastasis outside the liver, four of eight patients, or 50%, responded. It is also noteworthy that one patient responded to the combined therapy after failing both Adriamycin and radiation given conventionally. This suggests that at least in this case, a radiation–sensitizing effect occurred. While the number of patients treated is small, these results are promising enough that we plan to continue the trial with patients who are untreated and with disease confined to the liver.

One concern with this treatment approach is an enhanced radiation hepatitis caused by the potentiation of the radiation effect on normal hepatocytes by the Adriamycin. One report has suggested that this does occur, describing two cases of augmented acute postradiation hepatopathy after receiving Adriamycin concomitantly or subsequently to liver radiation (KUN and CAMITTA 1978). Using intra-arterial Adriamycin and concomitant hepatic irradiation, no significant hepatic toxicity was observed (FRIEDMAN et al. 1979). In our present and prior study, clinically significant acute hepatocellar dysfunction did not occur other than the transient mild elevations in the liver function tests mentioned above. Because of the short survival of most patients and the overlapping hepatocellular dysfunction caused by progression of the hepatoma, it is impossible to exclude the possibility that the treatment causes significant late hepatocellular dysfunction. The distinction between treatment-related hepatotoxicity, progression of underlying liver diseases, and progression of hepatocellular cancer may be resolvable by histological evaluation of hepatic tissue obtained by biopsy and postmortem in patients receiving this treatment. This is an aspect that will have to be monitored closely in future trials.

Other innovative and promising approaches to treating hepatocellular cancer have been reported and should be compared with the present trial. These include hepatic arterial infusion of chemotherapy alone or in combination with hepatic irradiation, hepatic arterial embolization or chemoembolization, and use of isotopically labeled antiferritin in conjunction with hepatic radiation and systemic chemotherapy.

Hepatic artery infusion of Adriamycin alone or in combination with other drugs has been reported by a number of groups. Doci et al. (1988) reported an overall response rate of 42% to Adriamycin alone, and Patt et al. (1988) reported a response rate of 70% to intra-arterial 5-fluorouracil deoxyribonucleoside, doxorubicin, and mitomycin. Friedman et al. (1979) reported that 6 of 13 patients responded to intra-arterial Adriamycin and 5-fluorouracil combined with whole liver radiation. Using chemoembolization of the hepatic artery, Sasaki et al. (1987) and Ohnishi et al. (1987) reported response rates of 65% and 57% respectively. Using hepatic radiation, concomitant bolus Adriamycin, and 5-fluorouracil, followed by radiolabeled antiferritin, Order et al. (1985) reported a 54% response rate. In the above reported studies, patients were generally selected with disease confined to the liver. If a response rate of approximately 50% can be confirmed for the use of hepatic radiation with concomitant infusion Adriamycin when the disease is confined to the liver, then it can be concluded that this approach gives comparable results to these other technically more complicated approaches.

References

Doci R, Bignami P, Bozzetti A, Bonfanti G, Audisio R, Colombo M, Gennari L (1988) Intrahepatic chemotherapy for unresectable hepatocellular carcinoma. Cancer 61: 1983–1987

Falkson G, Coetzer BJ (1986) Application and results of different chemotherapy regimens in primary liver malignancies. In: Herfarth C, Schlag P, Hohenberger P (eds) Therapeutic strategies in primary and metastatic liver cancer. Springer, Berlin Heidelberg New York (Recent Results in Cancer Research, vol 100, pp 103–111)

Friedman MA, Volberding PA, Cassidy MJ, Resser KJ, Wasserman TH, Philips TL (1979) Therapy for hepatocellular cancer with intrahepatic arterial adriamycin and 5-fluorouracil combined with whole liver radiation: an NCOG study. Cancer Treat Rep 63: 1885–1888

Ihde DC, Kane RH, Cohen MH, McIntyre KR, Minna JD (1977) Adriamycin therapy in American patients with hepatocellular carcinoma. Cancer Treat Rep 61: 1385–1387

Kun LE, Camitta BM (1978) Hepatopathy following irradiation and adriamycin. Cancer 42: 81–84

Nagasue N, Yukaya H, Hamada T, Hirose S, Kanashima R, Inokuchi K (1984) The natural history of hepatocellular carcinoma, a study of 100 untreated cases. Cancer 54: 1461–1465

Ohnishi K, Sugita S, Nomura F, Iida S, Tanabe Y (1987) Arterial chemoembolization with mitomycin microcapsules followed by transcatheter hepatic artery embolization for hepatocellular carcinoma. Am J Gastroenterol 82: 876–879

Olweny CL, Katongole-Mbidde E, Bahendeka S, Otim D, Mugerwa J, Kyalwazi SK (1980) Further experience in treating hepatocellular carcinoma in Uganda. Cancer 46: 2717–2722

Order SE, Stillwagon GB, Klein JL et al. (1985) Iodine 131 antiferritin, a new treatment modality in hepatoma: a Radiation Therapy Oncology Group study. J Clin Oncol 3: 1573–1582

Patt YZ, Claghorn L, Charnsangavej C, Soski M, Cleary K, Mavligit GM (1988) Hepatocellular carcinoma–a retrospective analysis of treatments to manage disease confined to the liver. Cancer 61: 1887–1888

Rosenthal CJ, Rotman M, Bhutiani I (1986) Concomitant radiation therapy and doxorubicin by continuous infusion in advanced malignancies – a phase I–II study – evidence of synergistic effect in soft tissue sarcomas and hepatomas. In: Rosenthal CJ, Rotman M (eds) Clinical applications of continuous infusion chemotherapy and concomitant radiation therapy. Plenum, New York, pp 159–175

Sasaki Y, Imaoka S, Kasugai H et al. (1987) A new approach to chemoembolization therapy for hepatoma using ethiodized oil, cisplatin, and gelatin sponge. Cancer 60: 1194–1203

Sciarrino E, Simonetti RG, Le Moli S, Pagliaro L (1985) Adriamycin treatment for hepatocellular carcinoma. Experience with 109 patients. Cancer 56: 2751–2755

Vogel CL, Bayley AC, Brooker RJ, Anthony PP, Ziegler JL (1977) A phase II study of adriamycin (NSC 123 127) in patients with hepatocellular carcinoma from Zambia and the United States. Cancer 39: 1923–1929

Zum Winkel K, Wieland C, Weischedel N (1986) Therapeutic strategies in primary and metastatic liver cancer: indication and results of external radiation therapy. In: Herfarth C, Schlag P, Hohenberger P (eds) Therapeutic strategies in primary and metastatic liver cancer. Springer, Berlin Heidelberg New York (Recent Results in Cancer Research, vol 100, pp 289–297)

Subject Index

List of Contributors

JAMES D. AHLGREN, MD
Associate Professor of Medicine
Division of Hematology-Oncology
The George Washington University
Medical Center
2150 Pennsylvania Avenue, NW
Washington, DC 20037
USA

JEAN-PHILIPPE AUSTIN, MD
Department of Radiation Oncology
Charity Hospital of New Orleans
1532 Tulane Ave.
New Orleans, LA 70140
USA

HASSAN AZIZ, MD
Associate Professor
Radiation Oncology
SUNY Health Science Center at
Brooklyn
450 Clarkson Avenue
Brooklyn, New York 11203
USA

GEORGE R. BLUMENSCHEIN, MD
Arlington Cancer Center
906 W. Randol Mill Road
Arlington, TX 76012
USA

MICHEL A. BOILEAU, MD
Bend Urology Associates
2275 N.E. Doctor's Drive
Bend, OR 97701
USA

GARY V. BURTON, MD
Department of Medicine
Louisiana State University Medical
Center
P.O. Box 33932
Shreveport, LA 71130-3932
USA

JOHN E. BYFIELD, MD, PhD
Medical Director
Radiation Therapy Associates
Medical Group
3550 Q Street, Suite 106
Bakersfield, CA 93301
USA

WARREN H. CHAPMAN, MD
Professor Urology
University of Washington Medical
Center
1959 N.E. Pacific Street
Seattle, WA 98195
USA

KWANG CHOI, MD
Associate Professor
Radiation Oncology
SUNY Health Science Center at
Brooklyn
450 Clarkson Avenue
Brooklyn, New York 11203
USA

LAWRENCE R. COIA, MD
Fox Chase Cancer Center
Associate Professor Radiation
Oncology
University of Pennsylvania School of
Medicine
Central & Shelmire Aves.
Philadelphia, PA 19111
USA

C. NORMAN COLEMAN, MD
Professor and Chairman
Joint Center for Radiation Therapy
Harvard Medical School
50 Binney Street
Boston, MA 02115
USA

MORTON COLEMAN, MD
Clinical Professor of Medicine
Cornell University Medical Center
407 East 70 Street
New York, NY 10021
USA

CAROLINE COLLINS, MD
Assistant Professor, Medical
Oncology
University of Washington Medical
Center
1959 N.E. Pacific Street
Seattle, WA 98195
USA

JEFFREY CRAWFORD, MD
Department of Medicine
Duke University Medical Center
Durham, NC 27710
USA

IAN CROCKER, MD
Department of Medicine
Duke University Medical Center
Durham, NC 27710
USA

BERNARD J. CUMMINGS, MBChB,
FRCPC
Department of Radiation Oncology
Princess Margaret Hospital
500 Sherbourne Street
Toronto, M4X 1K9
Canada

RONALD DeCONTI, MD
Professor
Division of Medical Oncology
Albany Medical College and Veterans
Administrations Center
47 New Scotland Ave., A-52
Albany, NY 12208
USA

ALFRED DiSTEFANO, MD
Arlington Cancer Center
906 W. Randol Mill Road
Arlington, TX 760 12
USA

EVAN B. DOUPLE, PhD
Radiobiology Laboratories
Dartmouth-Hitchcock Medical Center
Hanover, NH 03756
USA

JADRANKA DRAGOVIC, MD, FRCP (C)
Henry Ford Hospital
Dept. of Radiation Oncology
2799 West Grand Boulevard
Detroit, MI 48202-2689
USA

Dr. med JÜRGEN DUNST
Department of Radiation Therapy
University of Erlangen
Universitätsstraße 27
W-8520 Erlangen
FRG

PAUL F. ENGSTROM, MD
Vice President, Population Science
Department of Medical Oncology
Fox Chase Cancer Center
Central & Shelmire Aves.
Philadelphia, PA 19111
USA

RICHARD G. EVANS, PhD, MD
Professor and Chairman
Department of Radiation Oncology
University of Kansas Medical Center
39th and Rainbow Blvd.
Kansas City, KS 66103
USA

BARRY A. FIRSTENBERG, MD
Arlington Cancer Center
906 W. Randol Mill Road
Arlington, TX 76012
USA

DONNA GLOVER, MD
Chief Hematology – Oncology
Presbyterian Medical Center
39th and Market Streets
Philadelphia, PA 19104
USA

JOSE E. GOMEZ-YEYILLE, MD
Arlington Cancer Center
906 W. Randol Mill Road
Arlington, TX 76012
USA

STEPHEN GRABELSKY
Section of Hematology/Oncology
Presbyterian Medical Center
39th and Market Streets
Philadelphia, PA 19104
USA

KATHERINE GRIEM, MD
Assistant Professor of Therapeutic
Radiology
Rush-Presbyterian. St. Luke's
Medical Center
1725 W. Harrison St.
Chicago, IL 60612
USA

THOMAS W. GRIFFIN, MD
Professor and Chairman, Radiation
Oncology
University of Washington Medical
Center
1959 N.E. Pacific Street
Seattle, WA 98195
USA

PERRY W. GRIGSBY, MD
Associate Professor
Radiation Oncology Center
Mallinckrodt Institute of Radiology
Washington University School of
Medicine
510 S. Kingshighway
St. Louis, MO 63110
USA

GERALD E. HANKS, MD
Chairman, Department of Radiation
Oncology
Fox Chase Cancer Center
Professor and Vice-Chairman, Dept.
of Radiation Oncology
University of Pennsylvania School of
Medicine
Central & Shelmire Aves.
Philadelphia, PA 19111
USA

CELESTIA S. HIGANO, MD
Assistant Professor, Medical
Oncology
University of Washington Medical
Center
1959 N.E. Pacific Street
Seattle, WA 98195
USA

WILLIAM HRUSHESKY, MD
Professor
Division of Medical Oncology
Albany Medical College and Veterans
Administration Center
47 New Scotland Ave., A-52
Albany, NY 12208
USA

SAMUEL L. JAMPOLIS, MD
Arlington, Cancer Center
906 W. Randol Mill Road
Arlington, TX 760 12
USA

MADHU J. JOHN, MD
Director Radiation Oncology
Kaweah Delta Cancer Care Center
248 S. Floral
Visalia, CA 93291
and Associate Clinical Professor
University of California
San Francisco, CA 94143
USA

ELLEN L. JONES, PhD
Radiobiology Laboratories
Dartmouth-Hitchcock Medical Center
Hanover, NH 03756
USA

DWIGHT KAUFMAN, MD, PhD
Radiation Oncology Branch
National Cancer Institute
National Institutes of Health
Bldg. 10, Room B3-B69
Bethesda, MD 20892
USA

THOMAS J. KEANE, MBChB, MRCPI,
FRCPC
Department of Radiation Oncology
Princess Margaret Hospital
500 Sherbourne Street
Toronto, M4X 1K9
Canada

JOHN P. KELLY, MD
Arlington Cancer Center
906 W. Randol Mill Road
Arlington, TX 76012
USA

BRUCE F. KIMLER, PhD
Professor and Director,
Radiation Biology Laboratory
Department of Radiation Oncology
University of Kansas Medical Center
Kansas City, KS 66103
USA

TIMOTHY J. KINSELLA, MD
Professor and Chairman
Department of Human Oncology
University of Wisconsin
School of Medicine Clinical Cancer
Center
K4/312-600 Highland Avenue
Madison, WI 53792
USA

WUI-JIN KOH, MD
Assistant Professor, Radiation
Oncology
University of Washington Medical
Center
1959 N.E. Pacific Street
Seattle, WA 98195
USA

ROSELLEN LANNING, RN
Medtronic, Inc.
7000 Central Ave. NE
Minneapolis, MN 55432
USA

VICI LISTON, RN
Department of Radiation Oncology
University of Kansas Medical Center
Kansas City, KS 66103
USA

JACOB J. LOKICH, MD
Chief of Neoplastic Disease
New England Baptist Hospital
Medical Director
Boston Cancer Center
125 Parker Hill Avenue
Boston, MA 02120
USA

NORMA L. LOWE, PhD
Alpha Therapeutics Corporation
5555 Valley Boulevard
Los Angeles, CA 90032
USA

JOSE R. MARTI, MD
Associate Professor of Surgery –
SUNY
Chairman of Surgery
The Brooklyn Hospital
121 Dekalb Avenue
Brooklyn, NY 11201
USA

JAMES B. MITCHELL, PhD
Head, Radiation Biology Section
Radiation Oncology Branch
National Cancer Institute
National Institutes of Health
Bldg. 10, Room B3–B69
Bethesda, MD 20892
USA

R. BRIAN MITCHELL, MD
Joint Section of Hematology/
Oncology
The University of Chicago
5841 S. Maryland Avenue, Box 420
Chicago, IL 60637
USA

ROBERT A. MORANTZ, MD
Brain Tumor Institute
2316 E. Meyer Boulevard
Kansas City, MO 64132
USA

MOHAN NUTHAKKI
Department of Medical Oncology
State University of New York
SUNY Health Science Center at
Brooklyn
Brooklyn, NY 11203
USA

ROBERT K. OLDHAM, MD
Director
Biological Therapy Institute
Hospital Drive
Franklin, IN 37064
USA

ANTHONY R. PAUL, MD
Department of Radiation Oncology
Fox Chase Cancer Center
Central & Shelmire Aves.
Philadelphic, PA 19111
USA

CARLOS A. PEREZ, MD, FACR
Professor
Director, Radiation Oncology Center
Mallinckrodt Institute of Radiology
Washington University School of
Medicine
510 S. Kingshighway
St. Louis, MO 63110
USA

LOUIS POTTERS, MD
Department of Radiation Oncology
State University of New York
SUNY Health Science Center at
Brooklyn
Brookly, NY 11203
USA

LEONARD R. PROSNITZ, MD
Professor and Chairman
Department of Radiation Oncology
Duke University Medical Center
Durham, NC 27710
USA

MARK J. RATAIN, MD
Assistant Professor of Medicine and
Clinical Pharmacology
Joint Section Hematology/Oncology
The University of Chicago
5841 S. Maryland Avenue, Box 420
Chicago, IL 60637
USA

A. MICHAEL RAUTH, PhD
Division of Physics
Ontario Cancer Institute
Princess Margaret Hospital
500 Sherbourne Street
Toronto, M4X 1K9
Canada

SETH REINER, MD
Department of Radiation Oncology
SUNY Health Science Center at
Brooklyn
450 Clarkson Avenue, Box 1211
Brooklyn, NY 11203
USA

TYVIN A. RICH, MD
Associate Professor
Uni. of Texas System Cancer Center
M.D. Anderson Hospital and Tumor
Institute
6723 Bertner Drive
Houston, TX 77030
USA

C. JULIAN ROSENTHAL, MD
Professor of Medicine and Oncology
SUNY Health Science Center at
Brooklyn
450 Clarkson Avenue
Brooklyn, NY 11203
USA

MARVIN ROTMAN, MD
Professor and Chairman
Department of Radiation Oncology
SUNY Health Science Center at
Brooklyn
450 Clarkson Avenue
Brooklyn, NY 11203
USA

ANTHONY H. RUSSELL, MD
Radiation Oncology Center
5271 "F" Street
Sacramento, CA 95819
USA

KENNETH J. RUSSELL, MD
Associate Professor, Radiation
Oncology
University of Washington Medical
Center
1959 N.E. Pacific Street
Seattle, WA 98195
USA

ANGELO RUSSO, MD, PhD
Head, Experimental Phototherapy
Section
Radiation Oncology Branch
National Cancer Institute
National Institutes of Health
Bldg. 10, Room B3–B69
Bethesda, MD 20892
USA

LEONARD SALTZ, MD
Division of Medical Oncology
Memorial Sloan Kettering Cancer
Center
1275 York Avenue
New York, NY 10021
and
Division of Hematology-Oncology
Cornell University Medical Center
407 East 70th Street
New York, NY 10021
USA

Prof. Dr. med. ROLF SAUER
Department of Radiation Therapy
University of Erlangen
Universitätsstraße 27
W-8520 Erlangen
FRG

LAWRENCE E. SCHEVING, MD
Professor
Department of Anatomy
University of Arkansas for Medical
Sciences
Little Rock, AR 77205
USA

HILLIARD F. SEIGLER, MD
Department of Surgery
Duke University Medical Center
Durham, NC 27710
USA

BEN SISCHY, MD
Clinical Professor of Radiation
Oncology
University of Rochester School of
Medicine and Dentistry and the
Daisy Marquis Jones Radiation
Oncology Center at Highland
Hospital
1000 South Avenue
Rochester, NY 14620
USA

PATRICK STAFFORD, PhD
Fox Chase Cancer Center
Assistant Professor Dept. of
Radiation Oncology
University of Pennsylvania School of
Medicine
Central & Shelmire Aves.
Philadelphia, PA 19111
USA

RICHARD S. STARK, MD
Director Medical Oncology
Interfaith Medical Center
555 Prospect Place
Brooklyn, NY 11238
USA

SAMUEL G. TAYLOR, IV, MD
Professor of Medicine
Section of Medical Oncology
Rush-Presbterian St.-Luke's Medical
Center
1725 W. Harrison St.
Chicago, IL 60612
USA

GARY B. THURMAN, PhD
Department of Biochemistry
Vanderbilt University
School of Medicine
Nashville, TN 37232-0146
USA

ANDREW T. TURRISI, III, MD
Associate Professor
Department of Radiation Oncology
University of Michigan
UH-B2C490, Box 0010
1500 E. Medical Center Drive
Ann Arbor, MI 48109
USA

TRIBHAWAN S. VATS, MD
Professor and Chief
Section of Pediatric Oncology
Department of Pediatrics
University of Kansas Medical Center
Kansas City, KS 66103
USA

NICHOLAS J. VOGELZANG, MD
Associate Professor of Medicine
Joint Section of Hematology/
Oncology
The University of Chicago
5841 S. Maryland Avenue, Box 420
Chicago, IL 60637
USA

EVERETT E. VOKES, MD
Assistant Professor of Medicine and
Radiation Oncology
The University of Chicago Medical
Center
5841 S. Maryland Ave., Box 420
Chicago, IL 60637
USA

REINHARD VON ROEMELING, MD
Assistant Professor
Division of Medical Oncology
Albany Medical College and Veterans
Administration Center
47 New Scotland Ave., A-52
Albany, NY 12208
USA

HENRY WAGNER, Jr., MD
Assistant Professor
Division of Radiotherapy
Albany Medical College and Veterans
Administration Center
47 New Scotland Ave., A-52
Albany, NY 12208
USA

CLARE WEILER, RN
Section of Hematology/Oncology
Presbyterian Medical Center
39th and Market Streets
Philadelphia, PA 19104
USA

MARCIA L. WILLS
Radiobiology Laboratories
Dartmouth-Hitchcock Medical Center
Hanover, NH 03756
USA

WALTER G. WOLFE, MD
Department of Surgery
Duke University Medical Center
Durham, NC 27710
USA

PETER YI, MD
Department of Medicine
Cornell University Medical Center
407 East 70th Street
New York, NY 10021
USA

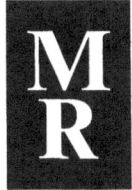

Medical Radiology

Diagnostic Imaging
and
Radiation Oncology

Series Editors:
L. W. Brady, M. W. Donner, H.–P. Heilmann, F. Heuck

This series recognizes the demand for an international state-of-the-art account of the developments reflecting the progress in the radiological sciences. Each volume conveys an overall picture of a topical theme so that it can be used as a reference work without taking recourse to other volumes.

The contents of the volumes concentrate on new and accepted developments in a manner appropriate for review by physicians engaged in the practice of radiology.

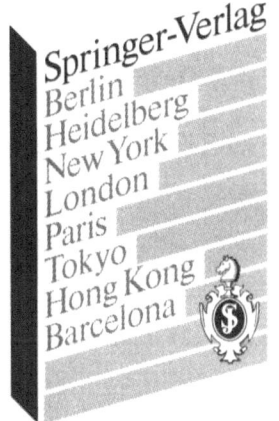

Springer-Verlag
Berlin
Heidelberg
New York
London
Paris
Tokyo
Hong Kong
Barcelona

C. W. Scarantino (Ed.)

Lung Cancer

Diagnostic Procedures
and Therapeutic Management
with Special Reference to Radiotherapy

1985. XI, 173 pp. 42 figs. Hardcover.
ISBN 3-540-13176-0

H. R. Withers, University of California, Los
Angeles, CA; L. J. Peters, University of Texas,
Houston, TX (Eds.)

Innovations in Radiation Oncology

1987. XVII, 329 pp. 111 figs. Hardcover.
ISBN 3-540-17818-X

G. E. Laramore, University of Washington,
Seattle, WA (Ed.)

Radiation Therapy of Head and Neck Cancer

1989. XII, 237 pp. 123 figs. Hardcover.
ISBN 3-540-19360-X

J. H. Anderson, The Johns Hopkins University,
Baltimore, MD (Ed.)

Innovations in Diagnostic Radiology

1989. XIII, 213 pp. 144 figs. some in color.
Hardcover. ISBN 3-540-19093-7

R. R. Dobelbower Jr., Toledo, OH (Ed.)

Gastrointestinal Cancer

Radiation Therapy

1990. XV, 301 pp. 76 figs. 90 tabs. Hardcover.
ISBN 3-540-50505-9

E. Scherer, C. Streffer, University of Essen;
K.-R. Trott, London (Eds.)

Radiation Exposure and Occupational Risks

1990. XI, 150 pp. 32 figs. 55 tabs. Hardcover.
ISBN 3-540-51174-1

S. E. Order, The Johns Hopkins University,
Baltimore, MD; S. S. Donaldson,
Stanford University, Stanford, CA

Radiation Therapy of Benign Diseases

A Clinical Guide

1990. VIII, 214 pp. 103 tabs. Hardcover.
ISBN 3-540-50901-1

R. Sauer, University of Erlangen-Nürnberg,
Erlangen (Ed.)

Interventional Radiation Therapy Techniques – Brachytherapy

1991. XII, 388 pp. 193 figs. 162 tabs. Hardcover.
ISBN 3-540-52465-7

E. Scherer, C. Streffer, University of Essen;
K.-R. Trott, Medical College of London (Eds.)

Radiopathology of Organs and Tissues

1991. Approx. 500 pp. 169 figs. 5 tabs.
Hardcover. ISBN 3-540-19094-5